Guided Reflection

A narrative approach to advancing professional practice

Guided Reflection
A narrative approach to advancing professional practice

Second edition

Edited by Christopher Johns

WILEY-BLACKWELL
A John Wiley & Sons, Ltd., Publication

This edition first published 2010
First edition published 2002
© 2002, 2010 Blackwell Publishing Ltd

Blackwell Publishing was acquired by John Wiley & Sons in February 2007. Blackwell's publishing programme has been merged with Wiley's global Scientific, Technical, and Medical business to form Wiley-Blackwell.

Registered office
John Wiley & Sons Ltd, The Atrium, Southern Gate, Chichester, West Sussex, PO19 8SQ, United Kingdom

Editorial offices
9600 Garsington Road, Oxford, OX4 2DQ, United Kingdom
2121 State Avenue, Ames, Iowa 50014-8300, USA

For details of our global editorial offices, for customer services and for information about how to apply for permission to reuse the copyright material in this book please see our website at www.wiley.com/wiley-blackwell.

The right of the author to be identified as the author of this work has been asserted in accordance with the UK Copyright, Designs and Patents Act 1988.

Library of Congress Cataloging-in-Publication Data

Guided reflection : a narrative approach to advancing professional practice / edited by Christopher Johns. – 2nd ed.
     p. ; cm.
   Rev. ed. of: Guided reflection / Christopher Johns ; with contributions from Aileen Joiner . . . [et al.]. 2002.
   Includes bibliographical references and index.
     ISBN 978-1-4051-8568-4 (pbk. : alk. paper) 1. Nursing–Philosophy. 2. Self-evaluation.
3. Self-knowledge, Theory of. 4. Holistic nursing. I. Johns, Christopher. II. Johns, Christopher. Guided reflection.
   [DNLM: 1. Philosophy, Nursing. 2. Mentors. 3. Nursing Assessment–methods. 4. Nursing Care–psychology. 5. Nursing Evaluation Research–methods. 6. Self Assessment (Psychology) WY 86 G946 2010]
   RT84.5.J6363 2010
   610.7301–dc22

                                                                                                    2010001842

A catalogue record for this book is available from the British Library.

Set in 10/12 pt Sabon by Toppan Best-set Premedia Limited
Printed and bound in Malaysia by Vivar Printing Sdn Bhd

1 2010

Contents

Preface

This book reveals narrative as a journey of self-inquiry and transformation towards self-realisation – a way of enabling health care practitioners to research self in the context of their clinical practice within a community of inquiry. Self-inquiry, through skilled and dedicated guidance, *is seeing what is and going beyond it* towards self-realisation, however that might be known. As Anderson (1996) notes:

> 'If one has not seen what is, how can we go beyond it?' Unfortunately, academic practice shows little or no understanding of 'seeing what is' in the context of genuine self-inquiry. (Words in quotations by Krishnamurti)

It is not an easy journey for the path is strewn with barriers. Issues of force, tradition and embodiment lie in wait to constrain the erstwhile practitioner. We may lack commitment, tired and burnt out from working within seemingly uncaring environments and trapped in our own complacency and ritualised patterns of practice. Seeing self in the reflective mirror may simply be too uncomfortable. Caught in the glare of guided reflection many practitioners will scurry back to their dark caves of habitual practice. Yet, others, intrigued by new vistas, will grasp the opportunity of reflection as an opportunity to liberate themselves from the shackles of habitualised practice to realise their visions of self and practice – to take themselves seriously as practitioners who have been entrusted by society to care. This is no casual agenda, for failure to care adds to suffering when the demand is to ease it. This must be the quest of all practitioners, to know and realise self as caring within everyday practice.

The narrative approach in this book builds upon the ideas set out in the first edition published in 2002. Since then, my insights on narrative have been continuously tested through my own and my students' narratives. New programmes developed at the University of Bedfordshire have been formally constructed around narrative. Most significant is the master's in clinical leadership (now MSc in Leadership in Healthcare Practice) commenced in February 2002 whereby students construct narratives of being and becoming the leader they desire to be commencing on the first day of the programme. In 2005, I established the school of guided reflection and narrative inquiry to create a focus for doctoral work using narrative. Over this time, the reflective turn moved naturally into a narrative turn and now into the performance turn, marking a distinction between representing lived experience as narrative to presenting it as performance.

The narratives in this book explore the way practitioners do make a difference and the way this difference can be nurtured. Practitioners must be committed to what they do and accept responsibility for ensuring they are most effective, challenging habitual ways of viewing and responding to practice situations. By placing self at the core of the learning process of self-inquiry, commitment and responsibility are foremost in the reflective lens.

Narrative is not primarily an intellectual pursuit. Rather, it is a genuine endeavour to become better at what we seek to do. For health care practitioners this must mean becoming most effective in our caring and healing practices. It is both our destiny and responsibility if we choose to walk this path. If narrative of self-inquiry is riddled with contradiction as a research process then that is no more than a reflection of life itself. As reflective practitioners we learn through experience. We can never eradicate contradiction because as our understanding deepens, deeper contradictions emerge.

The post-modern turn may dissect our taken for granted ways and partial views of being in the world yet it can feel detached like a cold blade dissecting a living body. In doing so it can lose sight of the practical focus of self-inquiry to realise self-realisation.

Structure of the book

The book is set out in 17 chapters. Chapters 1–5 set out the narrative approach in which I unfold and explore the various influences that have guided my thinking about the nature of narrative as self-inquiry and transformation towards self-realisation. These chapters in themselves contribute to my continuous reflection on working within reflective practices as therapist, educator and researcher over a 20-year period. In this sense, the chapters are partially written as a personal narrative of my own journey of realisation. Within these five chapters are exemplars taken from my students' narratives at both master's and doctoral levels.

As I emphasise throughout, narrative is not prescribed. The ideas I set out and indeed the ideas I do not set out, are no more than tentative paths to consider and follow mindfully, if at all. Yet, we do need some guidance to get going, no more so than a skilled guide and peers within a community of inquiry. These things are not done so well alone or without a skilled guide. Guides must have a strong narrative pedigree, for narrative is only learnt and honed through the doing and reflecting on it. If someone offers a formula, you know you are in the wrong place. Narrative is not learnt from books or theories. It just doesn't work that way.

Guided reflection is the weaving of two strands of *being* and *becoming*. *Being* is the reflection of the practitioner's clinical practice as known through reflection. The stories written in a reflective journal or shared in guided reflection. *Becoming* is the reflection of the practitioner's journey from where she[1] is at now to where she wants to be as known by looking back through the unfolding series of reflected-on experiences to perceive self as transformed or not. The perception is given form by drawing on appropriate markers. Guided reflection unfolds and weaves the practitioner's unique pattern of being and becoming in narrative form.

This idea of knowing as being was inspired by Doug Boyd (1974). He wrote, in relation to his experience with Rolling Thunder, a Western Shoshone Native American medicine man, who believed that understanding could only be experienced, juggled and pieced together until the person knows it is right. It cannot be verbally communicated. You sort of have to dwell wisely and intently with narrative and it reveals its insights and patterns. It is as if the body gets to know the dance as a natural thing, something

---

[1]I have used 'she' for practitioner and 'he' for guide throughout for ease of reading.

less thought about but lived. This takes time it and like most creative things it cannot be prescribed or rushed.

A Feminist slant (Chapter 5) is developed from the first edition (Chapter 2, pp. 40–44). Since writing the first edition, I have come more to realise the blend between the masculine and feminine within narrative. I invited Colleen Marlin, Professor of English at Centennial College in Toronto, to write the empathic poems to give voice to the self-harm patients within *Jane's rap* (Chapter 13). Such were the power of these voices, both masculine and feminine, that I invited her to contribute to the idea of 'writing as woman' – no easy task considering the way woman in intellectual writing has been socialised within dominant patriarchal patterns of learning that privileges rationality and order. 'A feminist slant' endeavours to address this domination, asserting the legitimacy of a narrative scholarship and academic form that most reflects the contradictory, complex and multi-patterned lived experience – an issue I pick up on when I explore the nature of the coherent narrative (Chapter 15). Colleen writes as she travels on a train. She uses the metaphor of 'backyards', which she views from the train for a feminist perspective in contrast to 'frontyards', which may characterise more masculine narrative – all appearance and orderly.

What follows is a collection of narratives that illuminate the narrative approach. It is the skill of the narrator to turn the apparent mundane, the ordinary into something extraordinary, in ways that grip the reader's attention. Each narrative offers a deep insight into everyday practice and invites the reader to relate to the narrative in terms of her own experiences. In this way the narratives intend to be deeply both challenging and informative, and open a reflective space for readers to dwell and consider their own experiences. It is the value of reflective texts to open spaces for dialogue and learning.

From the first edition I have omitted the three narratives[2] that I had constructed based on extensive notes that I had recorded verbatim during guided reflection sessions with the practitioners. Although I had given these notes and the constructed narrative back to the practitioners for verification, the narrative was my version.

With hindsight, I know better now. Either I should have written my own narrative of guiding these practitioners and guided them to write their own stories if they had been appropriately motivated. Whilst they verified my notes, they were my interpretations. What else were they thinking, feeling, acting that was significant that was not revealed in the guided reflection sessions?

'Awakenings' (Chapter 6) has been retained from the first edition. I edited this narrative from Aileen Joiner's reflective assignments whilst undertaking the 'Becoming a reflective and effective practitioner' programme at the University of Luton. In her narrative, Aileen, drawing inspiration from 'Demian'[3] by Herman Hess (1969) describes herself as a seeker rather than a scholar, and that this search is found in her experience rather than in books or gazing at stars. This seeking enters her blood as she begins to listen to her body where she finds meaning. Reflecting Demian, Aileen continues:

> Mine is not a pleasant story, it does not possess the gentle harmony of invented tales; like the lives of all men who have given up trying to deceive themselves, it is a mixture of nonsense

---

[2] These three narratives are:
- Striving to realise leadership;
- Becoming available within the hustle of a medical ward;
- Realising the therapeutic relationship with head and neck cancer patients and families.

[3] This was mis-spelt as Damian in the first edition.

and chaos, madness and dreams. The life of everyman is a way to himself, an attempt at a way, the suggestion of a path. ... Each individual, who is himself an experimental throw from the depths, strives towards his own goal. We can understand each other; but each person is able to interpret himself to himself alone.

I was going to omit Aileen's narrative, but I couldn't because, as the words above illuminate, her work profoundly reflects the spirit and quest of reflection, as a moment for reflection on reflection and as an exemplar of setting out a (hermeneutic) background.

I have also retained Yvonne Latchford's narrative (Chapter 7) simply because it illuminates the idea of a critical social science as she strives in unison with her client to find voice and gain participatory competence whereby both she and her client can overthrow their perception of oppression and realise more satisfactory lives for Yvonne as a practitioner and for her client as a mother. In editing the narrative, in the light of narrative experience, just a few changes were made to the narrative form, such was its initial excellence. Whilst the references are now dated to government and health visiting, the same issues still haunt health visiting today as it continues to be marginalised as a profession within an health agenda that seemingly does not value health protection beyond its obvious rhetoric. Such (unhealthy) contradiction has become seemingly ingrained within the health visitor's persona.

Maria Fordham has been a doctoral student since 2005. She is now weaving her narrative towards completion and examination. Her chapter comprises two pieces of narrative taken from the whole narrative that are reflexively linked. She shows the profound nature of her work with homeless people and the struggle to be heard in political corridors. Using the metaphor of a 'net', her work is an exemplar of social action in the way stories can be used to empower and change people. Maria has revolutionised homelessness care in Bedford through her work. She is also a talented story-teller, weaving words, art and poetry into poetic prose.

'Climbing walls' (Chapter 9) was my first directed performance with my dance and theatre colleagues, Amanda Price, April Nunes Tucker and Antje Diedrich. It has been performed in public theatre to good acclaim. It is an experiential work exploring the idea of performance developed from reflective journals. The performance narrative tells my story of journeying with a woman experiencing breast cancer treatment over the first six months following her diagnosis.

April, Amanda and Antje (Chapter 10) reflect on this performance juxtaposed with theoretical ideas about performance. Can there be a theory of such performance? We think not, yet we have learnt much doing it. With the emergence of the performance turn and performance ethnography, such issues require appreciation as we move narrative and curriculum into a performance turn. Perhaps the most significant issue in the performance turn is the idea of SHOW NOT TELL. This is a profound appreciation, that reflective practice intends to show people another way rather than tell them about another way. Performance enables people to embody learning by listening with their whole self.

'More than eggs for breakfast' is a line taken from a Tony Hancock script when he commenced journalling. The narrative (Chapter 11) sets out John-Marc Priest's journey of being and becoming the leader he desires to be within a hospital emergency department. This narrative is one of 40 or more similar narratives written by students on the MSc in Leadership in Healthcare Practice programme at the University of Bedfordshire (www.beds.ac.uk/rpf). The programme is an exemplar of creating a community of inquiry. Students commence their narratives from day one, using dialogue from taught modules to inform their journey. John-Marc's narrative was chosen to represent his type of narrative because of his novel use of time within the narrative and because it is so well written. Here, I have included the performance I constructed/edited from his original narrative and first performed in Toronto, 2008, at the Reflective Practice Conference hosted by Centennial College.

I extensively edited Jane Groom's narrative on working with self-harm patients in A&E (Chapter 12), which was included in the first edition of the book. I wanted to keep this narrative in the new edition because it demonstrates the way reflective practice can lead to profound change. In editing the narrative I developed my own voice of Jane's guide – so I could use the narrative as an exemplar of guiding reflection. From this new narrative I constructed *Jane's rap*, reducing her 10 500-word narrative into 4000 words. As noted previously, I invited Colleen Marlin to write the empathic poems. Feedback from performances to date endorse the narrative as powerful in confronting normal uncaring practices. So the performance turn gathers pace through my own work and collaboration with others. It is profound turn that influences narrative construction and moves narrative into overt social action. I sense we are just at the beginning of this adventure.

The idea of social action is linked to the relationship between narrative and its audience (Chapter 14). Whilst narratives of self-inquiry have an intrinsic value for recording the narrator's own journey of self-realisation, there is also the idea of using narrative as social action. 'Audiencing' explores some ideas about this relationship between narrator/performer and audience. Narratives of self-inquiry, not least for academic scrutiny, need to be coherent and ethical. I have taken an approach (Chapter 15) that positions coherence as a whole within the hermeneutic spiral of being and becoming. So whilst aspects of coherence such as rhizomatic validity can be explored, such exploration is always against a background of whole coherence. Hence, there can be no specific criterion of coherence that stands alone. Coherence is essentially irreducible. Again this is an experiential idea as I endeavour to find meaning in coherence. Ethics as always is controversial with experiential work.

Lei Foster is another doctoral student. His piece 'An accidental tourist' (Chapter 16) is a reflection on his journey. As with all Lei's work it is both clever and witty, and helps at the end of such a book to gain a sense of perspective. And finally, I pause for my own brief reflection (Chapter 17), both a summing up and opening towards new horizons. Nothing is certain within this book, narrative is always an adventure and yet as self-inquiry nothing could be more vital if we take ourselves seriously as practitioners. Research becomes lived day by day. Everything becomes meaningful as practitioners become mindful through reflection. The real stuff.

Christopher Johns
May 2010

Reference

Anderson A (1996) Introduction. In: Krishnamurti J. *Total freedom: The essential Krishnamurti*. Harper Collins, San Francisco, pp. xi–xiv.

List of contributors

Antje Diedrich
Senior Lecturer in Theatre and Course
Leader for BA English and Theatre
University of Bedfordshire
Bedfordshire
UK

Maria Fordham
Specialist Public Health Nurse – Homelessness
Bedford Primary Care Trust
Bedford
UK

Lei Foster
Mental Health Nurse
Bedford Community Mental Health Team
Bedfordshire and Luton Mental Health and
Social Care Partnership NHS Trust
Bedfordshire
UK

Jane Groom
Lead Nurse
Accident & Emergency
Kettering General Hospital NHS Trust
UK

Christopher Johns
Professor of Nursing
Reflective Practice Forum
University of Bedfordshire
Bedfordshire
UK

Aileen Joiner
Senior Team Manager
Learning Disability Service
Milton Keynes General Hospital NHS Trust
UK

Yvonne Latchford
Counselling Student
(formerly Health Visitor)

Colleen Marlin
Professor of English and General Education
Centennial College
Toronto, Ontario
Canada

April Nunes Tucker
Lecturer in Dance
University of Bedfordshire
Bedfordshire
UK

Amanda Price
Principal Lecturer in Theatre
University of Bedfordshire
Bedfordshire
UK

John-Marc Priest
Emergency Registered Nurse
Vancouver Island Health Authority (VIHA)
Victoria, BC
Canada

Chapter 1
The basic scheme

Christopher Johns

> The philosophical assumptions that underlie a 'method', and whether those assumptions are consistent with the researcher's own view, seem to me to be at the necessary starting point of inquiry. (Koch 1995:827)

The basic scheme is quite simple – that people can learn through their everyday experiences to become who they want to be. This requires a vision and perhaps some guidance along the journey. The journey is written as narrative. The narrative might then be read or performed in public spaces for dialogue and social action.

What started as scribbling in a journal one evening becomes a performance in a public theatre. Such is the dramatic potential of such inquiry. Nothing can be more significant to a professional, no matter what discipline, than his or her own performance. When we are mindful enough, practice becomes a narrative unfolding. In this way self-inquiry research is something lived, unfolding moment by moment. It becomes a profound way of being in the world.

In the first edition of this book, I opened Chapter 1 with the words 'Guided reflection is a process of self-inquiry to enable the practitioner to realise desirable and effective practice within a reflexive spiral of being and becoming'.

Since I wrote these words over eight years ago, the world has turned. The *reflective turn* has evolved into the *narrative turn*. As I gain greater insight into narrative construction and form, I appreciate that guided reflection is part of the process of narrative, albeit the most vital. Appreciating this turn, I have substituted *narrative* for *guided reflection*. I also prefer to talk of the research as a *journey* of being and becoming, not as a *process*, as if it were being manufactured.

I now describe *narrative as a journey of self-inquiry and transformation towards self-realisation*. The emphasis on *self-realisation* acknowledges that this journey is about being and becoming. It shifts from an outward focus on realising desirable practice to an inward focus on realising self.

Narrative

This is a book about narrative. Wikipedia informs that:

> A narrative is a story that is created in a constructive format (written, spoken, poetry, prose, images, song, theater or dance) that describes a sequence of fictional or non-fictional events.

It derives from the Latin verb *narrare*, which means 'to recount' and is related to the adjective *gnarus*, meaning 'knowing' or 'skilled'. (Ultimately derived from the Proto-Indo-European root *gn[oline]-*, 'to know'.) The word 'story' may be used as a synonym of 'narrative', but can also be used to refer to the sequence of events described in a narrative. A narrative can also be told by a character within a larger narrative. An important part of narration is the narrative mode.

Ideas help to sense and shape meaning but as I shall reveal, narrative can be only known through living and reflecting on it. The idea of *living or being* narrative reflects an ontological perspective in contrast with an epistemological perspective concerned with ideas and *doing* narrative. The ontological is a higher level of consciousness. Mattingly (1994:811) writes:

> Narrative plays a central role in clinical work, not only as a retrospective account of past events, but as a form healers and patients actively seek to impose on clinical time.

Narrative, through reflection, nurtures mindfulness. Narrative is mindful practice, mindful research, mindful teaching. Hence the more I reflect on my experience, the more aware I become of those things in my practice. It is a spiral that feeds itself leading to higher level of consciousness, towards enlightenment.

Practice, whatever its nature, is always uncertain, unpredictable, a mystery unfolding simply because human encounter is unique. It has not been lived before. As experts, claiming knowledge, we may think we know but knowing can never be certain with human encounter (Johns 2009a). As such, we must hold our ideas and frameworks loosely for their value to inform each encounter. Research is like this, something lived, a mystery unfolding. An over-reliance on method – 'this is how you should do this' resists play, forcing things into a certain shape and in doing so distorting the truth. Truth needs to find its own expression. This is so obvious yet people cling to method as if their life hangs upon it.

There is no 'correct' method to guarantee true results (Lather 1986). Methodology is no longer bound by the prescribed rules and boundaries of positivist thinking. Instead, the current era of post positivism allows a multiplicity of methods in order to make sense of human experience (Bentz and Shapiro 1998).

My approach to narrative inquiry is informed by diverse influences woven into a coherent pattern. Since first formulating this research approach, I have continued to dialogue with diverse methodological influences – exploring and playing with these influences in terms of the 'whole' as if within a hermeneutic cycle where understanding of the whole deepens. Working on my own narratives, and more recently on performances, and working with students at both master's and doctoral levels, has enabled me to dialogue with these diverse philosophical ideas from a practical level for, sensing and relishing the subtlety of their nature.

Perhaps as a defensive gesture I adhere to the idea that narrative inquiry is *always* experiential. It is *never* certain. However, philosophical and theoretical ides do help shape the path and guide the steps along it. They have a utility – what is their value to inform me? So whilst there is no formula to construct narrative, guidelines are helpful, notably the idea that self-inquiry narrative is always reflexive and coherent. Mighty words indeed. Perhaps other people's approaches to narrative do not make this demand. Hence when we talk of narrative we must be clear what we are talking about given the diverse usage of this word.

To reiterate – there is no formula. Like a mountaineer feeling his way along the edge of a crevice, the narrator pays attention to each step along the way with care because the terrain is unknown, a mystery unfolding. Ideas can be like crevices where you plunge and lose your way. We can get lost in method or what Janesick (2003:65) describes as *methodolatry*:

> a combination of the words method and idolatry to describe traditional researcher's preoccupation with selecting and defending methods to the exclusion of the actual substance of the story being told.

We hold a vision of self and practice, and each step is mindfully taken along the narrative path towards realising the vision as something lived. It is called 'the plot'. Weinsheimer (1985:6–7) citing Gadamer (1974) writes:

> Everywhere where one has to come across something which cannot be found by learning and methodical alone – that is, everywhere where invention emerges, where something is owing to inspiration and not methodical calculation – there it depends on ingenium, on genius (TM:50).[1] Thus it is clear why Gadamer avows any attempt in TM to 'develop a system of regulations that could describe or even direct methodical procedures of human science' (TM:xvi) Such an endeavour would be futile, for there is no art or technique onto things/ there is no method of stumbling.

Stumbling seems to me the perfect descriptor for inventing my approach to narrative inquiry. No doubt if I was to retrace my journey I would do it differently. I would have found other influences that would have been equally persuasive. Hence, those practitioners whom I guide are urged to find their own paths, even as they are informed by my own. I emphasise to hold all ideas lightly because the footsteps of others can lead into blind alleys if you are not mindful enough.

Consider the following description of narrative by Art Bochner (2001:134–135):

> I see narrative inquiry as a turn away from as well as a turn towards … the narrative turn moves away from a singular, monolithic conception of social science toward a pluralism that promotes multiple forms of representation and research; away from facts and toward meanings; away from master narratives and towards local stories; away from idolizing categorical thought and abstracted theory and toward embracing the values of irony, emotionality, and activism; away from assuming the stance of the disinterested spectator and toward assuming the posture of feeling, embodied and vulnerable observer; away from the writing essays and toward telling stories.

Bochner inspires and fuels revolution to break out of conformity that chokes the imagination and stifles creative work. He opens the possibility that research is legitimately art not science (and the intellectual and political crisis of legitimacy!). He sets up narrative as a movement away from a *monolithic conception of social science towards a pluralism*. Of course, he also sets up the problematic of pluralism notably – well these words are all well and good but how does it all fit together and work in coherent ways? The challenge is to move from reflections on experience to telling stories, to constructing narratives and then perhaps to performing them within an agenda of social change.

---

[1]TM is 'truth and method' (see references).

Table 1.1 Methodological framework, version 1 (*c.* 2002)

Critical social theory	Hermeneutics	Phenomenology
Evolutionary consciousness	Guided reflection: A co-developmental and collaborative research process	Literature
Dialogue		Ancient and spiritual wisdom
Empowerment theory	Reflective and supervision theory	Feminism

Hermeneutic cycle/Kosmos/Gestalt

Table 1.2 Methodological framework, version 2 (*c.* 2006)

Critical social science and empowerment	Hermeneutics and dialogue	Narrative inquiry
The feminist slant	Guided reflection as a journey of self-inquiry and transformation	Ancient and spiritual wisdom
Auto-ethnography (autobiography)	Reflective theory	Chaos theory

Table 1.3 Methodological framework, version 3 (*c.* 2009)

Hermeneutics	Performance studies and performance ethnography	Buddhist psychology
Critical social science Empowerment theory Collaborative theory	Narrative is a journey of self-inquiry and transformation towards self-realisation	Guided reflection and narrative theory
Auto-ethnography and autobiography	Feminist slant	Chaos theory

So, in constructing narrative I put on my pluralistic hat (well I think it is a pluralistic hat – would I know one if I saw one?) and begin to weave diverse influences into a methodological pattern that shifts as I come to better understand these influences in themselves and their synergy as a pattern. I then attempt to weave these ideas within a patterned whole. My understanding of this pattern continues to evolve as I engage the ideas in practice and read more widely (see Tables 1.1–1.3). Bourdieu's *Sketch for a self-analysis* (2007) lies invitingly on my desk, as yet unread.

Understanding of ideas must always tentative because of their deep philosophical nature and the inevitable partiality of interpretation as I engage with these ideas within my own experience of narrative, assimilating and simmering such ideas within my narrative knowing. A slow cook to get full flavour.

Collaborative research

Narrative as self-inquiry resonates with collaborative research theory (Reason 1988). Collaborative inquiry exists when all participants contribute to the design and management of the research as a mutual process of co-inquiry, negotiated social action and personal development. It intends a harmonising of power within the relationship in order for dialogue to flourish. Nice idea, yet easier said then done. People's shared backgrounds do not necessarily lend themselves to collaborative work within prevailing bureaucratic health care service cultures characterised by an emphasis on a tradition of authority that has imposed subordination and dependency.

In writing my narrative as a complementary therapist, I am telling my own story in relationship with those with whom I practice. I am not telling their story, even though I show an empathic detail about their lives. I obscure identity and even write fiction to protect the identity of those I relate with in my stories. Using my judgement I inform people that I reflect on my practice as routine and construct narrative that may at some time be published or performed. It is an extension of the caring relationship. Practice becomes narrative, empowering and healing for practitioners and patients (Colyer 1996; Kralik *et al.* 2001).

Beginnings

Let me turn the clock back to the beginning. In 1989, in my role as lead nurse at Burford Community Hospital, I commenced a project to facilitate practitioners to realise holistic practice as set out in the hospital vision (Johns 1998, 2009b). I entered into guided reflection relationships with practitioners whereby I would guide their learning through the experiences they disclosed in the sessions. These sessions were about an hour long and held every two to three weeks. My agenda was to fulfil my assumed leadership role to enable practitioners to become effective practitioners. Through the project we came to appreciate deeper the nature of holism, the holistic practitioner role, those things that constrained its realisation – either embodied within the practitioner or embedded in organisational systems and patterns of relationships, and guided reflection as collaborative inquiry.

On moving to university in 1991 I developed curriculum grounded in reflective practice that fundamentally shifted the relationship between practice and theory. Now we learnt through stories informed by theory as appropriate. Practice was a hook to hang the theory hat on. Theory became more meaningful and more easily assimilated within personal knowing. Assignments were narratives of transformation.[2] The first guided reflection dissertations were constructed.[3] In 2004 I commenced the MSc in Leadership in Healthcare Practice programme whereby students constructed narratives of being and becoming the leader they desired to be.[4] The programme itself became a community of inquiry to guide this work. In this way teaching and research became one.

In 2003, in my role as visiting professor at City University I started working with Louise Jarrett, guiding her PhD narrative of being a spasticity nurse (Jarrett 2008). In 2005 I created the School of Guided Reflection and Narrative Inquiry at the University of Bedfordshire, recruiting Lei Foster and Maria Fordham (see Chapters 16

---

[2] Several of these narratives are published in the third edition of *Becoming a reflective practitioner* (Johns 2009b).
[3] Jane Groom and Yvonne Latchford's narratives are examples of this work (Chapters 12 and 7, respectively).
[4] John-Marc's narrative is an example of the leadership narratives (Chapter 11).

and 8, respectively). In 2007, I began working with Amanda Price, April Nunes and Antje Diedrich, dance and drama teachers at the University of Bedfordshire, as co-supervisors expanding the community of inquiry into an inter-disciplinary approach, and most significantly fuelling the performance turn. The Community of Inquiry meets for four hours every four weeks throughout the year, supplemented by two three-day intensives. The intensives were created primarily for overseas students to join the community. A Google group enables continuous dialogue within the community. In 2009 I launched the Reflective Practice Forum website[5] to open dialogue with a wider world.

Reflection

At the core of narrative inquiry is reflective practice. Intellectually I describe it as:

> Being mindful of self, either within or after experience, as if a mirror in which the practitioner can view and focus self within the context of a particular experience, in order to confront, understand and move toward resolving contradiction between one's vision and actual practice. Through the conflict of contradiction, the commitment to realise one's vision, and understanding why things are as they are, the practitioner can gain new insight into self and be empowered to respond more congruently in future situations within a reflexive spiral towards self-realisation. The practitioner may require guidance to overcome resistance or to be empowered to act on understanding. (Adapted from Johns 2009b)

I write *within a reflexive spiral towards self-realisation* in contrast with earlier descriptions where I stated *within a reflexive spiral towards developing practical wisdom and realising one's vision as praxis* (Johns 2006). This adaptation reflects the idea that reflection is more about 'who I am' and less about 'what I do', although the two are intrinsically linked – as 'what I do' is reflected in 'who I am'.

Whilst I have written extensively elsewhere on the nature and method of reflective practice (Johns 2009b), I would emphasise a number of key points:

- Reflection is essentially concerned with being in the world (ontological) rather than doing (epistemological);
- Becoming mindful of self is the quintessential quality of reflective practice as something lived, more than merely a technique to learn through experience;
- Reflection is always being mindful in practice or on practice, i.e. that the act of reflection on experience is an experience in itself;
- The reflective outcome is insights that enable people to live more effective, more desirable, and more satisfactory lives;
- Reflective practice is energy work – nurturing commitment, dissipating anxiety, realising power, finding meaning, becoming vision, enabling healing, knowing self;
- Guidance (in guided reflection) is collaborative dialogue towards creating better worlds.

Personal knowing

Knowing through reflection is subjective and contextual. Such knowing is the very stuff of professional practice, the knowing that practitioners use in everyday practice in

---

[5] www.beds.ac.uk/rpf

response to the complex and indeterminate issues that practitioners face (Schön 1987). Schön described professional practice as the swampy lowlands where there are no pre-scribed answers to the situations of human–human encounter. Schön claimed a new epistemology of professional practice, which gave primacy to personal knowing in con-trast with the high hard ground of technical rationality that was of limited use to prac-titioners. Personal knowing is largely tacit. Being tacit is not easily expressed in words. Practitioners know more than they can say (Schön 1983). Reflection taps the tacit, lifting it to the surface so to speak. Such learning is subliminal, cultivating personal knowing and the intuitive response within future experiences. It is only by looking back over reflected-on experiences that the practitioner becomes aware of the insights she has gained.

Dreyfus and Dreyfus (1986), in their model of skill acquisition appropriated by Patricia Benner (1984) in her work on expert practice, suggest that people do move along a continuum from novice to expert without consciously being aware of being reflective. In becoming an expert the practitioner shifts from a reliance on linear models of decision making to intuition based on prior experience, suggesting that reflection occurs naturally on a subliminal level because people do seem to learn through experience. I assume that reflection speeds this natural learning process. Intuition is seeing and responding to a situation as a whole as if the self is part of that whole rather than outside it.

Through reflection I may come to understand some things rationally, but applying that into practice is another matter as embodied responses shape my response.

Pinar (1981:180–181) asserts that:

> All knowing begins in intuition. It is the medium through which the qualities of situation become discerned, conceptualised and articulated. Intuition is the representation and medita-tion of situation and self. Thus, it behoves us to be interested in knowing how to cultivate the intuitive capacity, and to begin to utilise language to render our intuitions sensitively, hence more accurately.

The work of Ken Wilber is grounded in an integrated model of evolutionary conscious-ness that seeks to integrate partial and seemingly contradictory views of the nature of consciousness and knowing. Wilber (1998) set out four quadrants of knowing (Figure 1.1). Each quadrant or paradigm has its own rules for generating knowing and its own rules for deciding whether such knowing is valid. In health care, the right hand paths

	Interior (left hand paths)	Exterior (right hand paths)
Individual	Upper left Subjective knowing Personal (I)	Upper right Objective knowing Behavioural fit (IT)
Collective	Cultural fit (WE) Inter-subjective knowing Lower left	Social fit (IT) Inter-objective knowing Lower right

Figure 1.1 Four quadrant view of knowing. (Wilber 1998)

have been dominant with its demand that knowledge should be observable and generalisable. Wilber refers to this type of knowledge as 'IT' knowledge that seeks to predict and control life by reducing things into parts and seeking cause and effect type relationships between them, even situations associated with the human sciences. From this perspective 'I' knowing tends to be dismissed pejoratively as anecdote.

Upper left quadrant

This is the quadrant of reflective or personal knowing, revealing the subjective and contextual world of 'I'. It reveals a perception of self that is not observable and therefore the reader or listener is at least partially reliant on the truthfulness of the writer or narrator. I say 'partially' because readers always project a meaning into the text based on their own experience. Hence truthfulness is always mediated.

Knowing in the left hand path makes no claim to generalisability because human life is not predictable. Each event is unique and life is constantly changing, even ourselves.

Only from the perspective of personal knowing can the practitioner meaningfully dialogue with knowledge constructed within the other paradigms and assimilate such knowledge into their personal knowing.

Upper right quadrant

However, if the writer was observed within a particular situation, the observer would pick up certain signs to provide specific information about the writer's state of mind, behaviours and the such like, enabling the observer to draw certain conclusions of the 'facts' of the matter based on verified criteria. This 'objective' or 'abstract' perspective may bear little semblance with the narrator's reflection of the event, using as it does a different language.

Lower left quadrant

As the narrator reflect on 'I', he or she inevitably positions 'I' within relationships with others, revealing patterns that shape the everyday world or what Wilber (2000:143) describes as 'the shared cultural worldspace necessary for the communication of any meaning at all'. People do not live in isolation from others, but share a world that is largely pre-governed by cultural norms that strongly, albeit unwittingly, shape the way people think, feel and behave within situations. Reflection gives access to understanding these patterns of relationship and the way the individual is both shaped by and shapes such patterns.

Lower right quadrant

Practice can be viewed objectively as *systems* within a complex machine that governs all aspects of social life. An over-emphasis on systems, then the human factor becomes lost within the system, *the ghost within the machine* (Koestler 1976) where humans are reduced to objects to be manipulated as parts within the machine. This is very apparent in health care organisations that are primarily governed by their self-demand for smooth running. Reflection helps the 'I' to appreciate systems for their value in supporting clinical practice.

Through reflection the 'I' can dialogue with the other quadrants as appropriate to integrate apparently diverse ways of knowing within personal knowing. Wilber (1998) urges caution because the subjective path has tended to be aggressively reduced into the objective path. As he acerbically writes:

> But when you have finally finished reducing all 'I's and all 'we's to mere 'Its', when you have converted all interiors to exteriors, when you have turned all depth into shiny surfaces, then you have perfectly gutted an entire kosmos. You have completely stripped the universe of all meaning, of all value, consciousness, depth and discourse – and delivered it dried and desiccated, laid out on the marble slab of a monological gaze. (Wilber 1998:22)

Ruth Morgan (2004) writes:

> Wilber's image here of dried and desiccated theory, shallow and depersonalised, is strong, and helps to balance the years of training that taught me only to value definitive, empirical research. His words are liberating, and inspire me to continue to challenge positivist dominance, to trust intuition, acknowledge feelings, and free myself from the restraints and limitations of depersonalised practice.

Reflection is opening a transformative space. It is not simply an internal, introspective process, purely for the benefit of the reflector. It has social and political repercussions affecting the wider community in ways that serve human interest (Boud *et al.* 1985). Our changed perspectives only have relevance in context with the life we share with others. As a political activity, reflection becomes part of an emancipatory process in its capacity to identify and release self and others from the irrational, unjust and repressed.

The influence of a critical social science

Jack Mezirow (1981:223) writes:

> Our meaning structures are transformed through reflection, defined here as attending to the grounds (justification) for one's beliefs. We reflect on the unexamined assumptions of our beliefs when the beliefs are not working well for us, or where old ways of thinking are no longer functional. We are confronted with a disorientating dilemma, which serves as a trigger for reflection. Reflection involves a critique of assumptions to determine whether the belief, often acquired through cultural assimilation in childhood, remains functional for us as adults. We do this by critically examining its origins, nature, and consequences.

Mezirow's words suggest that reflection is 'critical' in the sense of a critical social science. I prefer to think of reflection as depth. We can scratch at the surface of experience purely in terms of problem solving without disturbing the deeper currents of affairs that determine the conditions that support the problem. We don't go out of our depth because these deeper currents are dangerous. Mezirow (1981) described this as critical consciousness leading to perspective transformation, another word to describe insights.

We learn to think about our thinking that caused the problem in the first place. Going deeper we reveal the way power is played out in practice. Going deeper we reveal the way power is constructed and maintains a certain political order. Going deeper we acknowledge our own oppression and our loss of integrity. Going deeper we drown in our misery, for we are indeed in murky depths.

My description of reflection reflects the tenets of a critical social science as a process of enlightenment, empowerment and emancipation (Fay 1987), what I colloquially refer to as the 3Es even as I prefer to term these three movements as understanding, empowerment and transformation (Table 1.4).

Critical social science takes the perspective of enabling people to rise up and overthrow their oppression in order to live more satisfactory lives. Governed by dominant social forces, practitioners are largely unable to take control of their own professional practice and realise their therapeutic potential (Buckenham and McGrath 1983). Roberts (1982, 2000) labels nursing as an oppressed group socialised into a subordinate role that traps them by fear into their oppression and makes them unable to take action, often denying or rationalising their own oppression. And yet, as the practitioners' narratives in the book reveal, oppression quickly surfaces through reflection. An understanding and commitment to realise one's therapeutic destiny, and with the challenge and support of guidance, practitioners are empowered to take action towards a better state of affairs, as revealed in transformation – albeit a chipping away rather than revolution. My leadership in health care programme has an overt revolutionary camaraderie to storm the barriers that constrain transformational leadership within transactional organisations.

Fay (1987) labels these barriers as force, tradition and embodiment. They are buried deep within each of us, suggesting that we are not radically free to change ourselves and certainly not from any rational perspective. Within the UK's National Health Service (NHS), it is tempting to project this oppression emanates from others: managers, 'the system', and the oppressive culture of the NHS. Yet, as Wilber (1998) reminds us, oppression also comes from within; denying voice to the feelings and anxieties that surface, denigrating intuition and closing a doorway to transformation. Developing a positive identity by respecting and valuing intuition within a nursing framework can help to liberate this oppressor within (Roberts 2000) and open the door to transformation.

To overcome oppression, the practitioner must understand it, to appreciate its nature, the way it is patterned within normal relationships and organisational structures. Only

Table 1.4 Typology of enlightenment, empowerment and emancipation (Fay 1987)

Enlightenment (understanding)	Enlightenment is understanding why things are as they are. It is a critical process of deconstruction, of peeling away the layers of experience to reveal the conditions that govern why people respond as they do. These conditions are embodied within self and embedded within the fabric of practice in ways that reinforce the embodied conditions through ways of relating.
Empowerment	Empowerment is having the understanding, commitment and courage to take appropriate action towards changing the way things are in order to realise self's own interests. Empowerment acknowledges the limits of rationality to bring about change, and the positive energy required to take appropriate action in ways that may incur resistance from more powerful others whose interests may be threatened.
Emancipation (transformation)	The realisation of self's best interests as a consequence of taking appropriate action.

then can the practitioner act to transform the situation towards realising a better state of affairs in line with her vision of practice. Of course, the practitioner may see self as oppressed, simply because that is the normal state of affairs. She may be dissatisfied and frustrated; and that is the spark for reflection to germinate the struggle for liberation and in doing so, the reflective spiral of being and becoming is developed as one thing inexorably leads to another in the awakened self (Freire 1972).

From this perspective, empowerment *is* the cornerstone of reflection, the critical edge to reflection to free ourselves from oppressive forces in order to relieve our misery. Perhaps in our frantic world it is easier to defend against anxiety than face up to such strong emotions where there are no easy answers. As such, reflection may create a crisis for practitioners as normal coping mechanisms are exposed as incongruent with achieving desirable work. Given insight into 'their condition' may exacerbate a sense of frustration ultimately leading to a personal crisis where self-doubt about competence and de-masked ways of coping become redundant. Yet with enlightenment the practitioner can view the scenario unfolding, almost as an observer, and accept that things do not necessarily change quickly.

Cox *et al.* (1991:387) write:

> As we come to expose these self-imposed limitations, then the focus of our reflection shifts towards new action, towards the ways in which we might begin to reconstruct and act differently within our worlds.

However, exposing these 'self-imposed limitations' may not necessarily be easy or comfortable. It may be difficult for practitioners to see beyond themselves because of 'habits of mind' that act as barriers (Margolis 1993). Margolis refers to the way paradigms are maintained and shifted. Where particular habits of mind need to be shifted for change to take place they constitute a barrier. However, as noted, a practitioner's own best interests may be distorted because of competing dominant power discourses that she has internalised and taken for granted as normal. Practitioners may feel more comfortable adhering to false beliefs or 'false consciousness' defined by Lather (1986:264) as 'the denial of how our common-sense ways of looking at the world are permeated with meanings that sustain our disempowerment'. Similarly Mezirow (1981) viewed reflection as the means to enable practitioners to penetrate 'false consciousness' through perspective transformation. He defined this as:

> The emancipatory process of becoming critically aware of how and why the structure of psycho-cultural assumptions has come to constrain the way we see ourselves and our relationships, reconstituting this structure to permit a more inclusive and discriminating integration of experience and acting upon these new understandings. (Mezirow 1981:6)

Psycho-cultural assumptions are those norms and prejudices embodied within individuals and embedded within practice settings that lead people to see and act in the world in certain ways. Mezirow (1981:7) writes of 'disorienting dilemmas' and how the 'traumatic severity of the disorienting dilemma is clearly a factor in establishing the probability of a transformation'. It is this sense of disorientation or trauma that brings the person to pay attention to the experience, although a more deliberative stance can be developed as the practitioner becomes increasingly sensitive to herself in the context of what they are trying to achieve. Street (1992:16) drew the conclusion from her critical ethnography of nursing practice that:

The confrontation with experience through reflection and of the meanings and assumptions which surround it, can form a foundation upon which to make choices about future actions based on chosen value systems and new ways of thinking about and understanding nursing practice.

Hermeneutics

Hermeneutics is the art of understanding text (Gadamer 1975). With self-inquiry, the text is our lived experiences. As such, the practitioner must stand back far enough from the text enough to move into a subjective-objective dialogical relationship with it. The art of dialogue is to know and suspend our assumptions and judgement so as to see things with clarity.

Hermeneutic spiral

Understanding evolves from a dialectical process of moving between the parts and the whole within the hermeneutical spiral. Gadamer (1975:167, cited in Weinsheimer (1985:40)) writes:

Understanding is always a movement in such a (hermeneutic) circle, for which reason the repeated return from the whole to the parts and vice versa is essential. In addition, this circle continually expands itself in that the concept of the whole is relative and the inclusion in ever larger contexts alters the understanding of single parts.

Weinsheimer (1985:40) adds:

The universe of discourse, like the physical universe, is constantly expanding. Thus the hermeneutic circle, in which truth is understood as the conclusive reconciliation of whole and part, might better be conceived as a hermeneutic spiral, in which truth keeps expanding. That is, the whole truth never *is* but always *to be* achieved.

Within one experience everything about practice and self would be revealed if we pulled it apart enough. Reflective method first seeks to reveal what is significant within the experience (written as a spontaneous story – see Chapter 2), pulling this significance out for scrutiny against the background of the whole, opening a dialogue between the whole and the parts, and always with the view to learn, and in so doing, deepening and expanding the hermeneutic spiral of being. It is both as simple and profound as that.

Wilber (1998:1) alludes to the hermeneutic spiral:

We move from part to whole and back again, and in that dance of comprehension, in that amazing circle of understanding, we come alive to meaning, to value, and to vision: the very circle of understanding guides our way, weaving together the pieces, healing the fractures... lighting the way ahead – this extraordinary movement from part to whole and back again, with healing the hallmark of each and every step, and grace the tender reward.

Wilber's language is always tinged with a sense of grace, as he acknowledges that such work is implicitly spiritual. His words have poetic resonance, reflecting that narrative, like life itself, is finding expression to flowing with meaning. Hermeneutics is not primarily seeking understanding *of* the movement of experience but *is* the movement or flow of experience. Yet I recognise a risk in identifying hermeneutics as a 'method' in a traditional sense. It may suggest a linearity and structure that belies the circular, seamless, fluid nature of this reflexive, reflective approach to inquiry. I would suggest though that the hermeneutic circle accommodates this fluidity. Zukav (1979) urged us not to see hermeneutics as a concept to fit into but as a descriptor of inquiry into mystery, a kind of dance.

In his critique of Gadamer, Weinsheimer (1985:35) writes:

Historical understanding sees every moment of history, including its own, as ineluctably factical and particular, immersed in having been, and never finally determined as an instance of a general concept under which it could be conclusively subsumed, but always awaiting interpretation and always exceeding it.

Now, the subtlety of these words may have alluded me, but the practitioner always positions self as a movement within the flow of history, seeking to find meaning in experience situated within a background of past experiences. In finding meaning, the 'who' of practitioner changes, not simply what she does.

It is an event of being that occurs. But this event changes who she is in such a way that she becomes not something different but rather herself. (Weinsheimer 1985:71)

A resonance with Buddhism, in that one finds oneself through reflection, a self that is already there but a self obscured by false consciousness. It is as if we have to lift the blanket to see our true selves. But would we recognise our true selves? I think so, because lifting the blanket is peeling away the layers of false consciousness.

The practitioner does not stand outside tradition. Indeed she is determined by tradition. Yet by understanding tradition, she can see how it applies to her experience and can learn from it – indeed, this is how tradition and practice changes – the way a tradition determines itself from within – that is, for the way understanding alters it precisely by belonging to it. Indeed, tradition can only be understood in relation to its application to the present. Without applying learning to future experience there can be no understanding. In other words, understanding is something lived not merely an idea. As such reflection is always lived, a way of being in the world rather than an intellectual technique or learning approach.

Weinsheimer (1985:182) writes:

It is possible to become more aware of our own historical situation, the situation in which understanding takes place. Having such awareness does not mean that once the situation has become more fully conscious, we can step outside it, any more than seeing our own shadow means we can outrun it. Rather our shadow moves along with us. The situation of understanding can also be called our horizon. It marks the limit of everything that can be seen from a particular point of view, but the idea of horizon also implies that we can see beyond our immediate standpoint.

Reflection is a way of appreciating and moving beyond one's own horizon through understanding. The idea of 'horizon' is visual in contrast with 'perspective'. Becoming more aware is becoming mindful of self within experience. In becoming mindful, the practitioner makes conscious her prejudices that shape perception. Here a guide is helpful to provoke. In provoking, the guide offers his own horizon towards co-creating meaning (see Chapter 3).

Gadamer (1975:263) writes:

> If understanding always means coming to an understanding, then it always involves two – and two different – participants. The ideal is not that one party should understand the other but rather that they should reach an understanding between them. This *between* is the true locus of hermeneutics.

The suspension of beliefs, judgements, prejudices and the like within dialogue reflects what Gadamer (1975) refers to as pre-knowledge; the way people dialogue through a lens of personal concerns. These personal concerns are shared within a *tradition* that characterises society. Tradition has a powerful impact on the way people view the world largely because it is pre-reflective. It is most powerfully reflected in the prejudices people hold and which govern their responses to the world. Given the powerful impact of prejudice and tradition on the way people respond to the world, the reflective effort is to surface and understand the way the practitioner's prejudices create contradiction with what is desirable. It goes without saying then, that the practitioner must suspend her preconceptions.

Background

Heidegger (1962) terms *background* as a pre-reflective state that leads people to respond to others in certain ways. Heidegger (1962) noted that the researcher's background will inevitably influence understanding simply because they exist in the world. Heidegger's idea of fore-structure gives structure to background (Table 1.5). It has three aspects; fore-having, fore-sight and fore-conception. It isn't simply descriptive, but reflective, enabling the writer to consider carefully who they are, where they are coming from and what they are moving towards, and to enable readers to appreciate better where the narrator is coming from in drawing out significance and insights from the text.

The background is an introductory personal statement. It sets the boundaries to the narrative space. The significance of background usually emerges slowly through the transformative journey in context of the experiences being shared.

Table 1.5 Fore-structure as background

Fore-having	All interpretation must start with fore-having – something we have in advance. I interpret this to mean that the writer sets out their past experiences that influence the way they are in the world. How their being has been shaped. These experiences often stem back to childhood, through training and positions held. This is not easy considering who we are has largely been taken for granted.
Fore-sight	There needs to be something we see in advance. I interpret this to mean how the person views self in the context of their practice (and life), the assumptions, values, fears they hold – relating to how the present moment shapes intention.
Fore-conception	The narrator already has expectations as to what he will find out – fore-conception. This relates to expectations and projections that influence what the writer anticipates, driven by a vision that is held tentatively because often a vision is merely words. What such words mean as lived is the project.

- What is my vision that guides me forward?
- What aspects of my past are influencing how I am now?
- How do my circumstances now shape me?

As the practitioner begins to reflect and consider ideas such as vision, history, and influences on actions, then she can begin to connect with her history. Only then does history make sense in the light of who I am now.

Buddhist psychology and ancient wisdom

I have been a Buddhist these past nine years. Buddhist ideas have slowly soaked into my skin and permeated my being, inspiring and influencing my approach to reflective practice. Why I became a Buddhist is immaterial except perhaps to say that the Buddha's central message of acknowledging and easing suffering resonated deeply with my practice as a nurse and complementary therapist working with people facing death.

People suffer and lead unsatisfactory lives trapped in the samsaric world chasing pleasure and avoiding pain, poisoned by craving, aversion and ignorance. However, there is a gate along the wheel of life where they can shift, if mindful enough, into a spiral towards enlightenment, where suffering can be eased to lead a more satisfactory life in realising one's vision as a lived reality. The gate lies between the junction of feeling and acting on the feeling. The gate is open if I am mindful enough, leading to insight and changing how I am in the world.

My self-image as a complementary therapist is the Bodhisattva, flowing with wisdom and compassion in response to ease suffering. To be wise is to be mindful. The ultimate expression of reflective practice is mindfulness. Mindfulness is being present to self within the moment, with clarity, without judgement.

Goldstein (2002:89) notes:

> Mindfulness is the quality of mind that notices what is present without judgment, without interference. It is like a mirror that clearly reflects what comes before it.

The idea of being without judgement, without interference, is very significant, as if being mindful is a precursor for making good judgements based on clear understanding; a precursor for wisdom. Pinar (1981) challenges us to be aware of the smudges on the mirror that distort the way we perceive self. Hence to learn, we must be aware of the smudges and then to clean the mirror to see with clarity, without distortion.

Previously I have described 'being mindful' as holding a vision within that moment, that being mindful is intentional, a movement towards transforming self towards realising one's vision as a lived reality (or enlightenment). Another aspect of being mindful is *apramada* – being aware of negative mental events that are destructive (*sangharakshita* – know your mind) – what I describe as the guard at the gate of the senses. In summary, mindfulness has these three aspects – of being present now, of being aware of the path ahead, and of being aware of how the past impacts on now. In being present now, the Buddhist sees all things as impermanent, ever changing, free from attachment to self and ideas, and that life is unsatisfactory, that it causes suffering because of ignorance (what is described as the three *lakhanas*).

Mindfulness is traditionally developed through meditation, using the breath to concentrate the mind and develop insight. Through reflection, the practitioner learns to pay attention to self within the context of her practice. She will be more aware of those things she writes about when she returns to practice, including herself, her senses, her thought patterns, her emotions, her responses, her energy, her anxieties and the such like, and also her vision (Why am I here? What am I trying to achieve?). The development of self-consciousness is vital for the development of reflexivity.

Bringing the mind home

It may be difficult cognitively for the practitioner to focus on self, especially if the self is well defended from looking in, fearful of what might be unearthed. As such the practitioner and her guide may benefit from contemplative practices such as meditation to help her tune into 'who I am' and become more present to self to bring the mind home prior to reflection or prior to any clinical moment. This can be done by just paying attention to the breath, and flowing the breath in and out, clearing the mind of thoughts and unwanted feelings. It relaxes, energises and focuses mind, body and spirit, a mind that is often scattered in so many places.

Rinpoche (1992:31) notes:

> We are fragmented into so many different aspects. We don't know who we really are, or what aspects of ourselves we should identify with or believe in. So many contradictory voices, dictates, and feelings fight for control over our inner live that we find ourselves scattered everywhere, in all directions, leaving nobody at home. Reflection then helps to bring the mind home. (p. 59)

and yet, how hard it can be to turn our attention within! How easily we allow our old habits and set patterns to dominate us! Even though they bring us suffering, we accept them with almost fatalistic resignation, for we are so used to giving in to them.

Rinpoche's words help balance the image of reflection as a cognitive activity. The ancient wisdom keepers know the secrets of the universe and consciousness, whilst the theorists grasp for explanation. Reflection is where the Buddhist and quantum theorist collide in the way they talk of the whole and the relationships between things. Spending a few minutes 'quiet time' before a session relaxing and focusing self will also help establish guided reflection as a special place for reflection, creating a sense of connection between the practitioner and her guide. It will also help the guide to be more aware of her own concerns and the need to suspend these for effective dialogue and co-creating meaning.

Framing the pursuit of self-realisation within Buddhism, or indeed any other faith, the search for self-realisation is a spiritual journey. Perhaps another way of saying self-realisation is the search for wholeness, and putting Buddhism aside, the idea of writing as search for wholeness is compelling. It is enabling self to become present to self, a self that has become distracted in so many ways. Presence is at the very centre of what nurses do ... to be fully present to another one must first be fully present to self. So writing can bring us home to ourselves.

Bentz and Shapiro (1998) draw together Buddhist thinking with Western thinking in their *Mindful inquiry in social research*, which resonates with my own thinking. They blend Buddhism with phenomenology, critical social science and within the spiral of mindful inquiry. They position mindful inquiry as a necessary approach as the fabric of modernity is torn apart in an increasingly complex world.

They set out a number of values that underpin 'mindful inquiry':

- Human existence, as well as research, is an ongoing process of interpreting both one's self and others, including other cultures and subcultures;
- All research involves both accepting bias – the bias of one's own situation and context – and trying to transcend it;
- We are always immersed in and shaped by historical, social, economic, political, and cultural structures and constraints, and those structures and constraints usually have domination and oppression, and therefore suffering built into them;
- Knowing involves caring for the world and the human life that one studies;
- The elimination or diminution of suffering is an important goal of or value accompanying inquiry and often involves critical judgement about how much suffering is required by existing arrangements;
- Inquiry often involves the critique of existing values, social and personal illusions, and harmful practices and institutions;
- Inquiry should contribute to the development of awareness and self-reflection in the inquirer and may contribute to the development of spirituality;
- Inquiry usually require giving up the ego or transcending self, even though it is grounded in self and requires intensified self-awareness;
- Inquiry may contribute to social action and be part of social action;
- The development of awareness is not a purely intellectual or cognitive process but part of people's total way of living their lives.

Bentz and Shapiro's work is centred on the posture of the researcher rather than as a methodology for undertaking research, suggesting that research is both moral and spiritual. Indeed, the transformation of self into higher consciousness towards self-realisation *is* spiritual (Wilber 1998). The idea that inquiry is social action leads into a deeper exploration of self-inquiry within the influences of autobiography and autoethnography.

First nations

In 1996, rummaging in a small Cambridge bookshop with Dawn Freshwater, I pick up *Earth Dance Drum* by Blackwolf and Gina Jones. It is truly an inspirational text on reflective practice, offering a poetic sense of reflection as movement through ritual dance.

I am caught by the idea of Bimadisiwin (Jones and Jones 1996:47):

Bimadisiwin is a conscious decision to become. It is time to think about what you want to be. The dance cannot be danced until you envision the dance, rehearse its movements and understand your part. It is demanding for every step needs an effort in becoming one with the vision. It takes discipline, hard work and time. Decide to be an active participant in your life journey. It is rewarding. Embrace the joy your vision brings you, it is yours to hold forever. It is freeing, for its frees the spirit. It releases you to become as you believe you must.

Believe in the vision of you
Practice the vision
Become the vision

Buddhist and First Nations' ideas are essentially ways of being in the world; they were not formulated cognitively. These ideas help to balance a Western cognitive approach grounded in rationality – itself an ironic twist from Schön's idea of overturning a technical rationality in favour of a personal knowing that determines practice, to emphasise reflection is essentially grounded in an ontology of *who we are* (Johns 2005) in contrast with an the epistemological perspective, which whilst significant, is concerned with ideas about reflection and doing reflection as some technique to be applied.

Autobiography and autoethnography

Self – the elusive 'I' that shows an alarming tendency to disappear when we try to introspect it. (*Oxford Dictionary of Philosophy* 1996)

Self-inquiry is at the core of autobiography and autoethnography. Pinar (1981:184) captures the essence of autobiography as movement:

We write autobiography for ourselves, in order to cultivate our capacity to see through the outer forms, the habitual explanations of things, the stories we tell in order to keep others at a distance. It is against the taken-for-granted, against routine and ritual we work, for it is the regularized and habitual which arrest movement. In this sense we seek a dialectical self-self relation, which then permits a dialectical relationship between self and work, self and others. … one falls back on oneself – rather than on the words of others – and must articulate what is yet unspoken, act as midwife for the unborn. One uncovers *one's domain assumptions*, one's projections – not in order to wipe the slate clean but in order to understand the slate of which one is the existential basis, the basis which makes knowing possible.

Dialectical relationships resonate with dialogue, commencing with self and then, like pebbles tossed into the still water, rippling out to embrace all situations and relationships, peeling away the surface layers to reveal the concealed taken-for-granted that constructs unwitting lives, enabling the practitioner to come to a reflexive awareness of self. From this awareness comes movement to move beyond existing understandings. Pinar's language resonates with critical social science yet on a personal level as if suggesting that *one's domain assumptions* constrains one's possibilities – the idea of a self not yet born. As Pinar (1981) continues:

What we aspire to when we work autobiographically is not adherence to conventions of a literary form. Nor do we think of audience, of portraying our life to others. *We write autobiography for ourselves*, in order to cultivate our capacity to see through the outer forms, the habitual explanations of things, the stories we tell in order to keep others at a distance. It is against the taken-for-granted, against routine and ritual we work, for it is the regularized and habitual which arrest movement. [Emphasis added]

When I first engaged with reflection, I saw it as self-inquiry in order towards realising a vision of practice and of self. Pinar's words do not reflect this quest. He suggests autobiography is understanding what exists or existed. He does suggest that this understanding opens a path to move beyond but he doesn't say move beyond to what. Perhaps simply getting in better shape.

Reflecting on Pinar's words, 'We write autobiography for ourselves', I want to add a proviso – 'although others may read it'. Narratives are to be read and performed, to engage and challenge others. They are always written for more then just ourselves, although I would agree with Pinar if he had said that narratives are written *primarily* for ourselves. Reflection is always concerned with *self*-realisation.

Pinar asserts that the focus of autobiography is *the felt problematic*. The emphasis on *felt* suggests that autobiography is not simply a rational approach, but perceptive, responsive to situations and intuitive, without formulaic approaches on how to do it. Leaps of the imagination to be tested.

Autoethnography

Discovering autoethnography I spontaneously felt at home such was the resonance. Clough (2000:282) writes:

> Autoethnographic writing has been nothing so much as the work of a subject self-consciously reflecting on the process of knowing self and other – that is knowing one's place in relationship to the other.

Ethnography is the study of culture whereby the researcher is immersed within another's culture in order to study it as if from within the culture rather than as a stranger to it. It is only by experiencing culture every day can it be appreciated. The researcher is immersed in his or her own culture.

Ellis (2004:xix) defines autoethnography as:

> Research, writing, and method that connect the autobiographical and personal to the cultural and social. This form usually features concrete action, emotion, embodiment, self-consciousness, and introspection portrayed in dialogue scenes, characterization, and plot. Thus, it claims the conventions of literary writing.

Linking the personal to the cultural and social suggests that autoethnography reveals and critiques social conditions that govern the personal, a personal that is traumatised, characterised by trauma stories that reflect issues of gender, class, abuse, race, prejudice, hatred and oppression, and triggered by rage and a 'disturbed' subjectivity – narratives that reveal and heal wrapped into an experimental intellectual covering where the personal becomes political and the political becomes personal, an image drawn from autoethnographic accounts from the USA.

Holman Jones (2005:767) cites Oleson (2000:215) that 'rage is not enough' – the challenge to move from rage to progressive politic action, to theory and method that connect politics, pedagogy and ethics to action in the world. In other words, feelings trigger reflection on some unsatisfactory aspect of life and culture, and that the revelation in coherent narrative form must move to social action that confronts and changes culture for the better.

Clough (2000) argues that the critique of traditional ethnographic writing is grounded in a reconfiguration of nature, culture and technology, both a reflection of and a response to what Bentz and Shapiro (1998) note as the 'post-modern turn', suggesting we are living at a historical turning point, when modern myths no longer offer adequate explanations, leading to a crisis in ways of knowing and opening a contested space for ways of knowing and what counts as truth.

In line with this, Holman Jones (2005) views autoethnography as a radical democratic politics – a politics committed to creating space for dialogue and debate that instigates and shapes social change. Again shades of a critical social science. Emotions are important to understanding and theorising the relationship among self, power and culture and that narrative/performance is a palpable emotional experience for the writer/performer. It is writing the body. Hence narratives themselves must be written in deeply engaging and shocking ways to make their point *if* social change is the agenda. The narrator is transformed in the process of self-inquiry.

What differentiates autoethnography from narrative as self-inquiry and transformation is reflexivity. Autoethnography is not so much something being lived through as a looking back on a situation. It does not seem to have an overt agenda of self-inquiry towards self-realisation in tune with a vision of self or practice. Stories help us create, interpret, and change our social, cultural, political and personal lives. Autoethnographic texts point out not only the necessity of narrative in our world but also the power of narrative to reveal and revise that world, even when we struggle for words, when we fail to find them, or when the unspeakable is invoked but not silent (Holman Jones 2005).

The performance turn

And as if narrative was not enough stimulation, I am turned by performance.

> As we move beyond ethnography as description to consider its performative potentials, we open a space for conceptual flowering. (Gergen and Gergen 2002:12)

I suppose this chapter is about conceptual flowering, shaping ideas into a coherent whole. To reiterate – narrative is the representation of the journey towards self-realisation. Along the journey, barriers that constrain self-realisation are encountered – barriers that are embodied within self and embedded in social structures. The practitioner seeks to understand these barriers in order to understand them and shift them, changing these conditions and self as necessary to realise self. Not an easy task given the resistance of these barriers firmly embedded as they are within self and society. There is no rational approach, just finding new paths through experience. As such the personal is always social, cultural, political and vice versa.

Performance shifts narrative into a new domain, from representation of self to presentation of self. Denzin (2003:9/14) writes that performance is an act of intervention, a method of resistance, a form of criticism, a way of revealing … agency … performances make sites of oppression visible. Narrative also does this, but performance does it in a different way – engaging the audience in a lived experience of their own within an agenda to use the performance as social action towards change, however slight.

I know that reading a narrative and listening to a narrative are different experiences. Some years ago I read a narrative as a conference paper. I had given this paper to a number of delegates to read some weeks before. In the ensuing dialogue these 'readers' commented that the experience of listening to the narrative was different from reading it. In what way? The reading was more heart-felt. People tend to listen with their hearts and read with their heads. As I envisaged reading narrative, I began to write them differently – the reason why my narratives struggled for publication acceptance – so that people were reading words meant to be listened to! And with a critical eye that revealed prejudice to what a scholarly paper should look like. A significant insight.

I take some refuge in the words of Gergen and Gergen (2002:18) (ethnographically speaking):

but given the twin assumptions that scholarship is inherently the work of the rationally engaged mind, and that words are the finest expression of rational deliberation, the visual media are typically treated as secondary to the more important craft of writing. It is high time to challenge the prevailing logo-centrism of this tradition, not only with visual media but also with the entire range of communicative expression at our disposal.

At this time I was simply reading my narrative, often against a background of images and music to heighten and contrast the impact of words. I was not self-conscious of 'performing it'.

Langellier (1999:127) writes:

> Performance is the term used to describe a certain type of particularly involved and dramatized oral narrative. Of special importance is how performance contributes to the evaluative function of personal narrative – the 'so what'.

I realised that the difference between reading a narrative and performing a narrative was primarily my self-consciousness of the impact of the performance on the audience. So I began to write performances from the narratives. The scripts were no longer the same as I learnt that performance is a stylised form of narrative that seeks to make dramatic impact to make certain points that aim at disrupting the normal state of social affairs. In other words, the personal became political. This is what I understand by *performativity*. Langellier (1999:135) writes that performativity:

> Articulates and situates personal narrative within the forces of discourse ... which makes cultural conflict concrete and accessible – to become aware of performance as a contested space, problematizing identity and contextual assumptions. ... The personal in performance implies a (performative) struggle for agency ... without performativity personal narrative risks being a performance practice without a theory of power to interrogate what subject positions are culturally available, what texts and narrative forms are privileged, and what discursive contexts prevail in interpreting experience.

Langellier's words reflect the critical social science agenda. I resonate with the idea of contested space – that the performer opens this space for dialogue – and so performance must always have this space built in, otherwise it is merely a performance that lacks performativity. It lacks the 'so what'. So, performance is texted to reveal the 'critical' relationships between people grounded within a specific situation, with the intention of triggering self-inquiry and transformation within the audience about their own lives. The performer crafts a dialogical space to disturb public life.

Ellis and Bochner (1996:28) write of the desire for the audience to engage on some level in a self-conscious reflexivity on their own relation to the experience. Turner (1988) writes of enabling the audience to draw back upon themselves self-consciously.

Performance of possibilities

Alexander (2005) drew my attention to Sonyi Madison's (1998) idea of the performance of possibilities. I could see that narratives were narratives of possibility and resistance – that they opened the path of what was possible and revealed the resistance to that path. Such conceptualisation offers a neat way of summarising the critical social science agenda. Hence the reader or listener can ask – to what extent is this narrative a narrative of possibility and resistance?

Madison (1998, cited in Alexander (2005:430–1)) sets out a number of criteria to appreciate her stance on possibility:

- 'The performance of possibilities functions as a politically engaged pedagogy that never has to convince a predefined subject – whether empty of full, whether essential or fragmented – to adopt a new position. Rather, the task is to win an already positioned, already invested individual or group to a different set of places, a different organization of the space of possibilities.
- The performance of possibilities invokes an investment in politics and "the other", keeping in mind the dynamics of performance, audience and subjects while at the same time being wary of both zealots and cynics.
- The performance of possibilities takes the stand that performance matters because it does something in the world. What it does for audience, the subjects, and those engaged in it must be driven by thoughtful critique of assumptions and purpose.
- The performance of possibilities does not accept being heard and included as its focus, but only as a starting point. Instead, voice is an embodied historical self that constructs and is constructed by a matrix of social and political processes. The aim is to present and represent subjects as made and makers of meaning, symbol, and history in their fullest sensory and social dimensions. Therefore, the performance of possibilities is also a performance of voice wedded to experience.
- The performance of possibilities as an integrative field aims to create or contribute to a discursive space where unjust systems and processes are identified and interrogated. It is where what has been expressed through the illumination of voice and the encounter with subjectivity motivates individuals to some level of informed and strategic action.
- The performance of possibilities motivates performers and spectators to appropriate the rhetorical currency they need, from the inner space of the performance to the outer domain of the social world, in order to make a material difference.
- The performance of possibilities necessitates creating performances where the intent is largely to invoke interrogation of specific political and social processes so that art is seen as consciously working toward a cultural politics of change that resonates in a progressive and involved citizenship.
- The performance of possibilities strives to reinforce to audience members the web of citizenship and the possibilities of their individual selves as agents and change makers.
- The performance of possibilities acknowledges that when audience members begin to witness degrees of tension and incongruity between a subject's life-world and those processes and systems that challenge and undermine that world, something more and new is learned about how power works.
- The performance of possibilities suggests that both performers and audiences can be transformed. They can be themselves and more as they travel between worlds – the spaces that they and others actually inhabit and the spaces of possibility of human liberation.
- The performance of possibilities is moral responsibility and artistic excellence that culminates in the active intervention of unfair closures, remaking the possibility for new openings that bring the margins to s shared centre.
- The performance of possibilities does not arrogantly assume that we are exclusively are giving voice to the silenced, for we understand they speak and have been speaking in space and places often foreign to us.

- The performance of possibilities in the new millennium will specialize in the wholly impossible reaching toward light, justice, and enlivening possibilities.'

As I dwell within these criteria I begin to explore their meaning for my own work. I recognise that my own narratives lack this political intention. I am beginning to rectify this, nurturing my political consciousness reflected in more recent performances such as *My mum's death* (Johns 2009c) and *Jane's rap* (see Chapter 11). Like all ideas, Madison's ideas of possibility and resistance requires the reader to consider and critique in applying to their own work. I ask my students to consider Madison's criteria whilst observing performance, offering a context much easier than an abstract review. Dialogue enables a play of ideas, evolving into a gradual weaving into meaning. The hermeneutic spiral at play. Considering Madison's criteria seems to interrupt the flow of meaning; it demands looking at each criterion as a part rather than grasping the whole of the performance. The criteria become a checklist and yet deepen appreciation of performance as possibility.

Self-inquiry as chaos

Wheatley (1999:118) writes about a chaotic view of order:

> When we concentrate on individual moments or fragments of experience, we see only chaos. But if we stand back and look at what is taking shape, we see order. Order always displays itself as patterns that develop over time.

Self-inquiry is essentially chaotic in its quest to find meaning and gain insight through the maze of lived experience. Yet self-inquiry doesn't seek to impose order, rather it seeks to pattern the myriad of meanings within the complexity and uncertainty of human service practice. Self-inquiry is guided by the intention to realise a vision of practice. This is the strange attractor that patterns meaning. The reflective practitioner stretches to move beyond personal and organisational boundaries in the quest to realise self. As she moves away from the centre where it feels safe and secure because things do not change, the practitioner comes to realise that practice *is* chaotic. Chaos is the creative edge. It is confidently stretching into the unknown, encouraging the practitioner to let go of any need to impose control on experience and to being open to the possibilities of her own practice. It is liberation from the demand of the Newtonian machine for control and predictability.

Wheatley (1999) in her exploration of the world of chaos and complexity finds there is no analytical language for explaining things at the quantum level. Technical analysis is inadequate to understand and embrace the wholeness of human life. Wheatley (p. 141) finds it necessary to move beyond traditional ways of knowing into the realm of sensation described by the German philosopher Heidegger as a 'dwelling consciousness'. This is a realm in which analytical skills are put to one side and intuition and sensation are called on in their place. In traditional science, the scientist creates a question and then interrogates the subject in order to draw a conclusion. The art of 'dwelling consciousness' demands that we move away from interrogation to receptivity, that we 'dwell with the phenomenon and feel how it makes itself known to us' (Wheatley 1999:141). With greater appreciation of the ultimately random, irrational world of existence, reflection is a way of drawing the self together from the turmoil of daily life. Johns (2002:11) describes it as a 'space of stillness that enables the practitioner to reconstitute the wholeness of experience'. Sadly modern life has developed such a momentum that without discipline there is no time to reflect or be still. Lack of meaning has little impact until tragedy draws us to a halt. Then we find we cannot ignore the human need for self-reference and meaning (Wheatley 1999).

Self-inquiry is finding pattern both within practice and as a way of looking back on practice, shaping the reflexive narrative through meaning and insights.

References

Alexander BK (2005) Performance ethnography. In: N Denzin and Y Lincoln (eds.) *The Sage handbook of qualitative research* (third edition). Sage, Thousand Oaks, pp. 411–442.

Benner P (1984) *From novice to expert*. Addison-Wesley, Menlo Park.

Bentz V and Shapiro J (1998) *Mindful inquiry in social research*. Sage, Thousand Oaks.

Bochner A (2001) Narrative virtues. *Qualitative Inquiry* 7:131–157.

Boud D, Keogh R and Walker D (1985) Promoting reflection in learning: a model. In: D Boud, R Keogh and D Walker (eds.) *Reflection: Turning experience into learning*. Kogan Page, London, pp. 18–40.

Bourdieu P (2007) *Sketch for a self-analysis* (transl. Nice R). Polity Press, Cambridge.

Buckenham J and McGrath G (1983) *The social reality of nursing*. Adis, Sydney.

Clough P (2000) Comments on setting criteria for experimental writing. *Qualitative Inquiry* 6:278–291.

Colyer H (1996) Women's experience of living with cancer. *Journal of Advanced Nursing* 23:496–501.

Cox H, Hickson P and Taylor B (1991) Exploring reflection: knowing and constructing practice. In: G Gray and R Pratt (eds.) *Towards a discipline of nursing*. Churchill Livingstone, Melbourne.

Denzin N (2003) *Performance ethnography: critical pedagogy and the politics of culture*. Sage, Thousand Oaks.

Denzin N and Lincoln Y (2003) *Strategies of qualitative inquiry* (second edition). Sage, Thousand Oaks.

Dreyfus H and Dreyfus S (1986) *Mind over machine*. Free Press, New York.

Ellis C (2004) *The ethnographic I*. AltaMira Press, Walnut Creek.

Ellis C and Bochner A (1996) *Composing ethnography: alternative forms of qualitative writing*. AltaMira Press, Walnut Creek.

Fay B (1987) *Critical social science*. Polity Press, Cambridge.

Freire P (1972) *Pedagogy of the oppressed*. Penguin, Harmondsworth.

Gadamer HG (1975) *Truth & method* (transl. Barden G and Cumming J). Seabury Press, New York.

Gergen K and Gergen M (2002) Ethnographic representation as relationship. In: A Bochner and C Ellis (eds.) *Ethnographically speaking*. AltaMira Press, Walnut Creek, pp. 11–34.

Goldstein J (2002) *One dharma*. Rider, London.

Heidegger M (1962) *Being and time* (transl. Macquarrie J and Robinson E). Harper & Row, New York.

Holman Jones S (2005) Autoethnography: making the personal political. In: N Denzin and Y Lincoln (eds.) *The Sage handbook of qualitative research* (third edition). Sage, Thousand Oaks, pp. 763–792.

Janesick V (2003) The choreography of qualitative research design: minuets, improvisation, and crystallization. In: N Denzin and Y Lincoln (eds.) *Strategies of qualitative inquiry* (second edition). Sage, Thousand Oaks, pp. 46–79.

Jarrett L (2008) From significance to insights. In: C Delmar and C Johns (eds.) *The good, the wise and the right clinical nursing practice*. Aalborg Hospital, Arhus University Hospital, Aalborg.

Johns C (1998) *Becoming an effective practitioner through guided reflection*. PhD thesis, Open University.

Johns C (2005) Balancing the winds. *Reflective Practice* 5:67–84.

Johns C (2006) *Engaging reflection in practice: a narrative approach*. Blackwell Publishing, Oxford.

Johns C (2009a) Journeying with Alice: some things I don't know for certain. *Complementary Therapies in Clinical Practice* 15:133–135.

Johns C (2009b) *Becoming a reflective practitioner* (third edition). Wiley-Blackwell, Oxford.

Johns C (2009c) Reflection on my mother dying: a story of caring shame. *Journal of Holistic Nursing* 27:136–140.

Jones B and Jones G (1996) *Earth dance drum*. Commune-A-Key, Salt Lake City.

Koch T (1995) Interpretative approaches in nursing research: the influence of Husserl and Heidegger. *Journal of Advanced Nursing* 21:827–836. Used with permission.

Koestler A (1976) *The ghost in the machine*. Random House, New York.

Kralik D, Koch T and Telford K (2001) Constructions of sexuality for midlife women living with chronic illness. *Journal of Advanced Nursing* 35:180–187.

Langellier K (1999) Personal narrative, performance, performativity: two or three things I know for sure. *Text and Performance Quarterly* 19:125–144.

Lather P (1986) Issues of validity in open ideological research: between a rock and a soft place. *Interchange* 17:63–84.

Madison S (1998) Performance, personal narratives, and the politics of possibility. In: S Dailey (ed.) *The future of performance studies: visions and revisions*. National Communication Association, Annandale, pp. 276–286.

Margolis H (1993) *Paradigms and barriers: how habits of mind govern scientific beliefs*. University of Chicago Press, Chicago.

Mattingly C (1994) The concept of therapeutic 'employment'. *Social Sciences and Medicine* 38:811–822.

Mezirow J (1981) A critical theory of adult learning and education. *Adult Education* 32:3–24.

Morgan R (2004) *Becoming a transformational leader*. Unpublished MSc in Clinical Leadership. University of Luton, Luton.

Oleson V (2000) Feminisms and qualitative research at and into the millennium. In: N Denin and Y Linoln (eds.) *Handbook of qualitative research* (second edition). Sage, Thousand Oaks, pp. 215–255.

Oxford Dictionary of Philosophy (1996) Blackburn S, Oxford University Press, Oxford.

Pinar W (1981) 'Whole, bright, deep with understanding': Issues in qualitative research and autobiographical method. *Journal of Curriculum Studies* 13:173–188.

Reason P (1988) *Human inquiry in action. Developments in new paradigm research*. Sage, London.

Rinpoche S (1992) *The Tibetan book of living and dying*. Rider, London.

Roberts S (1982) Oppressed group behaviour: implications for nursing. *Advances in Nursing Science* 5:21–30.

Roberts S (2000) Development of a positive professional identity: liberating oneself from the oppressor within. *Advances in Nursing Science* 22:71–82.

Sangharakshita (1998) *Know your mind*. Windhorse, Birmingham.

Schön D (1983) *The reflective practitioner*. Avebury, Aldershot.

Schön D (1987) *Educating the reflective practitioner*. Jossey-Bass, San Francisco.

Street A (1992) *Inside nursing: a critical ethnography of clinical nursing practice*. State University of New York Press, New York.

Turner V (1988) *The anthropology of performance*. PAJ Publications, New York.

Weinsheimer J (1985) *Gadamer's hermeneutics. A reading of truth and method*. Yale University Press, New Haven.

Wheatley M (1999) *Leadership and the new science. Discovering order in a chaotic world.* Berret-Koehler, San Francisco.

Wikipedia. Narrative. http://en.wikipedia.org/wiki/Narrative (accessed 3 October 2010).

Wilber K (1998) *The eye of spirit: an integral vision for a world gone slightly mad.* Shambhala, Boston. www.shambhala.com. Used with permission.

Wilber K (2000) *Sex, ecology, spirituality: the spirit of evolution.* Shambhala, Boston.

Zukav G (1979) *The dancing wu lui masters.* William Morrow, New York.

Chapter 2

Constructing the reflexive narrative

Christopher Johns

I construct narrative through six dialogical movements within the hermeneutic spiral of being and becoming (Figure 2.1). Within each dialogical movement I am mindful of coherence; that reflexivity can be adequately demonstrated within the whole, that the reader is persuaded that the narrative is authentic or worthy (Mishler 1990).

Whilst I offer the practitioner/researcher the six dialogical movements to guide her narrative construction, I must emphasise that this framework is not a formula for constructing narrative. It is a heuristic, opening a creative and coherent space for the practitioner to explore and yet feel supported.

> Heuristic – allowing a person to discover or learn something for themselves.
> (*Compact Oxford English Dictionary* 2005:474)

Narrative is only known through doing it and reflecting on the doing of it. Texts on narrative are available and offer perspectives that are useful to inform the practitioner. I previously described the six dialogical movements as the 'six layers of dialogue' (Johns 2006). On reflection, I came to better appreciate that each layer is not a discrete layer, but constantly in motion, flowing into and merging with the other layers in complex patterns. I have always made a significant distinction between description (the first dialogical movement) and reflection (the second dialogical movement). Yet the distinction, whilst initially helpful in recognising the importance of rich description as research data, ultimately becomes a hindrance because practitioners, having internalised the reflective model, naturally weave description and reflection. Hence *movement* seems a more appropriate descriptor – suggesting flow, progression, connection and pattern, as the self-inquirer is drawn into the hermeneutic reflective spiral of being and becoming towards understanding. The hermeneutic spiral represents the whole of experience against which issues of seeming significance are pulled out as a focus for developing insights but always in context of the whole. Understanding is always contextual, deepening understanding of the whole.

Whilst there is an order between the movements they are not linear especially for the 'expert' narrator, who blends the movements in seamless unity. However, for the 'novice', the movements may be more linear, as she seeks to find order not yet embodied.

1. Dialogue with self to write a rich descriptive story of a particular experience (*story text*) that pays attention to detail involving all the senses

2. Dialogue with the story text as an objective and disciplined process (using a model of reflection) to gain insights, producing a *reflective text*

3. Dialogue between the *text* and other sources of knowing in order to frame emerging tentative insights from the text within the wider community of knowing

4. Dialogue between the text's author and a guide(s) to check out, deepen and co-create insights

5. Dialogue with the emerging text to weave the pattern of insights into a coherent and reflexive narrative; producing a *narrative text*

6. Dialogue with others (through published text, performance and play) towards consensus of insights and social action; producing an *evolving text*

Hermeneutic spiral

Figure 2.1 The six dialogical movements

Dialogue

At the core of self-inquiry narrative is dialogue. Bohm (1996) notes that the meaning of dialogue is derived from the Greek word *dia-logus* – a stream of meaning flowing through and between us (p. 6). And this is exactly what we seek in narrative. Narrative is then the representation of derived meaning.

Dialogue can take place within self, between self and text, and with others. Bohm suggests that dialogue requires:

- The intention to work towards consensus (with others) to create a better world;
- The suspension of one's assumptions;
- The non-attachment to ideas and being open to possibility;
- Proprioception of thinking (knowing where thinking is);
- Treating all people in dialogue with respect;
- Knowing the rules of dialogue.

Intention to create a better world reflects an idea of holding a vision of self and practice that is essentially good. Indeed the universal health care agenda must be towards creating a better world. The idea that it is not would itself be a contradiction with the idea of health. Dialogue is the art of creating conversations. As Tufnell and Crickmay (2004:41) write:

Creating becomes a conversation when we enter into a dialogue with whatever we are doing. In this conversation we are drawn along in the moment by moment flow of sensation, interchange and choice, rather than following a predetermined intention or idea. Conversations grow as we listen and explore – a constantly shifting process of discovery that changes in momentum, rhythm, clarity or chaos as we work.

The first dialogical movement

Before we can reflect, we must first access our experiences. I sit at the computer wondering how do I write my stories? Remembering a moment ... the look on her face, a word said, a tear, the feeling I feel inside, a sad smile, the smell of curry, a picture on the wall, the dance of the trees outside the window ... so many signs to trigger my story. Reflection is awakening to self. With effort and appropriate guidance, practitioners can liberate themselves from the limiting habits and views that constrain self-realisation. It is a search for wholeness.

Experience is our raw data, the stuff we dwell within to find meaning and draw insight. Put simply, experience is the way an individual perceives self and others within the context of a particular event or series of events. Such a view is deeply subjective. This writing or journalling of experience tells the unfolding story; it requires rich description, paying attention to detail within the experience, drawing on all the senses – touch, sight, sound, taste, smell and consciousness. In doing so, the practitioner's senses are heightened. She becomes more awake, more alive, more open, more aware of coming to self through these avenues. It is a making sense of the complexity of the terrain of everyday practice – 'a broken and uneven place, heavily inscribed with habit and sedimented understandings' (Lather 1993;674).

Journalling is a mirror in which we can see our self in relationship within the particular experience – a broad canvas in which one can pay attention to and position self within the contextual forces that pattern experience. Journalling gives the practitioner voice to find and express self; feelings, thoughts, guilt, whatever. It is an opening to self that challenges those censors that might otherwise quieten self, a private confession, revealing those things to self that might otherwise be unsaid even to self. Not just things that disturb sleep at night but things that also bring satisfaction that might otherwise remain unacknowledged in the habitual taken-for-grantedness that characterises so much of life. As Manjusvara (2005:10) considers:

> The practice of writing takes us to the heart of ourselves and makes it palpable how alive with possibilities we really are.

I know practitioners who find journal writing easy and natural whilst others struggle to express their experience, especially in written form as if some censor is at work in their minds limiting their potential. If you have never written about self before it may feel strange, even threatening. The mirror is not always kind especially if we create false impressions of ourselves. Hence writing requires effort, honesty and perseverance. It also requires meaning; that writing is a movement towards something worthwhile. Writing is confrontational and begins to loosen the self from its bondage.

I tend to write my journal in a factual way to recapture something of the moment, usually straight onto the computer, sometimes referring to notes scribbled earlier in my journal, scribbled words that capture words spoken. I prefer to write in the present tense to better capture the moment. I like the computer because I can move words around later as I seek to find the flow between words. But first just let the words come as a spontaneous flow in rich description, paying attention to as much detail as possible, pursuing signs, running off on tangents.

In my workshops, practitioners are always astonished with the amount they write. Revealing the storied self. Putting together the pieces of self, of life itself. A creative, restorative act. Tufnell and Crickmay (2004:41) write:

> We come to know more of what matters in our lives, less through an in-tuned search for self, than in conversation, in relationship to what is around us. We rarely know what currents flow beneath what we are doing and feeling. The impulses, instincts and intuitions that impel our thoughts and actions are as animals moving in the shadows of our everyday awareness. As we create we discover events, characters, places, sights and sounds, whose significance we cannot quite define, yet whose presence makes more visible what is moving through our lives. Creating is a way of listening and of trying to speak more personally from within the various worlds we inhabit. It is a way of discovering our own stories, refreshing and reawakening our language and giving form to the way we feel.

Journalling is creating. Knowing I am going to write a story prompts me to be mindful, pay more attention to what is unfolding moment to moment within practice. It always seems remarkable how much detail the body absorbs. To write I find a quiet eddy out of the fast current of life, to pause, muse, to clear and let go of the mind and open the body to pay attention to the experience, to create a space where I can get back into the experience with all my senses. It is much more than a cognitive exercise of recall. It is as if I seek to dwell within the situation as a witness. In this way I tap into the 'right side of my brain and stir the centres for imagination, creativity, perception, intuition. These qualities of self are not just useful for reflection but are also pivotal in developing clinical expertise.

Teaching reflection, I first invite practitioners to write spontaneously for 20 minutes, not to take their pen of the paper or pause to think too much about what they are writing. I intend to move them beyond the rational mind into their deep wells of intuitive knowing, letting submerged thoughts and feelings rise to the conscious surface and find expression. People are often surprised by what emerges, how one thing has tangentially led to another. Leaps of connection.

Okri (1997:22) writes:

> Do not distain the idle, strange, ordinary, nonsensical, or shocking thoughts which the mind throws up. Hold them. Look at them. Play with them. See where they lead. Every perception or possibility has its own life-span: some have short lives, others keep on growing, and many are open to infusions of greater life …

When the 20 minutes have passed, some practitioners have not written about what they had initially intended. When practitioners try to reflect before they write description they often seem to get caught up in the situation, and struggle to free their self enough to write. Like trying to run before you can walk. Writing itself creates space to see self more clearly but sometimes the entanglement seems too tight. Then I might suggest going to the window and writing about what can be seen, describing something neutral to loosen the mind and body. Often practitioners are weighed down with deep-seated experiences that stem back many years, and feel the urge to write about these experiences. Without doubt, writing is a way of healing (DeSalvo 1999). DeSalvo cites Mark Doty (1996) 'what is healing, but a shift in perspective?' (p. 3). From the old English word 'haelen', healing is to make whole – as if writing can help us return to a sense of being whole – bringing the self fully home.

Writing is a making sense at a deeper, embodied level of knowing than the conscious mind. It is tuning into learnt patterns of being, and so, imperceptibly, the writer begins to re-pattern. As we pay attention to these things in writing, so we expand our attention span within practice itself. Again, Okri (1997) writes:

> There is an inner part of us for ever obscured, for ever mysterious, which is the most alive during the process of composition. And that inner part, that inner glow, is timeless, and it functions beyond time. It drinks from deep waters. It has the stillness and the dance and the radiance of the firmament.

Journalling may seem relatively simple but it requires discipline to get down to do it. And that is just the beginning of the reflective process. In busy worlds there may seem more important and enjoyable things to do. This is especially so if we view journalling as a task. But if we can see that journalling is writing our self, then nothing should be more significant then this first step of self-inquiry towards realising self.

Cox *et al.* (1991:379) write 'there are no rules, no right or wrong ways of journaling'. People tell their stories as best they can. Over time they will develop a certain style that suits them. Just do it and see where it takes you. You might write a story or just a few words, or simply scratch the paper with your feelings. Consider also what constrains your writing.

Commitment and practice are vital before we seek perfection (Manjusvara 2005) – the commitment to become the most effective practitioner. Those to whom we offer service to deserve nothing less. If we are tired or burned out then we turn away from the reflective mirror – it can be too painful to contemplate self, to remind ourselves of our responsibility. We may not value this approach to learning and research, being caught up in more 'scientific' approaches where the 'I' is buried in the objective demand. I meet many practitioners who say they cannot write, or are harsh critics of what they do write, as if protecting themselves against failure. We need to tame our inner critics who strip us of confidence and make us feel unworthy. Setting time limits such as 20 minutes is helpful, because it encourages focus on getting words on paper rather than the quality of the words written.

Description enables the practitioner to articulate the way she intuitively responds within often complex situations:

> drawing on their own private data base, immediate and persuasive, which informs them of the truth value of any particular concept (Spence 1982:212).

Writing is opening the doors of perception. In doing so, Okri (1997:21) urges us to approach writing with:

> the spirit of play, of foreplay, of dalliance, doodling, messing around – and then, bit by bit, you somehow get deeper into the matter. But if you go in there with a businessman's solemnity or the fanaticism of some artistic types you are likely to be rewarded with a stiff response, a joyless dribble, strained originality, ideas that come out all strapped up and strangled by too much effort.

Ruth Morgan (2005) writes:

Journalling is a means of writing reflectively about meaningful events as a way of listening and paying attention to one's own 'heartbeat of experience' (Johns 2000:45). The discipline of writing journal acts as a trigger to reflective contemplation of the day's events. It also provides a means of collecting data on self, which Street (1995) argues is a responsible way of developing personal practice.

The exercise of writing regular entries has proved an ongoing struggle for me. Faced with home and work pressures, journal keeping has felt an extra burden and a low priority. I am conscious that the time I have allotted and the infrequency of my entries have not done justice to the clear benefits of the exercise. Reflective writing brings everyday experiences events into focus enabling the journal to act as a midwife, giving birth to new understanding Pinar (1981).

My own experience has consistently proved the value of this. Regardless of the brevity of time allowed, I find the process of journalling consistently enlightening. My writing tends to take place during unplanned, quiet moments at home and I am frequently amazed by the insights that just a few minutes of focused reflection can achieve. Today I wrote briefly about a clinical supervision session with Ellen in which I was acting as supervisor, triggered by a distant feeling of unease:

> 'May 2005 – Ellen spoke of the difficulties she was having with another member of staff. Initially I thought this was a helpful session but now as I look back I recognise how I took over the conversation and led the conclusions. The unhealthy relationship she described did not surprise me as its effects are obvious and causing problems for other members of staff. I can see that my strong (and rather irritated) feelings on the subject led me to give solutions rather than allow Ellen to consider her own. My responses now echo back at me sounding managerial and uncompromising ...'

These insights surprised me since I had not recognised them earlier. Ellen had been tearful during the session causing me some disquiet but that had been erased by the business of the remainder of the day. Through writing reflectively on this event, my future ways of responding are challenged and changed. The possibility of journal writing is to write freely and without censure.

Looking back my early entries clearly served as a cathartic process as I struggled with the doubts and insecurities of a change of job and role. Further entries represent the highs and lows of many experiences and demonstrate my struggles as a leader within a complex, unpredictable environment. I cannot go so far as to give my journal the title of 'friend' (Street 1995) but it is certainly proving a loyal and faithful companion on my leadership journey illuminating the shadows and shining a guiding light ahead.

In the narrative construction chapter of her master's dissertation Susan Brooks (2004:28–31) writes:

Data was collected and analysed by means of journaling to chronicle and reflect upon a multitude of experiences encountered in daily practice. Journal writing, as a means to facilitate learning, is a technique endorsed by many writers (Boud *et al.* 1985; Hahnemann 1986; Street 1995; Wong *et al.* 1995; Johns 2002).

It is essentially the recording of experiences and snaring of moments and this process formed the basis of research into self, providing the necessary data to facilitate reflective analysis and determine systematic and rational change (Street 1995; Moon 2004). Street (1995) records that journal writing has the capacity to deconstruct the relationships between thought and action, knowledge and practice, values and assumptions, and the individual and society. Hahnemann (1986) sees the journal writing process as intensely personal when she writes that it involves the use of highly complex cognitive processes and enables the writer to define oneself and one's beliefs and to make one's voice heard. Journal writing is not presented as an easy task and it posed some notable challenges, challenges that became quickly obvious to me from the outset. Having never attempted to keep a reflective journal before – the journey ahead seemed a little daunting as evidenced by the first recorded entry that reflects the fear that I experienced at that time.

> 'March 2002 – Today I start my journal. What shall I write? I'm really worried about this whole thing – will I get time to do it – will I want to do it – will I do it right? If I'm honest in it will it matter if others read it? Reflective practice, reflective practice – what is it really? I think I know but I don't think I've ever really done it properly. I feel so uncertain about everything at the moment and a bit scared and threatened. I don't feel I know anything about myself really and I suppose I just do what I do to fit in. I need to get over this and get on with it – pull yourself together Sue – you know you can do it.'

In retrospect, my first journal entry clearly reveals my initial uncomfortable reactions to the prospect of journal writing. I had doubts about my capacity to write, felt threatened by having to face myself on paper, questioned my ability to manage my internal censors that may inhibit complete honesty and held the naïve assumption that there is a correct way to keep a journal – all classic reactions to journaling (Street 1995).

These initial fears were quickly dispelled as the value of my journal soon became evident. After I while, it seemed to become a powerful emancipatory tool in giving my innermost thoughts voice. I was the only person with access to the journal and, possibly because of this, it became a very cathartic experience to write. As the process continued, I soon recognised that I did not need to confront all the chaos of my personal or professional life at any one time and became more discriminatory about the events that I considered worthy of deeper reflection and subsequent action (Street 1995). The journal became, in a sense, my auto-biography containing both positive and less than positive experiences – a non-hagiographic record of my daily life. My journal had, after just a few months on the course, become a silent but very powerful and challenging teacher – perhaps more persuasive and influential than any human embodiment that I had met.

The following entry signifies just how my attitude had changed since that first entry at the start of the course.

> 'July 2002 – I read of a teacher today who got very excited about writing his journal. He wrote that he felt especially good about writing for himself instead of someone else. His written thoughts were entirely his own regardless of lack of style, format or academic expression. He had never written like this before and felt that he was really communicating with and understanding himself. That's just how I feel now and I wish I had started writing like this ages ago. To be unrestricted by structural rigour, academic expectations and the approval of others is so liberating!'

Ann Saunders (2006) writes:

I started to journal in an enthusiastic manner, I noted initially this included most of the day, as if I was trying to justify my salary rather than focus on one event. This was tiring and after a while found that my enthusiasm was eroding. I then narrowed it down to one event per day, shorter and more concise but became a haphazard event. I am encouraged by the words of Street (1992) who describes journalling as an unfamiliar activity for nurses as we historically write short accounts. After more 'nagging' by our tutor on the importance of this, I decided to use half an hour at the end of the working day, as coming home and doing it felt like a chore. Why then am I viewing self exploration, higher academic study and the potential of the benefit for self and others, a chore? It is I believe the division that I try to maintain between taking my professional hat off as I come home, and putting on the mother, wife, daughter hat. It is almost as though I have adopted the Newtonian view of life at work and the ontological theory at home, when in reality they both interlink to form my own lived reality. Or in Schön's (1983) terms a principle of technical rationality.

Journalling is open to interpretation as with all forms of communication. What I write in my journal is my perception of events. It may be inaccurate, my mental models, as Senge (1990) points out, may be biased due to my assumptions. I acknowledge this, but writing in a 'naïve' and spontaneous manner offers up these assumptions for examination. I concur with Woolf (1945) when she expresses the view that the writer is different from the self who later reads what is written. The experience of writing naïvely is to capture unknowingly, what later becomes evident on analysis. I could argue however that from the spoken word to the written word something may be lost in the ether. The spoken word can float away but the written words remains.

Why then, if my negativity still prevails, do I lean towards the writings of Street (1992) who challenges the views with which I aspire to? She argues that we must first recognise ourselves before we recognise others. However, in order to make sense of my newfound reality my journal has been a comfort, friend and critic enabling me to view situations from a variant slant. It has made me stand still and enabled me to select issues from the unending data that Wheatley (1999) describes as being barely noticeable in the fast pace of our lives.

As previously mentioned, I hesitated to write honestly and openly towards self. Street (1992) likened this to the recognition of the 'internal censor', which regulates, emotions, feelings and failings which flags them up to myself or others to criticise. The internal censor however, is also open to questioning through self, being honest and in recognising the need for truth. This is the practitioner's own responsibility and one is which I did not take lightly. As one continues to journal and the benefits become apparent, the unfolding moments are unveiled in greater depth and insight.

One morning I write:

The first shafts of light filter through the window, appearing from the side of the thick curtain that doesn't quite cover the window opening. Frost thick on the ground, the slate roof of the adjoining barn white, the meadow grass a faint green. The sky clear, lightening, the sun not yet risen beyond the distant peach coloured horizon. Nature is first contact, a reality check from the thoughts and dreams of the night – one dream quiet vivid, and yet as my dreams are always, so unreal, surrealist images, I can never capture them in written words … (my journal – 27 December 2008).

Sometimes I surprise myself with my writing. Writing transcends the rational mind, and as we write we stumble upon and discover images, metaphors, analogies and symbols that sharpen perception, hold meaning and 'open ourselves into intuition of which our rational side is barely conscious' (Manjusvara 2005:12).

The second dialogical movement: from description to reflection

We usually just look at the surface of life, thinking we can find meaning there, that is, if we think about meaning at all. So much is simply taken for granted. Yet when we work with peoples' lives, every moment is significant and should never be taken for granted. Every moment is a mystery unfolding if we can learn to pay attention. 'There are many things you don't know, because life is really unfathomable' (Katagiri 2008:10). Reflection enables you to plunge below the surface and leads you to touch the core of your life. It's not easy. But even so, you have to do it because who we need to become is important to us. Reflection provides a way of 'turning the mirror inwards' and 'learning to unearth our internal pictures of the world' (Senge 1990:9).

I pause from my writing. Description is exhausted. I can say no more, at least for the moment. In front of me is my 'story text'. I step back from the text in order to see it more clearly, to bring it into a more objective focus. Curious, I can now ask questions of my text, to converse with it and pull it open for its significance and meaning, to expose contradiction between my practice and my vision of desirable practice and open up the learning space.

Dewey (1933:35) writes:

> While we cannot learn or be taught to think, we do have to learn how to think well, especially how to acquire the general habit of reflecting.

Reflection is the conscious opening to experience, as if opening the lid on the rich descriptive text – 'OK – so what does it all mean?' 'What insights do I draw from this towards self-realisation?'

Describing reflection

I describe reflection as a window through which the practitioner can view and focus self within the context of her own lived experience in ways that enable her to confront, understand and work towards resolving the contradictions within her practice between what is desirable and actual practice. Through the conflict of contradiction, the commitment to realise desirable work, and understanding why things are as they are, the practitioner can become empowered to take more appropriate action in future situations within a reflexive spiral of being and becoming. The practitioner may require guidance to realise the potential of reflection.

The emphasis on *being* acknowledges the existential moment of the unfolding moment, whilst the emphasis on *becoming* acknowledges the transformative nature of reflection. Reflexivity is the looking back and seeing self as a changed person through the series of unfolding experiences that have been reflected on and learnt through. Many practitioners do not have a clear vision of desirable practice, although they easily sense contradiction as an affront to their beliefs. By exploring contradiction, the practitioner is challenged to articulate and confront her beliefs for their meaning in practice and congruence within a wider health care community.

Structured reflection

If I asked you to reflect on experience, you may be uncertain what this means. A number of 'models' have been constructed with the intention of guiding this process (Mezirow 1981; Boyd and Fales 1983; Boud *et al.* 1985; Gibbs 1988) to name a few. In my own work, I have analysed patterns of *guidance* dialogue with practitioners to construct the *Model for Structured Reflection* (MSR) (Johns 2009) to guide the practitioner to access the breadth and depth of experience for learning to take place.

The MSR sets out a pathway from significance to drawing insights. Significance lies on the surface of experience and as we peel away the skin and go deeper into the hermeneutic spiral guided by the MSR cues, we reveal insights.

Box 2.1   Model for Structured Reflection (15A edition)

(1) Bring the mind home
(2) Write a description of an experience that seems significant in some way
(3) What issues seem significant to pay attention to?
(4) How were others feeling and what made them feel that way?
(5) How was I feeling and what made me feel that way?
(6) What was I trying to achieve and did I respond effectively?
(7) What were the consequences of my actions on the patient, others and myself?
(8) What factors influenced the way I was feeling, thinking or responding?
(9) What knowledge did or might have informed me?
(10) To what extent did I act for the best and in tune with my values?
(11) How does this situation connect with previous experiences?
(12) How might I reframe the situation and respond more effectively given this situation again?
(13) What would be the consequences of alternative actions for the patient, others and myself?
(14) What factors might constrain me from responding differently?
(15) How do I NOW feel about this experience?
(16) Am I now more able to support myself and others better as a consequence?
(17) What insights do I draw towards self-realisation?

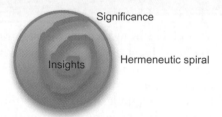

Significance

Insights

Hermeneutic spiral

Since its conception in 1990, the adequacy of the MSR to guide practitioners has been continually tested, and in response to feedback I have reflexively developed the model, culminating in the 15A edition (Box 2.1). The reflective cues prompt the practitioner to deconstruct her experiences in ways that lead to understanding and insights to influence future experiences towards self-realisation.

Commentary on the MSR

(1) The cue 'Bringing the mind home' is preparatory, reminding the practitioner/narrator to bring self fully present to the reflective moment through using the breath.

(2) The cue 'Focus on a recent experience that seems significant in some way' prompts the practitioner to write a description of experience as I have explored previously. This can be harder than imagined, especially when a practitioner commences reflection, simply because so much of experience is taken for granted. Usually something *significant* is associated with feelings because that is what brings the experience into consciousness. As practitioners become mindful, they tend to know which experiences are significant in terms of developing the reflexive narrative.

(3) The cue 'What issues seem significant to pay attention to?' prompts the practitioner to sift the description for significance. What is significant may seem obvious to the self-inquiry – after all, the narrator wrote it! However, scratching the surface of description reveals other, less obvious, significance, and as the inquirer goes deeper, more and more issues emerge as significant. Taken to its ultimate limits the whole

pattern of practice will be revealed, the way the single moment contains the whole. It is a question then of pulling out significance or 'parts' but always against the background of the whole – the hermeneutic spiral.

(4) The cue 'How were others feeling and why did they feel that way?' prompts the practitioner to pay attention to feelings of others within the situation. This cue helps to develop empathy, connection with others in terms of their experience. This is often difficult because we tend to see others through a lens of self-concern. So – how was the other truly feeling and what is the root of that? It is so easy to make surface assumptions as a projection of our own thoughts and feelings.

(5) The cue 'How was I feeling and what me feel that way?' prompts the practitioner to pay attention to their own feelings within the situation with a view to resolving any emotional tension that may impede clarity and interfere with realising desirable practice. Often feelings such as anger, guilt, frustration and sadness draw the practitioner's attention to experience. Feelings are gateways into our stories because they ripple and disturb consciousness. Like cream, such negative feelings rise to the surface of consciousness from the vast weight of experience that resides in the subconscious and which has never been consciously paid attention to precisely because it was uneventful. It leads to random reflection on disparate events.

Boud *et al.* (1985) highlight the way feelings influence the way things are perceived and hence the significance of paying attention to feelings within relation to taking action. They note:

> Of particular importance within description is the observation of the feeling evoked during the experience. On occasions our emotional reactions can override our rationality to such an extent that we react unwarily and with blurred perceptions. (Boud *et al.* 1985:28)

I question Boud *et al.*'s emphasis on rationality as the basis for learning when clearly feelings are so influential. Perception is simply what it is. It is not blurred by feelings. The expression of feelings is always cathartic. The issue is not so much removing them but accepting them as valid and harnessing this energy for taking positive action. One way to reflect is to write how one is feeling:

> 'I am angry'
> 'I feel guilty'
> 'I feel satisfied'

Then ask – why do I feel this way? With regard to negative feelings, the work of Pennebaker (1990) and DeSalvo (1999) indicates that the therapeutic impact of writing hinges around making connections between feelings and events. This is a significant insight to support the idea that guided reflection is a healing modality. Manjusvara (2005:21) offers a useful perspective:

> We can let go of our current ways of responding to ourselves and others and replace them with something better, entering a stream of ever more positive emotions and even greater creative energy.

(6) The cue 'What was I trying to achieve and did I respond effectively?' prompts the practitioner to reflect on her intention and the goals of her actions. This cue, more than any other opens up the sense of contradiction between intention and actuality.

The question of effectiveness is problematic – how might the practitioner appreciate her effectiveness? What criteria might she use to judge this? The cue nurtures responsibility for both self and other to be most effective. Our patients and those with whom we work should expect nothing less than this commitment.

(7) The cue 'What were the consequences of my actions on the patient, others and myself? prompts the practitioner to critique action in terms of consequences. I assume that all action is purposeful or intentional towards anticipated outcomes. But so many actions are reactionary to the moment, and may lead to unanticipated consequences, or consequences outside the normal scope of consideration, given that all things are connected. The cue is fundamental for the development of practical wisdom or phronesis – the ability to make wise judgement in the light of anticipated consequences. It goes to the core of effective practice and hence is the most vital of cues alongside 'was I effective'?

(8) The cue 'What factors influenced the way I was feeling, thinking or responding?' prompts the practitioner to identify and reflect on those forces embodied within self or embedded in the environment that influence the way the practitioner sees and responds to the world. It is a deceptive cue and difficult to penetrate simply because so much of 'who we are' is taken for granted. These forces can be summarised as 'force', 'tradition' and 'embodiment' (Fay 1987). I might also add 'theory' as a fourth force. Over time, I have drawn out common influences and incorporated them within the 'influences grid' (Figure 2.2). The grid acts as a checklist for the practitioner to consider the relevance of each point.

Cope (2001) writes of 'shadow maps', the concealed behaviours, thoughts and feelings that remain unidentified. Okri (1997) hints at these – 'the hidden selves of the stories' – but of course it is the story-teller who is really revealed, from the dark corners of the shadow maps. These lead us to establish defensive routines as a kind of protection. I think of the right side of my journal as the shadow side – it stands besides my explicit narrative; unseen, until the light of reflection exposes it. Guidance is often needed to confront and support the practitioner to move deep within self.

Conforming to normal practice/ habit? The weight of tradition		Negative attitudes and prejudice? Racism?	Expectations from others; knowledge to act in certain ways?
Limited skills/ discomfort/ confidence to act in new ways?			Fear of sanction? The weight of authority
Emotional entanglement/over identification?	What forces have influenced my decision making and actions?		Misplaced concern – loyalty to colleagues versus loyalty to patient? Anxious about ensuing conflict?
Need to be valued? Deeper psyche factors?			Knowledge to act in specific ways? The weight of theory
Wrapped up in self-concern? Pity? Stressed? Guilt? Frustration? Other feelings?	Time/priorities?		Expectations from self about 'how I should act' Doing what was felt to be right?

Figure 2.2 The influences grid

(9) The cue 'What knowledge did or might have informed me?' prompts the practitioner to reflect on whether I responded within the experience in the most effective way as indicated by theory, research findings, protocols and the suchlike. I describe this as theoretical framing – my ability to access and critique 'information' for its relevance to inform my actions and, as appropriate, to assimilate within my clinical practice.

From a reflective perspective, evidence is never accepted on face value. The reflective practitioner views all knowledge through a sceptical eye (Dewey 1933) for its validity and relevance to inform practice. Knowledge can only inform; it can never be predictive. It always needs to be interpreted for its relevance within the specific situation rather than applied as a prescription.

Libraries are lined with rows upon rows of books. Journal shelves are bulging. Health care is obsessed with 'evidence-based practice' – which puts a great strain on the practitioner to access and meaningfully apply such knowledge to her everyday practice. Making links between practice and theory is a daunting task for practitioners who lead busy lives and simply cannot find the time, even with the motivation, to explore the vast realm of journals and books.

(10) 'To what extent did I act for the good and in tune with my values?' – this cue prompts the practitioner to consider their decisions and actions from the perspective of ethics and values. Values are linked to integrity – that the practitioner always seeks to act according to her values. If these are compromised than she feels contradiction and unease. Hence the value of vision to enable the practitioner to be mindful of her values as lived within each moment. The nitty-gritty of reflection. The values practitioners hold are informed by ethics – the idea of acting for the good or in terms of what is the right thing to do. Often, such ethics are in themselves contradictory and lead to conflict.

Acting for the good can be critiqued using 'ethical mapping' (Figure 2.3).

The map focuses the practitioner to pay attention to multiple and competing perspectives about the particular situation, including her own. In this sense the practitioner positions herself 'in-between' (Parker 1997:22). Parker notes that 'a number of temporalities will intersect to create an uneasy space' (p. 22). This space 'in-between' is tense with potential and actual conflict about an unpredictable future. Where is each person coming from, what are their interests and agendas? Why are they responding as they do? The practitioner in mediating this space needs to be reflective of her own perspective and its

Patient's /family's position	Who had authority to make the decision/act within the situation?	The doctor's position
If there is conflict of perspectives/values – how might these be resolved?	The situation/dilemma	What ethical principles inform this situation?
The practitioner's position	Consider the power relationships/ factors that determined the way the decision/action was actually taken	The organisation's position

Figure 2.3 Ethical mapping (Johns 2009)

influence in mediating the other perspectives. From this perspective no one perspective is privileged, confronting authority claims for a dominant perspective. Mediation is given an objective edge by a claim on ethical principles to reflect on ethical decision making and consequent action. The map guides the practitioner to view these competing perspectives from diverse ethical perspectives and to review the interface between ethical principles and the ethics of the situation (Cooper 1991). Mediation reveals any conflict of interest and to consider ways in which any conflict might be resolved for the best. The map draws the practitioner's attention to explore issues around authority and autonomy to make decisions, and finally to examine the way the decision was actually taken in terms of power. The analysis of power ways of relating enables the practitioner to review herself in these terms and to consider ways of countering power in order for the best decision to be made.

However, as Rudge (1997:83) notes, citing Buchbinder (1994:30):

> Just as discourses reflect dominant positions, and prescribe 'what is said and to whom; and with regard to who is to be heard and thus empowered by given a voice, and who is to be silenced and hence disempowered', they do allow the possibility of alternative or *resistant* discourses. [Emphasis added]

From this perspective ethical mapping has the potential to facilitate discourse and shift taken for granted or hegemonic practices. It opens a Pandora's box. Ethical mapping intends to help practitioners 'see' the various contextual factors within any ethical decision. At each point within this 'map', the supervisor challenges the practitioner to understand and balance the dynamics towards making the 'right' decision within the particular circumstance.

Trail:

(a) Consider each perspective in turn commencing with the practitioner(s) own perspectives.
(b) Consider which ethical principles apply in terms of the best (ethically correct) decision.
(c) Consider what conflict exists between perspectives/values and how these might be resolved.
(d) Consider who had the authority for making the decision/taking action?
(e) Consider the power relationships/factors that determined the way the decision/action was actually taken.

(11) The cue 'How does this situation connect with previous experiences?' prompts the practitioner to consider the impact of past experiences on the way they perceived and responded to the present experience. It acknowledges that reflection is never an isolated event but a moment of paying attention within the endless flow of experiences. Every experience is informed by previous experiences. Are there patterns of behaviour evident? Do I keep falling into the stream? If I am looking back at the past (with regret, resentment, disappointment, longing, fond memory) then I am not looking forward to new possibilities.

(12) The cue 'How might I reframe the situation and respond more effectively given this situation again?' prompts the practitioner to shift from looking back at a situation to moving forward and anticipate the possibilities for responding differently, more effectively – to be creative and imagine new ways of responding within situations. Lateral thinking helps to pull open the mind's shutters, developing the creative and imaginative self and expanding the practitioner's repertoire of available and effective responses.

(13) The cue 'What would be the consequences of alternative actions for the patient, others and myself?' prompts the practitioner to consider potentially more effective ways to respond within a similar situation and then to choose the most favourable in light of its potential consequences. Imagining new ways of responding, of being, is like planting seeds in body to germinate under the right conditions (Margolis 1993). It prepares insights for action.

(14) The cue 'What factors might constrain me from responding differently?' prompts the practitioner to have a reality check. It cuts across any fantasy about how the practitioner would ideally respond to consider whether she has the resources to respond differently in tune with her values. I call this 'the reality wall' – the point where I must face reality because of factors embodied within me and reinforced within normal patterns of relating, which are likely to constrain me from responding in new, more desirable ways. It is vital to acknowledge that it is not easy to shift the realty wall, but that's okay – it is a real world and it's tough sometimes. I can understand the reality wall in the broad terms of tradition, authority and embodiment, whilst helping me to become empowered to act in more congruent ways. However, just because I can understand something doesn't mean I can change it. But understanding it *is* the first step towards changing it. I learn to plot, become strategic, devise tactics. I am resolute, committed and patient.

In my experience, these 'looking forward' cues are neglected perhaps because reflection is often perceived as looking back at events rather than looking forward and anticipating future situations. Yet these cues are vital for making the 'reflexive link' between experiences within the unfolding narrative.

(15) The cue 'How do I NOW feel about this experience?' prompts the practitioner to harness together the bits of energy dissipated within the reflective space and focus this energy to take positive action.

(16) The cue 'Am I now more able to support myself and others better as a consequence' prompts practitioners to reflect on their support systems within practice. The cue often exposes impoverished support systems and challenges the practitioner to develop more effective systems.

Insights

(17) The cue 'What insights do I draw towards self-realisation?' takes the practitioner full circle preparing the ground for the next experience where insights gained might be applied. Insights, by their very nature change people. They are not rational ideas, but embodied with the person's being, subtly or dramatically shifting the way the person perceives and responds to the world. They are profound and the links within the hermeneutic spiral and the basis of reflexivity.

Insights are moments of resistance and possibility – moments that resist development grounded in current reality and moments of possibility grounded in vision of self and practice. These insights are in constant creative tension that the practitioner seeks to resolve in order to live one's vision as a lived reality.

Table 2.1 The framing perspectives

Framing perspective	How has this experience enabled me to:
Vision (previously philosophical)	Confront and clarify my beliefs and values that constitute my vision of self and practice?
Role	Clarify and challenge my role boundaries, autonomy and 'power' relationships with others?
Reality perspective	Accept and understand that sometimes I cannot change things quickly because of forces within practice; whilst challenging and supporting me to become empowered to act in new, more congruent ways?
Theoretical	Access, critique and assimilate relevant theory within personal knowing in ways that enable me to make sense of my experience and inform my practice?
Problem	Focus, understand and explore new ways to solve particular problems in my practice?
Temporal (or reflexive)	Make connection between the present experience with past experiences whilst anticipating how I might respond in future situations?
Parallel process	Make connection between the learning process in supervision and clinical practice?
Reflexivity	Plot my emergence of self-realisation?

Framing perspectives

To create a way to pattern insights I developed 'framing perspectives' to guide the practitioner to sense the scope of potential insights (Table 2.1). To use the framing perspectives, the practitioner simply asks self, 'How has this experience enabled me to …'.

All experience is bounded by vision and role. Yet vision and role are always shifting as the practitioner moves towards self-realisation through her experiences. The constant review of 'vision' is essential in holding intentionality – giving purpose and direction to each moment. Holding the intention it is more realised. Role is simply a set of ideas that impose arbitrary limits on one's responsibility, autonomy and accountability. How these issues are played out are revealed through everyday experiences, notably the way tradition imposes normal hegemonic patterns of relating that constrain self-realisation. It is this understanding of current reality that is the focus of *reality perspective framing*. I call it the reality wall because practitioners get headaches banging their heads against it. Yet, as I constantly note, truly understanding current reality is the basis for change. In theoretical framing the practitioner connects her ideas emerging from her experience with theory-weaving them into her personal knowing and informing her insights. Put another way, experience is a hat to hang theory on – only then does theory make any sense and can be meaningfully applied within practice. This is the *third dialogical movement*, the dialogue with theory. Theory can be mapped to guide the practitioner to position and review herself within the theory. For example, the leadership students utilise the 'Thomas–Kilmann Conflict mode instrument' (1974) to position their actual and desired conflict management style. Another example is the development of voice as a metaphor for empowerment through the work of Belenky *et al.* (1986) (see Appendix 1 for a summary of some of these 'framing tools').

My vision of practice is to ease suffering. I do not seek to know suffering as a concept. Concepts close down possibility of experiencing simply because we then think we know what it is. It is the difference between an epistemological approach to clinical practice based on a conceptual knowledge and an ontological one based on experiencing leading to an embodied knowledge or personal knowing that is not so easily articulated. I sense the way theory is accepted uncritically, as if being published it has a built-in authority based on a positivist legacy that theory exists to predict and control practice. Hence practitioners' response to theory can be uncritical and passive. No theory can predict within the human–human encounter. All such encounters are mysteries unfolding. Even when we have experienced many similar situations, this particular one is unique. The non-critical application of theory to practice is to reduce people, including self, to the status of objects to be manipulated.

As I have alluded to throughout the book, sources of theory can be drawn from very diverse literary sources rather than from more traditional disciplinary theoretical texts. Indeed every book I read, I read for its potential to inform my narrative practice.

Through *problem posing*, the practitioner pulls out and frames what Mezirow (1981) describes as disorientating dilemmas that interrupt the flow of experience. Once framed, the practitioner can see the thing for what it is and focus her mind towards resolving it in tune with her vision. In this sense guided reflection is an action research process (Kemmis 1985) of problem identification, understanding, action and evaluation within the hermeneutic spiral.

Temporal framing is the key to reflexivity, guiding the practitioner to draw links between the present experience and past experiences whilst anticipating future experiences – the way experience loops together to give the narrative its distinct pattern, coherence and reflexive dimension. Parallel process framing seeks to appreciate the parallel nature of guided reflection and clinical practice. For example, the plot of Yvonne Latchford's narrative (Chapter 7) is the parallel growth of her own and her client's empowerment as inter-linking spirals that weave together. My guidance relationship with Yvonne is reflected within her relationship with Deidre. My response to Yvonne role models ways she can respond to Deidre. In parallel process framing these dynamics are surfaced and worked with consciously even though operate on a more subliminal level. This also reflects the way guided reflection and clinical practice mirror each other as holistic practices.

Reflection on using the MSR

The MSR *is not a prescription for reflection*. Nursing, in particular, has a culture of fitting experience to models rather than using models creatively to perceive the nature of experience (Johns and Graham 1996). As Emden (1991) suggested, adhering to a model (she used the model devised by Boud *et al.* 1985) may be unhelpful because it encouraged her to fit experience into arbitrary stages rather than using the model creatively. This is a legacy of the way many practitioners are socialised into a received knowledge of practice. From this view the model authoritatively defines the nature of reality although always from a partial view. From a reflective perspective, the value of any model is the extent it helps the practitioner see something in its wholeness rather than impose a rigid world view. A paradox of the MSR is that the cues might be perceived as fragmenting the holistic essence of experience, and yet practitioners often perceive experience as fragmentary. Rather than fragmenting experience, by using the MSR, the guide can enable the practitioner bring together the fragments of experience into a meaningful whole. Although there is a logical flow through the cues they are not intended to be sequential.

Whilst I advocate the use of the MSR, I also encourage the practitioner to chose a model that works best for them. Using a model is important because it gives reflection shape and rigour and hence helps to counter criticism that reflection lacks rationality. It is still a sign of our times that we have to try to justify our subjective processes.

By initially using the cues in an overt way, the practitioner integrates reflection within her consciousness until reflection becomes a natural process. Rather like choosing a pair of shoes, she tries various styles until one seems to fit. Whilst using the MSR may seem straightforward, many practitioners struggle with the idea of using a model of reflection and keeping a reflective diary.

Nina was a community nurse respondent within my PhD study. Donna was her guide. In their twelfth session (which took place after ten months of commencing the guided reflection relationship) Nina still struggled using the MSR.

Nina: I've tried to use the MSR for this experience from last session, but something else has happened. I wrote about that too but didn't use the model. I'm not quite sure about a couple of things. I seem to repeat myself. I shall see if you think it is a reflection or just a description. I'm concerned I'm not using it properly. My biggest problem I've got is paperwork. I find it difficult like care plans. What I find difficult is everything that is paper – there's a trend now that we have to write things down.

Donna: Hang on a moment. What are you saying? You mean the diary – you don't find it useful?

Nina: I don't know – it's helping me to think and therefore it is useful. Where I am finding it difficult is going through each section [of the MSR] knowing what to put where. I think I could get as much from just discussing it, not writing it down. The other experience I shared I just wrote down how I felt. I let it flow. I didn't use the model.

Nina resisted the model because it involved writing things down. She had a barrier with any sort of paperwork which she felt interfered with being with the patient. As it was, the description of the experience she read was muddled. Yet, the corner had been turned. In their next session Nina shared an experience using the MSR which led to a much deeper exploration of the experience. She reflected on how the structure had 'redefined my thinking'.

Donna was acting to reassure Nina when in fact she needed to guide Nina much earlier in the research process to become reflective. This can be done by using the MSR cues as a checklist at the end of the session or during a pause in the dialogue when either the guide or the practitioner feel uncertain about continuing the dialogue. Nina's comments reflect the way many practitioners try to fit experience into a model regardless of whether it is a model of reflection or a nursing model rather than use the model creatively as a way of seeing and making sense of experience. Whilst models of reflection, such as the MSR, can trigger additional thought they can also be simplistic and narrow the reflective process. I have deliberately not confined my writing to addressing concrete questions. However there are times when my head is spinning in a cross-wind of too many things to think through. On these occasions a structured approach has proved helpful in enabling me to unravel my thoughts and channel my reflections.

Dwelling with the text

Let the play of breeze flow through me without resistance …

Whilst exploring the MSR cues the practitioner dwells within the text (within the hermeneutic spiral) in her search for meaning and insights. Perhaps insights come dripping slowly or perhaps they come as moments of revelation. Whatever, it requires patience in scrolling down the text, as if turning over words to reveal hidden meanings, scrolling down the text through the familiar into new areas to explore until an insight is sensed, perhaps captured in a single word. I break the text into single lines and in doing so, making connections between words, revealing meanings buried between the lines. I change words and discover I am writing prose poetry, capturing meaning in metaphors and images.

Morgan (2005) writes:

> Unchallenged our preconceptions can develop into leaps of abstraction when we mistakenly translate inner assumptions into factual knowledge. The practitioner must be patient, spinning the experience around, shaking out nuggets of insight with each spin. Perhaps in the middle of the night or some weeks later, the insight will emerge. It is birthing process.

One technique to help the practitioner dwell within and scroll down the text is to create a right or left hand column depending on your preference to jot down the unspoken. Ruth Morgan (2005) preferred a left hand column! She writes:

> The left-hand column technique recommended by Senge (1990) is illustrated below in my journal entry of 2nd June 2004. I used this structure to clarify a situation that had irritated me that day and upset the sister on the ward.

WHAT I WAS THINKING	WHAT WAS SAID/DONE
	Sister X: I called for a doctor's visit to check the redness on patient R's sacrum.
The doctor will think we are pathetic for calling him.	*Me:* To call a doctor to look at that is absurd.
Surely she could have reassured the family herself. She's supposed to be an experienced nurse.	*Sister X:* The family were very anxious and wanted it seen by a doctor. I needed to cover myself.
This will reflect badly on me as a leader.	*Me:* I do not agree with calling the doctor. As nurses we should be reassuring the family. We are clinically competent to do so.

My thoughts in the left hand margin explain why I reacted so sharply to Sister X. My exasperation was not related to the clinical situation but to concerns around my own reputation. As a result I operated in pure advocacy laying the law down with no effort at finding the best argument (Senge 1990). Opportunities for learning and exploring other ways of working were lost in this dissatisfying exchange. Furthermore the hard working nursing sister was left feeling undermined and criticised. Journaling in this way clarified the issues sharply and enabled a further more productive discussion with Sister X.

Arts

Reflections can be expressed as painting, poems, dance and movement, photographs and the suchlike. I rarely use painting in my own reflections except in the art workshops I convene within the teaching programmes. I am more of a word person than a picture person. Art as a reflective medium does not appeal to all practitioners. Exploring their struggle, I get reasons such as 'not skilled at painting or poetry' as if they are going to be judged on artistic merit. Some people are uncomfortable 'playing' as if painting or art is something children do. Paramananda (2001:71) writes of the way people get trimmed as they grow up:

> We all start off with real heads full of space and imagination, but slowly, somewhere along the path that we call growing up, our heads get trimmed. We become caught up in the doings of this world, the realities of adult life, and we cut down to size.

We lose touch with the imagination and with it the creative and intuitive life. Instead we are caught up in the demand to be rational that seems to govern professional life. And yet, practice is performance, the greatest assets are perception, imagination, intuition, creativity – yet generally denigrated, these attributes are stunted. Art then, through reflection, enables the practitioner to value and develop these qualities. In doing so, the practitioner begins to use her whole brain again, recovering the wilted right side where these attributes are generally considered to reside. And at the end of the art workshops, the smiles are broad, the fears dispelled and a real sense of recovery and achievement are generally expressed.

Lei reflected on the way his painting had revealed so much about himself that normally he wouldn't reveal. He felt both vulnerable and elated at his revelation, surprised that his painting could be so revealing and cathartic. It seems as if our bodies hold dark secrets that can only find expression through the imagination, by-passing the censoring ego. Perhaps artists and art therapist know this well.

Spurling (1998:xix) writes in her biography of Henri Matisse:

> He [Matisse] said his portraits uncovered much that he could not have suspected at the start. 'To sum up, I work without a theory. I am aware primarily of the forces involved, and find myself driven forward by an idea which I can really only grasp little by little as it grows within the picture.' [Source uncited by Spurling]

And it is like that, the narrator doesn't quite know where the narrative will take her. She hangs onto the broad plot but the flow of meaning finds it own way as it unfolds, like the slow lift of thick morning mist to reveal the sun and the hills ahead.

I write poetry to capture meaning. Poetry enables me to touch the essence of the experience in fewer words that narrative, and by its nature lends itself to imagery. As noted above, one way to start writing poetry is to simply break down prose into single lines. The following example is taken from a new performance 'Dwelling with the ancestors' developed from a published narrative (Johns 2006:229):

> Early February. As I drive to the University I am mesmerised by the dance of the bare trees as they swirl in the wind against the rolling grey sky. A dervish dance, apparently chaotic rhythm yet perfect harmony, bending and flowing to the wind music. The tree naturally gives way to the forces and yet, so often, people like Edith resist life's forces and snap.

> The practitioner needs to appreciate the rhythm of the dance so as to synchronise rather than resist the dervish dance, what Newman (1999) describes as the rhythm of relating, by compassionately listening to the words and especially the silences between the words where empathy and connection become possible. Newman describes this as synchronised talk dance. She writes 'Such synchronisation has an effect of making the interactants feel good about what

they are doing and about each other'. (1999:227) And when the gusts and storms that blow is the patient's mood and talk, the practitioner, like the trees, must bend in the wind in graceful dance without resistance or else she too will surely snap. Then the connection is lost and caring perishes on the wind.

> Early February.
> The dance of bare trees as they swirl in the wind against the rolling grey sky.
> A dervish dance catches my imagination.
> Chaotic rhythm yet perfect harmony,
> bending and flowing to the wind music.
> The tree naturally gives way to the forces and yet,
> so often, people like Edith resist life's forces and snap.
> The practitioner needs to appreciate the rhythm of the dance
> so as to synchronise rather than resist the dervish dance.
> Newman (1999) describes this as the rhythm of relating,
> compassionately listening to the words,
> especially the silences between the words,
> where empathy and connection become possible.
> Newman describes this as synchronised talk dance.
> And when the gusts and storms that blow is the patient's mood and talk,
> I am like the trees,
> I must bend in the wind in graceful dance without resistance
> or else I too will surely snap.
> Then the connection is lost
> poise perishes on the wind
> in my struggle to hold myself upright.

Writing the prose poem opens up the words, and moves me into a more reflective mode than description. New images emerge as the imagination is stirred. In particular I pay attention to how I was feeling, reflecting the way writing poems stirs the senses. My original description was itself poetic. In breaking it down, I shift the perspective from caring perishes to poise perishes. Poise holds connection and yet is fragile to the gusts of the patient's suffering.

Writing my reflection as a poem captures something of the beauty, mystery and tragedy of caring, its light and its shadow. Words seem to emerge and flow from a spiritual source of creation. I am sometimes challenged – 'isn't it "soft" to write poems?' but such prejudice reflects ignorance grounded in left brain dominance that rejects the professional's expression of poetry. Writing narrative naturally challenges accepted ways of writing 'professional text'. I want to begin using paintings and photographs, perhaps collages in my narratives, even dance, to capture more exquisitely the passion, the beauty, the horror of my experience. I love the imagery in Louise Jarrett's collage:

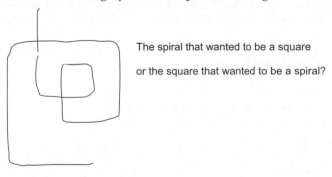

The spiral that wanted to be a square

or the square that wanted to be a spiral?

In an art workshop[1] we had been using Angeles Arrien's (1998) ideas of 'Signs of life – the five universal shapes and how to use them'. The exercise was intended to help the researchers look at themselves through these five shapes. The square represents stability whilst the spiral represented growth and change. Lou saw herself in tension between these two apparent opposites. She felt *square* but also strongly felt the pull of the *spiral*; she wanted to be spiral and less square. She came to realise that she could only spiral from the safety of the square. She came to appreciate that both shapes were vital to her. She could love the square again.

Art opens spaces for reflection beyond the mind. Recent studies (Cameron *et al.* 2008; Gaydos 2008) using art as reflection powerfully reveal the way art enabled practitioners and students to express their experience, revealing the potential of art to take the practitioner to deeper, more embodied spaces within self.

I pick up the idea of art as reflection further in Chapter 4 as I explore weaving the narrative.

References

Arrien A (1998) *Signs of life: the five universal shapes and how to use them.* Jeremy P Tarcher/ Putnam, New York.

Belenky M, Clinchy B, Goldberger N and Tarule J (1986) *Women's ways of knowing: the development of self, voice and mind.* Basic Books, New York.

Bohm D (1996) *On dialogue.* (Edited by L Nichol). Routledge, London.

Boud D, Keogh R and Walker D (1985) Promoting reflection in learning: a model. In: D Boud, R Keogh and D Walker (eds.) *Reflection: turning experience into learning.* Kogan Page, London, pp. 18–40.

Boyd E and Fales A (1983) Reflective learning: key to learning from experience. *Journal of Humanistic Psychology* 23:99–117.

Brooks S (2004) *A research study to examine self in being and becoming an effective clinical leader.* Unpublished dissertation MSc in Leadership in Healthcare Practice, University of Bedfordshire, Bedfordshire.

Buchbinder D (1994) *Masculinities and identities.* Melbourne University Press, Melbourne.

Cameron D, Phillips S, Sawh K and Wadey P (2008) Expressing voice and developing practical wisdom on social justice through art. In: C Delmar and C Johns (eds.) *The good, the wise, and the right clinical nursing practice.* Aalborg Hospital, Arhus University Hospital, Denmark, pp. 59–72.

Compact Oxford English Dictionary (third edition) (2005) Oxford University Press, Oxford.

Cooper M (1991) Principle-oriented ethics and the ethic of care: a creative tension. *Advances in Nursing Science* 14:22–31.

Cope M (2001) *Lead yourself: be where others will follow.* Pearson Education, London.

Cox H, Hickson P and Taylor B (1991) Exploring reflection: knowing and constructing practice. In: G Gray and R Pratt (eds.) *Towards a discipline of nursing.* Churchill Livingstone, Melbourne.

DeSalvo L (1999) *Writing as a way of healing: how telling our stories transform our lives.* The Women's Press, London.

Dewey J (1933) *How we think.* JC Heath, Boston.

Doty M (1996) *Heaven's coast.* Harper Collins, New York.

Emden C (1991) Becoming a reflective practitioner. In: G Gray and R Pratt (eds.) *Towards a discipline of nursing.* Churchill Livingstone, Melbourne.

---

[1] Facilitated by Lea Gaydos.

Fay B (1987) *Critical social science*. Polity Press, Cambridge.

Gaydos H (2008) Collage: an aesthetic process for creating phronesis in nursing. In: C Delmar and C Johns (eds.) *The good, the wise, and the right clinical nursing practice*. Aalborg Hospital, Arhus University Hospital, Denmark.

Gibbs G (1988) *Learning by doing: a guide to teaching and learning methods*. Further Education Unit, Oxford Polytechnic (now Oxford Brookes University), Oxford.

Hahnemann B K (1986) Journal writing: a key to promoting critical thinking in nursing students. *Journal of Nursing Education* 25:213–215.

Johns C (2000) *Becoming a reflective practitioner* (first edition). Blackwell Science, Oxford.

Johns C (2002) *Guided reflection: advancing practice* (first edition). Blackwell Publishing, Oxford.

Johns C (2006) *Engaging reflection in practice*. Blackwell Publishing, Oxford.

Johns C (2009) *Becoming a reflective practitioner* (third edition). Wiley-Blackwell, Oxford.

Johns C and Graham J (1996) Using a reflective model of nursing and guided reflection. *Nursing Standard* 11:34–38.

Katagiri D (2008) *Each moment is the universe: zen and the way of being time*. Shambhala, Boston.

Kemmis S (1985) Action research and the politics of reflection. In: D Boud, R Keogh and D Walker (eds.) *Reflection: turning experience into learning*. Kogan Page, New York.

Lather P (1993) Fertile obsession: validity after post-structuralism. *The Sociological Quarterly* 34:673–693.

Manjusvara (2005) *Writing your way*. Windhorse Publications, Birmingham.

Margolis H (1993) *Paradigms and barriers: how habits of mind govern scientific beliefs*. University of Chicago Press, Chicago.

Mezirow J (1981) A critical theory of adult learning and education. *Adult Education* 32:3–24.

Mishler G (1990) Validation in inquiry-guided research: the role of exemplars in narrative studies. *Harvard Educational Review* 60:415–442.

Moon J (2004) *A handbook of reflective and experiential learning: theory and practice*. Routledge, London.

Morgan R (2005) *Realising transformational leadership*. Unpublished dissertation MSc in Leadership in Healthcare Practice, University of Bedfordshire, Bedfordshire.

Newman M (1999) The rhythm of relating in a paradigm of wholeness. *Image: Journal of Nursing Scholarship* 31:227–230.

Okri B (1997) *A way of being free*. Phoenix House, London. Text extracts used with permission of The Marsh Agency Ltd.

Paramananda (2001) *A deeper beauty: Buddhist reflections on everyday life*. Windhorse Publishing, Birmingham.

Parker J (1997) The body as text and the body as living flesh. In: J Lawler (ed.) *The body in nursing*. Churchill Livingstone, Melbourne.

Pennebaker J (1990) *Opening up: the healing power of confiding in others*. Morrow, New York.

Pinar W (1981) Whole, bright, deep with understanding: issues in qualitative research and autobiographical method. *Journal of Curriculum Studies* 13:173–188.

Rudge T (1997) Discourses, metaphor and bodies: boundaries and the skin. In: J Lawler (ed.) *The body in nursing*. Churchill Livingstone, Melbourne.

Saunders A (2006) *Transforming self through transformational leadership*. Unpublished dissertation, Master in Clinical Leadership, University of Bedfordshire, Bedfordshire.

Schön D (1983) *The reflective practitioner*. Avebury, Aldershot.

Senge P (1990) *The fifth discipline*. Century Business, London.

Spence D (1982) *Narrative truth and historical truth: meaning and interpretation in psychoanalysis*. WW Norton & Co., New York.

Spurling H (1998) *The unknown Matisse: a life of Henri Matisse, volume 1 1869–1908*. Hamish Hamilton, London.

Street A (1992) *Inside nursing: a critical ethnography of clinical nursing practice*. State University of New York Press, New York.

Street A (1995) *Nursing replay*. Churchill Livingstone, Melbourne.

Thomas K and Kilmann R (1974) *Thomas–Kilmann conflict mode instrument*. Xicom, Toledo.

Tufnell M and Crickmay C (2004) *A widening field*. Dance Books, Alton.

Wheatley M (1999) *Leadership and the new science. Discovering order in a chaotic world*. Berret-Koehler, San Francisco.

Wong F, Keber D, Chung L and Yan L (1995) Assessing the level of student reflection from reflective journals. *Journal of Advanced Nursing* 22:48–57.

Woolf V (1945) *A room of one's own*. Penguin Books, London.

Chapter 3

Deepening insights

Christopher Johns

In the previous chapter I set out the concept of dialogical movement in constructing reflexive narrative and explored the first two movements. In this chapter I explore the third and fourth movements.

- Dialogue between the *text* and other sources of knowing in order to frame emerging tentative from the text within the wider community of knowing.
- Dialogue between the text's author and a guide(s) to check-out, deepen and co-create insights.

The third dialogical movement is the dialogue between emerging insights and the wider community of knowing to inform and deepen these insights.

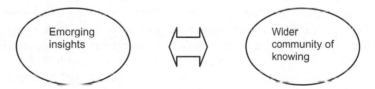

In this way, relevant knowledge is critiqued and assimilated into personal knowing, informing future experience. Such dialogue may be continuous, for example my persistent investigation into the nature of suffering and ways it might be eased. Returning to the same literature I read it differently in relation to particular experiences. Understanding is always deepening within the hermeneutic spiral of being and becoming. The development of guided reflection and narrative as a process of self-inquiry and transformation is, in a similar way, reflexively informed by a dialogue with a relevant literature. For example, the idea that reflection can really lead to a rational self-clarity or whether there is an inherent opacity to human life (Fay 1987). As such the understanding of one's own reality is always partial and flawed. In other words, both the authority of experience and knowledge is never taken on face value. Both are inherently viewed as problematic.

Guidance

The fourth dialogical movement is the dialogue between the narrator and guide(s) to check out and deepen the tentative insights emerging through the first three dialogical movements as a movement towards weaving the reflexive and coherent narrative. Whilst guidance is a continuous process, enhancing all levels of dialogical movement, it is at this fourth dialogical movement where guidance is most exact and influential.

Guidance is a vital and skilled role. Yet it is a potentially problematic role if the guide is inadequate to the task. As Dewey (1933:151) writes:

> A person needs to see for themselves, and he can't see just by being told, although the right kind of telling may guide his seeing and thus help him see what he needs to see.

So we are interested in the right kind of telling. The practitioner must be empowered to challenge the guide's authority (no matter its benevolent intent), and resist the intrinsic threat of the guide imposing an agenda and dominant meanings. The guide intends to enable:

- The practitioner/narrator to construct a coherent and reflexive narrative;
- The practitioner to realise desirable practice.

However, the guide is not neutral free. For myself, I have well-formed ideas about the nature of narrative, based on my developmental work in constructing narrative these past 20 years. I am mindful of my ideas pressing on me, mindful of any attachment to the idea that I am an expert in narrative inquiry or on easing suffering. This is where Buddhism helps me put things into perspective – the idea that as a guide my primary role is to be of service to the other. I know I could lead the practitioner up the proverbial garden path to a reasonable and perhaps predictable conclusion. But, if I did, the practitioner would miss the exploration of finding her own path.

But guides can lead you astray. They can lead you along a familiar and safe route limiting the breadth of view and take you away from the edges where the widest and most creative views are to be seen. It may be harder work than a prescriptive approach. You may get yourself into some difficulty but the rewards can be substantial. Journeying alone, against forces of authority that resist self-realisation, within institutionalised health organisations is tough work. Hence climbing alone can be arduous and tricky so it is vital to find the right guide who gives you enough rope to explore and yet is always at hand in case of difficulty to support you if you are in trouble. The good guide is not directive or judgemental. A balance is needed, reflected in the dialogue within the community of inquiry, where different routes can be explored and reflected on. When the terrain is too tough then a safer route can be taken.

Being directive and judgemental are projections of the guide's own covert agenda and imposition of values.

> The ancient masters
> Didn't try to educate people,
> But kindly taught them to not-know.
>
> When they think that they know the answers,
> People are difficult to guide.
> When they know they don't know,
> People can find their own way.
> Lao Tzu (1999 – part 65 translated by Stephen Mitchell)

In contracting the guided reflection relationship, the guide reveals his agenda and his intention to work collaboratively within a community of inquiry (if this exists). Greenwood *et al.* (1993:175) note:

> Participation is a process that must be generated. It begins with participatory intent and continues by building participatory processes into the activity within the limits set by the participants and the conditions.

Collaboration has to be *actively* constructed because it does not usually exist within normal relationships within clinical practice or academic institutions (despite rhetoric to the contrary). However, inequality of power (or force) is normal and hence may not be perceived as a problem that needs addressing within the research relationship. In my experience, inequality often seems grounded in a need for the guide to manage his anxiety for several reasons:

- The guide may identify with the practitioner's performance as a reflection of his own ability. If the research project is registered as a research degree, the guide may want *his student* to achieve a high grade and thus interfere with the agenda to manage this anxiety, especially if the practitioner is not performing well. This may encourage the guide to 'fix' problems for the practitioner rather than enable the practitioner to fix her own problems.
- The guide may feel constrained by the academic regulations to fit the research into some approved scheme of what a *normal* research project should look like.
- The guide may simply be attached to their own sense of expertise. As a consequence the guide flips into authoritative or parental mode; either critical at his naughty or rebellious child, or nurturing towards his suffering child.
- The guide may be caught up in his own or an agenda to shape the practitioner into an effective practitioner as determined by the organisation. This is more so, when the guide has firm ideas about the nature of what the practitioner seeks to realise. Guidance may then become focused on this technical agenda rather than the practitioner's emancipatory self-realisation, with an emphasis on product rather than process (Johns 2001).

The guide may not be aware of these issues. All is a contradiction within collaborative practice. Hopefully the practitioner is assertive enough to raise concerns with the guide – perhaps the main point of setting a contract is to open a space for continued dialogue about process including the guidance relationship. However, egos can be brittle.

The good guide tunes into the practitioner's pace and guides the practitioner to find the best research rhythm that has optimum momentum. Too fast and we can lose sight of detail along the way. If we do not dwell enough, interpretations are made too hastily. We miss things. Too slow, and we get stuck in a swamp of words and lose sight of the summit (Pirsig 1974). Like playing a guitar there is a rhythm to this work that we need to find and tune into. Reflection, by its very nature, enables one to 'be' the researchee, to find one's way along the narrow edge as something in itself rather than a barrier that must be traversed in order to reach the destination. Being and becoming *is* the research. The guide too, is being and becoming, learning.

In his research on empowerment of grass root community leaders in the USA, Kieffer (1984:27) emphasised the key role of the *external enabler* to support and challenge peoples' journeys of empowerment. In this respect, it is significant to acknowledge the power of the community of inquiry as mutual peer support alongside the particular role of the *acknowledged* guide. Most of the guidance I offer directly is participation within communities of inquiry. Practitioners read and share their stories, supporting, challenging, affirming each other. In reading their stories, gaining confidence, self-consciousness quickly drips away. Practitioners flourish in such a learning milieu.

In my research with ward sisters seeking to realise leadership through clinical supervision (Johns 2003), it was evident how isolated they were in practice. Individual supervision kept them isolated whereas group supervision might have created the conditions for ongoing peer support and mutual empowerment.

Contracting is the formal negotiation to establish the conditions for collaboration between the guide and practitioner. So, what makes a good guide? Because guided reflection is an intensely interpersonal process grounded in practitioner disclosure, the guide is someone who the practitioner *must* trust and feel confident in. Some degree of mutual attraction may be helpful. Ask yourself – what would attract you to a guide? Attraction is a deeply subjective experience! It is interesting to speculate whether it is important that the guide has an appropriate clinical background? As the reader will noted in the narratives, the focus of reflection is rarely on the 'technical' aspects of everyday practice. A good guide will always challenge the practitioner to access appropriate technical literature or steer the practitioner to access relevant sources for such information. Indeed, the resourceful guide can ask for copies of such material in order to expand his background and then use this literature to challenge the practitioner as appropriate. A guide with a similar background may be a disadvantage if the guide subsequently over-identifies with the practitioner's experiences or responds in the light of his own experiences. A lack of shared background will enable the guide to ask more naïve questions which may otherwise be taken for granted within a shared background. The guide's mind is less crowded with his own ideas.

On a more practical level can the guide (and practitioner) make the commitment to meet for regular sessions? Dedicated time is essential to sustain guided reflection relationships. I work with both individuals and groups. With individuals, I find a meeting for one hour every four weeks adequate over the period of the research. The advantage of individual meetings is that the work is focused and the sessions flexible to fit in with practitioner's own agendas. I always work individually with practitioners when I intend to write the narrative. I organise group guided reflection as a 'research school', which meets for three hours every three weeks. Practitioners who register for dissertations or research degrees are supervised through this school, which is supplemented by individual tutorials as required. The major advantage of a research school is that collaboration extends between students.

Group inquiry

Prior to each four-weekly community inquiry session, each practitioner is invited to 'post' on the community's Google group site a narrative that they would like to explore/read/ perform/dialogue with the community at the next session. Such work is a deeply creative process of connection with self and with the group, a movement along the hermeneutic tide, revealing ideas and possibilities that rise to the surface of consciousness, tentative, vibrant, possibilities along the creative edge, others relating, connecting, finding meaning in their own experiences, letting go of firm ideas, of projections, assumptions of what the text might mean, prejudices surface, doubts raised, self-esteem raw in the face of brutality, sense making, finding meaning, and then another return, another creative twist, nothing is firmly grasped, no concrete realities set.

After the group Bella says how stimulated she feels: 'This is what university should be about – creating creative moments.' It takes her back to her own undergraduate studies and the buzz she got from seminars (four to eight people), not from theory but just people sharing their ideas: 'I learnt more from that [than] from anything else ... indeed I think I only learnt from them.'

The community of inquiry is self-organising, unfolding patterns emerge within the group, constantly shifting amidst the laughter, the humour, the serious moments, the revelations. Is it possible that learning can be such fun and yet so disciplined, so productive? Without doubt, mutual support from other practitioners is probably the most sustaining force.

I reflect back on these insights with the group, the way we are working, to reinforce and nurture the pattern. The group is both stable and creative, finding the creative edge, security in connection. I notice the difference when I had supervised Lou Jarrett (in individual supervision) that with hindsight her disadvantage of not having peer support. And of course she was the pioneer, opening the frontier passages. Lou belatedly joined the group. She thrives in the peer support, as if she has come home to herself. She senses the others will have an easier passage. I think they do but because they are in this group not because Lou had walked a path before them.

The good guide is sensitive to the unfolding dynamics of the guided reflection relationship and able to surface and resolve any tension – what I term as 'pricking the bubble'. Otherwise the practitioner or the guide may become defensive and resort to game playing that undermines collaboration (Kadushin 1968). As I guide, I must always have a conscious mind-set to create the conditions for genuine collaboration within the guided reflection relationship and tuned into spotting what Whitehead (2004) terms *living contradictions*.

To reiterate, collaborative relationships are sacrosanct within narratives of self-inquiry. There can be no compromise. Failure to achieve collaboration must always be a contradiction that needs resolving. This is line with Freire's (1972) belief that empowerment should be a process of collaboration between groups rather than an outcome achieved by one powerful group for another less powerful group, or, in other words, where the powerful group retains control.

Within a collaborative relationship the researcher cannot adopt a detached or objective position. That the researcher can be objective is itself a distortion because of the way people always respond from a pre-reflective state (Heidegger 1962, in Dreyfus 1991:82/83). Hence, 'who I am' as a guide is necessary to appreciate. I need to be aware of my assumptions, values and the suchlike, and wary of its influence on the way I guide. Of course, as I shall reveal, such self-knowing is the paramount condition for dialogue. This point has widespread acceptance within collaborative research theory (Heron 1981) and feminist theory (see Acker *et al.* 1983; Paget 1983).

Paget (1983) recognised how the similarity between her own and her interviewees' life experiences influenced questions she asked and entered into her understanding and interpretation of the story being told. Paget points out her approach, which gave control of the interview process to the interviewee, establishing solidarity between them as they engaged in the shared task of trying to understand important life experiences.

Guidance is the balance of high challenge with high support underlined by *thick* trust. Only then can dialogue flourish. Cope (2001:152) notes that 'Trust is the oil that lubricates relationships'. The practitioner will sense when the guide is indifferent or judgemental, or imposing his own agenda. The consequence is a breakdown of 'collaboration'. Under these conditions, it might be hoped that the practitioner will raise her concern at this breakdown or even terminate the relationship. However, this may be difficult for the practitioner, especially if the guide has (unwittingly) assumed an authoritative role. I say unwittingly because even with good intent, people can slip into subordinate or authoritative modes of being. The practitioner may feel constrained in tackling interpersonal issues with the guide because she feels intimidated or have a misplaced concern about upsetting the guide or inviting sanction. Collaboration represents an equality of power and mutual responsibility. Yet it must be lived mindfully moment by moment rather than something taken for granted. Indeed, collaboration *is* lived, otherwise it doesn't exist.

Dialogue

Co-creating meaning is realised through dialogue. The guide and practitioner both need to know the rules as set out in Chapter 2:

- The intention to work towards consensus (with others) to create a better world;
- The suspension of one's assumptions;
- The non-attachment to ideas and being open to possibility;
- Proprioception of thinking (knowing where thinking is);
- Treating all people in dialogue with respect;
- Knowing the rules of dialogue.

Bohm (1996) viewed dialogue as a way to move through conflict by consensus and love – that people could set aside their assumptions and realise a common harmony. There is a nirvana idea about this that seems profoundly difficult to realise simply because people are caught up in self-interest. Yet, even so, it sets a path of possibility. Bohm conceived of dialogical groups as being around 40 people. However, he further writes:

> One can see that it is possible that this spirit of the dialogue can work in smaller groups, or one-on-one, or within the individual. If the individual can hold all of the meanings together in his own mind, he has the attitude of the dialogue. He could carry that out and perhaps communicate it to other people, both verbally and non-verbally, in principle this could spread. (Bohm 1996:29)

To dialogue within a group of 40 it would seem that each person in that group would need to hold the attitude of dialogue. In terms of realising desirable practice, dialogue is a core attribute of being.

At times the guide is more informative and directive, particularly in the early phase of narrative construction when the practitioner may be struggling to locate signposts to guide herself. However, as proprioception suggests, both people should be aware of these dynamics simply because the dynamics are themselves a constant focus of reflection. Suspension of one's assumptions, and not being attached to ideas and being open to possibility works for both guide and practitioner as they move towards co-creating insights. The guide is mindful of listening through filters of his own concerns and interests, or established ways of seeing things. These may block sensitive listening, or lead the guide to project a meaning prematurely, especially when what is being said 'fits' some scheme (Spence 1982).

Bohm's ideas on dialogue was strongly influenced by Krishnamurti's belief that dialogue could penetrate and transform the way people thought about issues, enabling new ways of seeing and responding to issues that could uproot the old ways of thought, freeing the mind from traditions and habits. In Krishnamurti's (1996:93) words:

> To inquire and to learn is the function of the mind. By learning I do not mean the mere cultivation of memory or the accumulation of knowledge, but the capacity to think clearly without illusion.

As such, the foremost intention of dialogue is the process of dialogue itself rather than its results. This requires careful listening. Yet to listen requires an awareness and suspension of personal ambition, dominant perspectives, values, defensiveness and weight of tradition. Bohm (1996) notes how thought is infiltrated with these notions. As such, dialogue requires people to be critically conscious of their own thinking so it does not corrupt the effort to find true meaning. Bohm calls this proprioception of thought in much the same way the body is aware of itself in space. This does not mean the listener has to agree with what is being said, but to understand what is being said without a sense of judgement in order to allow the dialogue to flow. Reflection is the way to access one's assumptions and see them for what they are. Yet this is profoundly difficult because our assumptions reflect 'who I am', and, as such, are taken for granted. Yet they are apparent as the root of all contradiction and contradiction is at the root of anxiety and emotion. This is the same for both guide and practitioner. The guide does not impose a meaning on the practitioner from his authoritative advantage. Yet neither does the guide simply accept the practitioner's interpretation. The aim of dialogue is to understand and challenge the perspective of others but always with the intention of moving towards a greater understanding that benefits humanity. Hence dialogue is always a movement towards consensus and harmony. Bohm (1996:4) writes:

> It is clear that if we are to live in harmony with ourselves and with nature, we need to be able to communicate freely in a creative movement in which no one permanently holds to or otherwise defends his own ideas.

To dialogue participants must be ready to drop old ideas and intentions towards making something in common or 'co-creating meaning'. The aim to dialogue is to reveal the paradoxes that exist within everyday practice – the contradictions between what is desirable to achieve and what is actually practised. Bohm refers to 'paradox' as the contradictions that exist in thought. For example, a practitioner may think she is good at listening to patient's problems. Indeed she has internalised this as a characteristic of a good nurse. Yet she is often intolerant of patients, which she rationalises in terms of the patient having a problem rather than herself. Bohm argues that the practitioner's thinking is dominated by a set of self-contradictory demands and needs that impede a solution. By paradox, Bohm suggests the self-contradictory thinking is exposed for what it is. This requires the suspension of the forces that govern the paradox, and highlights the fundamental need to set up conditions of trust in order for people to let go of their defences that sustain the paradox. This is to take people back to their values and the way values are contradicted within everyday practice. For example, Karen[1] believed she should have a positive regard for all patients and families and yet on a subconscious level she could not tolerate women who wanted to mother her. Dialogue, in pursuing the underlying reasons takes the person into deeper realms of self. It cannot exist, however, in the absence of a profound love for the world and for men (Freire 1972:62).

Bohm's work on dialogue reinforces the notion that who we are is embodied and governed by tradition over which people have little conscious control, and that the work of reflection is to reveal these conditions that lead to self-contradiction and paradox. Bohm writes (1996:67):

> What is called for, then, is a deep and intense awareness, going beyond the imagery and intellectual analysis of our confused process of thought, and capable of penetrating to the contradictory presuppositions and states of feelings in which the confusion exists.

Co-creating meaning

The creative point of guidance is co-creating meaning expressed as insights. Both guide and practitioner bring to the moment their respective 'horizons'. Through reflection the practitioner/narrator comes to some awareness of self that Gadamer (1975) describes as their 'horizon'. Weinsheimer (1985:182) writes:

> It is always possible to become more aware of our own historical situation, the situation in which understanding takes place. Having such awareness does not mean that once the situation has become more fully conscious, we can step outside it, any more than seeing our own shadow means we can outrun it. Rather our shadow moves along with us. The situation of understanding can also be called our horizon. It marks the limit of everything that can be seen from a particular point of view, but the idea of horizon also implies that we can see beyond our immediate standpoint.

Horizon is a metaphor to represent the person's normal vision and understanding. The practitioner's reflective effort is always to expand her horizon towards self-realisation within the hermeneutic spiral. The guide's role is a catalyst, and in doing so, the guide naturally expands his own horizons. Collaboration must lead to mutual growth. Weinsheimer (1985:178) notes (citing Gadamer 1975:279/263):

> If understanding always means coming to an understanding, then it always involves two – and two different – participants. The ideal is not that one party should understand the other but rather that they should reach an understanding between them. 'This between is the true locus of hermeneutics.'

Gadamer (1975) considered that people are always understanding and interpreting themselves in the context of their worlds and in light of their fore-knowledge, which, from the reflexive viewpoint, is always changing through experience. This looking back and seeing self as a changed person is the essential nature of reflexivity. It is not as some

---

[1]Karen was an associate nurse who worked with me in guided reflection research at Burford Community Hospital from 1989 to 1991.

end-point, but is always open and anticipatory to future experiences. As Gadamer (1975:216, cited in Weinsheimer 1985:156) writes:

> Every experience has implicit horizons before and after, and fuses finally with the continuum of experiences that are present before and after into the unity of the flow of experience.

Guidance is seeking to connect with the world of the practitioner. It is also the ground between the narrative and the narrative reader. Spence (1982:112) notes:

> We try to imagine how the person is experiencing the world – we are then in a better position to understand her/his choice of words and to respond to his/her particular shades and colours.

Why guidance

Co-creating meaning is the essential task of guidance. However, guidance is also necessary to create the conditions for successful co-creation. Perhaps first is the idea of prodding and waking people up to their experience. So many practitioners are asleep, complacent. Their practice has become routine, habitual, and mundane. They lack commitment and interest in what they do. O'Donohue (1997:122–123) reflects:

> People have difficulty awakening to their inner world, especially when their lives have become familiar to them. They find it hard to discover something new, interesting or adventurous in their numbed lives.

Guidance aims to kindle the practitioner's motivation, commitment, integrity and curiosity to their practice. It aims to rattle their cage and wake them up! So many practitioners are tired and burnt out. In response they turn away from the mirror of reflection because the image of themselves is difficult to face. But that is where guidance commences. Turn on the light!

So many experiences reflected on by practitioners are triggered by anxiety and breakdown when things no longer go smoothly. The practitioner's natural inclination is to defend against anxiety. Anxiety triggers defence mechanisms that prompt self-protection, notably rationalisation and projection. Gray and Forsstrom (1991:360) note how:

> The process of 'journalling' may sound simple and easy to execute, but at times it was extremely difficult. Mostly the incidents recorded were identified because there was an affective component. This may be related to feelings of our personal inadequacy to cope with the demands of the situation. Alone, it was emotionally painful to journal events that were largely self-critical.

Boud *et al.* (1985) describe how they constructed their model as something the student can do for themselves, but note that the 'learning process can be considerably accelerated by appropriate support' (p. 36) and that attending to feelings 'can be assisted by being encouraged' (p. 37). I am often asked, 'Aren't we all reflective?' I might say, 'Yes, but only to a certain depth.'

Mezirow (1981) distinguishes between reflection at consciousness and critical consciousness levels. At a critical consciousness level, the practitioner is aware and skilled to think about her thinking, mindful of her patterns of thinking, and mental models that are vital for learning as thinking governs responses to situations. As practitioners become more mindful, so they become more able to reflect at a deeper, more critical consciousness level, to become aware of and appreciate contradiction between their actual and desirable practice. It is an evolutionary process, enabling practitioners to become increasingly aware of contradiction within their practice and threats to their integrity. Practice ceases to be mundane.

The guide listens carefully and picks up cues, and reflects back his thoughts as questions, cuing the practitioner to explore issues more laterally, more deeply. It isn't easy for practitioners to see and appreciate those forces of authority, tradition and embodiment that constrain practice. Guidance challenges the practitioner to identify and consider the consequences of responding in new ways to practice situations. Trapped within the habitual patterns of their comfort zone, practitioners may defensively resist new ideas.

Guidance supportingly pulls away the practitioner's defensive responses as if a supportive hand across the messy and indeterminate swampy lowlands of practice (Schön 1987).

The balance of high challenge and high support!

High challenge and high support lead to empowerment and optimum learning. Too much challenge can overwhelm whereas too much support can lead to dependency and comfort. Guidance helps the practitioner to see with clarity. Okri (1997) urges an exploration into our innermost beings so that the hidden self does not emerge to haunt attitudes and dreams. It requires an honest gaze into the reflective mirror and the choice of 'the good eye and not the askew eye' (p. 65). The 'askew eye' can distort the picture so that reflection becomes warped by personal prejudices and assumptions.

Each situation is unique, a mystery unfolding. There is no formulaic response. It is so easy to get stuck in a rut and not even realise it! Holly (1989:71) suggests that:

> This voyage, like others which cover the most intriguing terrains, is not smooth, and deliberately setting off to explore what has become custom is not without its risks and discomforts as truths are challenged and the taken-for-granted questioned, and often found to be problematic.

The intention of a critical social science is not only to facilitate methodical self-reflection necessary to produce rational clarity, but to dissolve those barriers that prevent people from living in accordance with their genuine will (Fay 1987). Its aim is to help people not only become transparent to themselves but also to cease being mere objects in the world, passive victims dominated by forces external to them. Just because we can understand something differently does not mean we can change it. In response the guide supports the practitioner to 'live with and chip away these forces' as a process over time whilst keeping in focus a strong vision of what she wants to achieve. Like the sculptor chipping away with his hammer and chisel at the slab of grey rock, every stroke purposeful towards creating his beautiful image as a lived reality. There is a significant ethical dimension to pushing people against barriers they cannot overcome that the guided reflection researcher must be sensitive to.

Guidance supports the practitioner to face up to and harness anxiety as positive energy to take action. The guide facilitates energy exchange, enabling the practitioner to dissipate negative energy (anxiety) into positive energy necessary to take positive action to re-pattern or reorganise ways of being in the world that have broken down and led to the crisis prompting reflection. This idea has been developed by Prigogine and Stengers (1984) from the theory of dissipative structure (Newman 1994).

The guide acknowledges, supports and values the practitioner, injecting (to use a medical metaphor) the practitioner with courage and resolve, especially when the practitioner feels battered or helpless. Practitioners may perceive themselves as relatively powerless to change self (Robinson 1995), and need guidance to see new ways of being and ways of taking action to achieve this. Just because we come to understand things differently doesn't mean we can act differently. Powerful forces act to sustain the status quo (Smyth 1987). Menzies-Lyth (1988:62) noted how nurses tend to 'cling to the familiar even when the familiar has obviously ceased to be appropriate or relevant'. She made this deduction within the context of understanding how nurses protected themselves against anxiety. Perhaps one way this is achieved is by focusing objectively on the situation rather than subjectively as self within the situation. The guide points this out, confronting and supporting the practitioner with this avoidance. Guided reflection is not therapy although deep personal issues may arise as a consequence of reflection or may trigger anxiety. Of course, with self-inquiry, there is no boundary between the personal self and the professional self. Such boundaries are illusory and protective yet may hamper self-realisation. The extent the 'personal' is explored can never be prescribed. Just as the practitioner assesses their ability to respond within situations, so must the guide, and refer the practitioner to appropriate help as required. However, the guide must not draw his own illusory boundaries otherwise he will not be available to support the practitioner's self-inquiry. Put another way, the guide must be mindful enough of these dynamics to respond appropriately as supervisors of research and clinical practice.

Co-guidance is good practice. It widens the dialogical space, offering diverse views and possibility, especially when the background of the guides is diverse. For example, working with dance and theatre teachers at the University of Bedfordshire has added tremendous scope in terms of support for practitioners and most significantly, for myself, encouraging me to critically challenge my own perspectives. It is so easy to become complacent in one's own perspective.

Guidance is moral. It is always consensus to create a better world (Bohm 1996). As such, guidance continuously and consistently confronts the practitioner to act with integrity, infusing her with courage to act on her insights, especially when the will weakens or the threat of potential consequence freeze her. The guide supports the practitioner when she stumbles and fall against the hard face of reality, for without doubt, change is painful, like the small child learning to walk falls and bruises her knee yet she perseveres because she knows the gain is worth the pain (Rogers 1969). The guide is mindfully parental at times – 'this is good medicine'. I emphasise *mindfully* because of the risk of inadvertently responding parentally leading to critical and nurturing parental behaviours that diminish learning.

I recognise that in guiding others that I too can be dependent – needing someone to listen to my stories with *genuine* concern, especially when I am overwhelmed or persecuted. I need to know that my story matters to the guide so that my cry is heard across a wasteland when sometimes it seems that no one 'out there' cares. As Frank (2002) says 'Being heard I am *remoralised*' [emphasis added]. When so often practitioners have become demoralized working in harsh caring climates.

Stories are often long and complex. One part of a story can unfold to lead into further stories. Sometimes stories are told that unfold over weeks. A guide facilitates the practitioner to tell her story until she pauses. In the pauses, in the silence, the practitioner can hear herself. So the guide pauses rather than rushing to fill the space. Perhaps inquiring, 'What is significant?' The guide may then tentatively share what he perceives is significant- tentative rather than imposing significance.

If the story is traumatic, then the guide is cathartic – 'I can sense this is tough for you', 'I feel your anger', etc. – pulling the emotion up into dialogical space where it can be explored more objectively. This is not to deny or dismiss the emotion as 'negative' but to honour and accept the negative emotion as valid. The practitioner may feel a failure because of the way she feels. Feelings may not be expressed if she does not feel safe. This presents a huge paradox for the practitioner: 'I need to express my feelings but I cannot because it would show I am not coping and therefore a failure.' It is as if practitioners construct a stereotype of an ideal practitioner and then judge themselves harshly.

Jourard (1971) noted that failure to meet ideal self inevitably leads to self-alienation where the self is not available to use in therapeutic ways. As such feelings may be hidden within the story. Being cathartic pricks a tension bubble. It also enables the guide to reflect within the moment on the way he feels about the emotion. Does the guide feel comfortable working with strong feelings? Does the guide identify with the feeling or the situation around the feeling? If so, better to say something like 'I can feel this myself'. Working in this way with the practitioner is intense and intimate. I once described it as a 'this space between us a river of tears' (Johns 2004). Drawing out this energy is important because otherwise, it may be difficult for the practitioner to talk through the situation.

Guidance traps

As with all ideas there is a shadow side to guidance:

- The guide responds in ways that reflect organisational normal patterns of relating to either clinical or research guidance, reinforcing dependency and hierarchy. There is no place for authority and hierarchy is dialogue (Bohm 1996).
- The guide responds to 'fix it' for the practitioner rather than enabling the practitioner to pose and solve her own problems. This is likely when the guide views his own success as entangled with that of the practitioner or sees self as an expert leading to attachment to ideas and cut down of possibility. It can lead to a prescriptive/directive approach than a facilitative one, i.e. an issue of authority.
- The guide manipulates the research agenda to reflect his values and dominant perspectives. This can lead to 'moulding' whereby the guide 'shapes' the practitioner into an image of himself.

> Woe the academic's ego!
> For he has nowhere to go
> except up his own torso.

- The guide is anxious at the practitioner's revelations leading to inappropriate critical and nurturing parent patterns of response that breakdown the possibility of dialogue. This inevitably leads to thin trust.
- The guide is anxious because of his own limitations to guide self-inquiry and transformation, especially when he lacks experience of constructing of his own narratives of self-inquiry or where he is simply not mindful enough. In response, the guide may

hide behind a theoretical approach that denies the experimental nature of dialogue and creativity.

Ann Saunders (2006) reflects on guidance in constructing her leadership narrative. She writes:

The fourth level of dialogue concerns the belief that a guide is required to deepen the insight gained within extant theory. The reading and dialogue with the guide is the secondary level of interpretation, which enables me to remove the subjective perspective into a more objective frame. This belief is shared with Zen Buddhism, where students seeking enlightenment would travel from master to master in the hope that the dialogue would develop their awakening and furthering liberation. I smile as I compare the journey to University in a similar vein.

The role of the guide is instrumental in developing the insights of others who may lack cognitive, emotional, practical and ethical skills and in doing so empowers the individual. This is an interesting thought. Is it that we lack them? Or is it that we have not been encouraged to explore? By the very fact in doing so may reveal the flaws inherent in our world. Does that suggest we are damaged individuals? Gilbert (2001) would agree. He suggests the damaged individual is a product of traditional and rule bound organisations. Do I concur with this? That I lack the cognitive skills required? Evidence of this is found in my journal: 'Very cross. Fed up with being told what to do. One minute I feel I have some autonomy and the next hauled back in with a policy waved under my nose.' This would certainly attest to the fact that I felt powerless, damaged within the system that shaped me but did not have the cognition to extricate myself. Within group work through the course although presented in varying forms, others in the group could identify with this subtle form of power. The insights gained in this session, other sessions and the introduction of suggested reading material was empowering as well as liberating. As in the words of Gilbert (2001) guided reflection enables the practitioner to recognise the reality of their engagement in the health system. After all my organisation is hardly going to give me literature on the transactional culture by which they exert their power, if indeed it is transactional.

I mentioned earlier the word 'liberating'. I will expand on this. Our guided sessions were conducted away from the place of work, giving me the space I needed to stand back and able to express my views without fear of repercussions. It was another revelation. Our tutor highlighted that fear of sanction, fear of punishment was a transactional feature. I may have known I was fearful but I certainly had not thought of the mechanisms that were in place to control this. More evidence of lack of skill or wisdom. Covey (1989) discusses that clear guidance can bring true wisdom and may spark a cathartic release for self development and leadership. As mentioned in my introduction, I experienced friction between management and leadership. This was further reinforced when I related an experience in a group session. Acknowledging, by this time that some of my leadership was in part transactional. The tutor then further gently nudged me towards the realisation that I may have been acting in a critical parent mode. Looking at my journal, is there evidence of this: 'Another nurse came to tell on their colleague, more backbiting, like children.' Now that really sparked my journey, which not only led me back to my past and childhood, but highlighted the fact that it was within my future practice. It made a deep connection and one in which led to a focus on my emergence as a leader and will be continued in my narrative. Hence, I am on the path to cultivating wisdom as Zen Buddhism suggests is the way to enlightenment. The importance of guidance is as Johns (2004) believes, that had I not been guided, I may have laid the matter to rest. Hence, the importance of a guide cannot be fully emphasised. Had I not had a guide when I went to Egypt I would have missed the translation of the hieroglyphics and their meanings. In the same way had I not had a guide within this course I may have missed the significance of my insights. This does not mean I cannot continue with self-exploration, but as Boyd and Fales (1983) discuss, it guides the practitioner towards openness and lateral thinking.

Without doubt, guidance is vital towards gaining and deepening insight, enabling practitioners to wake up, to see beyond their normal selves, and, most vitally, to be open and receptive to new ways of being in the world, ways they may intrinsically resist because of embodiment. Guidance is the hallmark of scholarly work. It can never be a formula to follow. Mishler notes that (1990:422):

> Skilled research is a craft, and like any craft, it is learned by apprenticeship to competent researchers, by hands-on experience, and by continual practice. It seems remarkable, if we stop to think about it, that research competence is assumed to be gained by learning abstract rules of scientific procedure. Why should working knowledge be learned any more easily, or through other ways, than the competence required for playing the violin or blowing glass, or throwing pots?

References

Acker J, Barry K and Esseveld J (1983) Objectivity and truth: problems in doing feminist research. *Women Studies International Forum* 6:423–435.

Bohm D (1996) *On dialogue.* (Edited by L Nichol). Routledge, London.

Boud D, Keogh R and Walker D (1985) Promoting reflection in learning: a model. In: D Boud, R Keogh and D Walker (eds). *Reflection: turning experience into learning.* Kogan Page, London, pp. 18–40.

Boyd E and Fales A (1983) Reflective learning: key to learning from experience. *Journal of Humanistic Psychology* 23:99–117.

Cope M (2001) *Lead yourself: be where others will follow.* Pearson Education, London.

Covey S (1989) *The 7 habits of highly effective people.* Simon & Schuster, London.

Dewey J (1933) *How we think.* JC Heath, Boston.

Dreyfus H (1991) *Being-in-the-world. A commentary on Heidegger's being & time.* The MIT Press, Cambridge.

Fay B (1987) *Critical social science.* Polity Press, Cambridge.

Frank A (2002) Relations of caring: demoralization and remoralization in the clinic. *International Journal of Human Caring* 6:13–19.

Freire P (1972) *Pedagogy of the oppressed.* Penguin Books, London.

Gadamer H-G (1975) *Truth and method.* Seabury Press, New York.

Gilbert T (2001) Reflective practice and clinical supervision: meticulous rituals of the confessional. *Journal of Advanced Nursing* 36:199–205.

Gray G and Forsstrom S (1991) Generating theory from practice: the reflective technique. In: G Gray and R Pratt (eds.) *Towards a discipline of nursing.* Churchill Livingstone, Melbourne.

Greenwood D, Whyte W and Harkavy I (1993) Participatory action research as a process and as a goal. *Human Relations* 46:175–192.

Heidegger M (1962) *Being and time* (transl. Macquarrie J and Robinson E). Harper & Row, New York.

Heron J (1981) Philosophical basis for a new paradigm. In: P Reason and J Rowan (eds.) *Human inquiry.* John Wiley, Chichester.

Holly M (1989) Reflective writing and the spirit of inquiry. *Cambridge Journal of Education* 19:71–80.

Johns C (2001) Depending on the intent and emphasis of he supervisor, clinical supervision can be a different experience. *Journal of Nursing Management* 9:139–145.

Johns C (2003) Clinical supervision as a model for clinical leadership. *Journal of Nursing Management* 11:25–34.

Johns C (2004) *Becoming a reflective practitioner* (second edition). Blackwell Publishing, Oxford.

Jourard S (1971) *The transparent self.* Van Nostrand, Newark.

Kadushin A (1968) Games people play in supervision. *Social Work* 13:23–32.

Kieffer C (1984) Citizen empowerment: a developmental perspective. *Prevention in Human Services* 84:9–36.

Krishnamurti J (1996) *Total freedom; the essential Krishnamurti*. Harper Collins, San Francisco.

Menzies-Lyth I (1988) A case study in the functioning of social systems as a defence against anxiety. In: *Containing anxiety in institutions: selected essays*. Free Association Books, London, pp. 43–85.

Mezirow J (1981) A critical theory of adult learning and education. *Adult Education* 32:3–24.

Mishler E (1990) Validation in inquiry-guided research: the role of exemplars in narrative studies. *Harvard Educational Review* 60:415–442.

Newman M (1994) *Health as expanded consciousness*. National League for Nursing, New York.

O'Donohue J (1997) *Anan Cara: spiritual wisdom from the Celtic world*. Bantam Press, London.

Okri B (1997) *A way of being free*. Phoenix House, London. Text extracts used with permission of The Marsh Agency Ltd.

Paget M (1983) Experience and knowledge. *Human Studies* 6:67–90.

Pirsig R (1974) *Zen and the art of motorcycle maintenance*. Vintage, London.

Prigogine I and Stengers I (1984) *Order out of chaos*. Bantam, New York.

Robinson A (1995) Transformative 'cultural shifts' in nursing; participatory action research and the 'project of possibility'. *Nursing Inquiry* 2:65–74.

Rogers C (1969) *Freedom to learn; a view of what education might be*. Merrill, Colombus.

Saunders A (2006) *Transforming self through transformational leadership*. Unpublished Master in Clinical Leadership dissertation, University of Bedfordshire.

Schön D (1987) *Educating the reflective practitioner*. Jossey-Bass, San Francisco.

Smyth J (1987) *A rationale for teachers' critical pedagogy*. Deakin University Press, Victoria.

Spence DP (1982) *Narrative truth and historical truth: meaning and interpretation in psycho-analysis*. WW Norton & Co, New York.

Tzu L (1999) *Tao Te Ching* (transl. Mitchell S). Frances Lincoln, London.

Weinsheimer J (1985) *Gadamer's hermeneutics. A reading of truth and method*. Yale University Press, New Haven.

Whitehead L (2004) Enhancing the quality of hermeneutic research: decision trail. *Journal of Advanced Nursing* 45(5):512–518.

Chapter 4

Weaving the narrative

Christopher Johns

The first four levels of dialogue are dynamic movements creating the narrative pattern. Now, in the fifth dialogical movement, the narrator crafts the narrative, as if a complex jigsaw. What started as scribbling in a journal is transformed through reflection into reflective text and now, into narrative text.

Story text ──────▶ Reflective text ──────▶ Narrative text

Narrative patterns the practitioner's reflexive journey of self-realisation; a drama unfolding, revealing its insights. This pattern is shaped by the plot of the narrative (Fay 1987) – for the practitioner to realise her vision as a lived reality of self and practice, to become who self wants to be. For this type of narrative this is always the plot.

Plot gives narrative direction and focus (Mattingly 1994:813). Mattingly notes:

> It is the plot that makes individual events understandable as part of a coherent whole, one which leads compellingly towards a particular ending ... Any particular event gains its meanings by its place within this narrative configuration, as a contribution to the plot. This configuration makes a whole such that we can speak of the point of the story. Yet this is an always shifting configuration for we live in the midst of unfolding stories over which we have a very partial control.

Reflexivity

Reflexivity is looking back through the sequence of experiences incorporated within the narrative that plot the transformative journey towards self-realisation. Reflexivity is something dynamic, lived, through drawing out significance and insights that inform future experiences. Through constantly looking back, the practitioner/narrator patterns these insights into threads that weave through the narrative as developmental strands within the whole pattern of realising self. The result is a drama unfolding, moment by moment, moments of revelation. Reflexivity challenges the practitioner to find adequate ways to frame their self-realisation as a whole pattern. To reiterate, my vision of myself as a complementary therapist is to ease suffering. This is a very broad statement. What does it mean to ease suffering? The first question is – what is suffering? I might turn to the literature to inform me but suffering is not easily reduced to a scheme. I might say that suffering is a disruption of the human being that is unsatisfactory. Through my stories, people express their suffering in different ways but always it has this dimension of being human. So I can know and appreciate suffering as a whole phenomenon through story.

I might ask myself – what sort of person do I need to be to ease suffering? Through my stories I review my response to suffering. Am I effective in easing it? Yes, again through story, I can reflect on my responses to suffering and the response of the other to my response. I can make judgements about that. Could I be more effective in easing it? This question drives my reflective quest. Through my analysis of my own practice and the practices of others who desire to realise holistic practice (the holy grail of health care) I can explicate the characteristics of being a holistic practitioner in constructing the 'Being available' template as a means for knowing and monitoring the development of holistic practice (see Appendix 1).

Both Latchford (Chapter 7) and Groom (Chapter 12) used Kieffer's model of participatory competence (1984; see Appendix 1) to plot their journeys of becoming empowered, given the centrality of empowerment to transformation. John-Marc Priest (Chapter 11) used Schuster's characteristics of transformational leadership (1994; see Appendix 1) to frame the emergence of his leadership. These are only examples. Many other theories can be similarly appropriated to frame meaning and mark the reflexive transformational journey of self-realisation.

Having said that, the reflexive journey can be mapped through the narrative just within the sequence of experiences, where self-realisation is implied through the revelation and exploration of insights. Either way, if the narrative was being submitted for examination, the practitioner would summarise her transformative journey into a coherent pattern. This would also enable her to focus on particular insights that make a significant contribution to the idea of 'new knowledge' and the demand that a doctoral study is only worthy if it makes such contribution. Of course, this raises further issues of coherence (see Chapter 15).

To reiterate: reflexivity is a looking back, and seeing self emerge through a sequence of experiences and the insights gained that thread through the experiences. Each subsequent experience applies and reflects on the insights gained from the previous experience within the reflexive spiral towards realising one's vision of self and practice as a lived reality. Reflexivity is manifest as a process of looking back and seeing self transformed through the series of experiences. Dewey writes (1933:4–5):

> The successive portions of a reflective thought grow out of one another and support one another; they do not come and go in medley. Each phase is a step from something to something – technically speaking, it is a term of thought. Each term leaves a deposit that is utilised in the next term. The stream or flow becomes a train or chain. There are in any reflective thought definite units that are linked together so that there is sustained movement to a common end.

These *definite units* mark the reflexive developmental journey and pattern the narrative form. Each experience has a trace that informs the next experience even though such connections are not deliberately made or obvious because of the subliminal nature of reflexivity that is only revealed when looking back. Paget (1983:79) notes that:

> An exchange cannot be severed from the shared historical understanding which it pre-supposes without radically shattering its meanings. An exchange contains the meanings of what has already been said … isolating an exchange from its antecedents, those exchanges which already occurred and are pre-supposed, shatters a discourse process and undermines the unfolding complex and multi-meaninged construction of experience.

In other words, narrative only works because of reflexivity. This is not an easy idea to grasp when doing it, especially when the narrator commences constructing narrative, simply because experiences reflected on tend to be random and connection between them tenuous. As the narrator becomes more mindful, she begins to see threads emerging and learns to pay attention to particular experiences because they are linked to past experiences. This creates a gestalt view of the practitioner's *whole* experience unfolding over time whereby aspects of experience can be viewed against a background of the whole.

Frameworks can give the impression that experience is more orderly than it really is. In other words they impose an illusionary order. Experience is not an orderly affair with neat beginnings and endings amidst a smooth flow of logic. It is complex and contradictory. To adequately reflect experience, narrative must itself be a complex and contradictory affair; an unfolding drama of stories within stories. Hence narrative can only be constructed as an unfolding story rather than constructed at the end. As such, the guide and practitioner consciously construct the narrative by recording the dialogue of each session evolving from the previous session, layers upon layers woven together through the series of unfolding experiences. Within a good narrative the reader will sense the narrative is alive with a sense of movement through it, held together by the plot and the markers that monitor the journey of self being and becoming. It is edited, so nothing is superfluous. The qualities of courage, vulnerability and authenticity in the struggle to become should be transparent, adding to the sense of the narrative being alive. In contrast, narratives that lack flow and movement through them fail, despite many wonderful things being apparent within them.

The effort to reduce the complexity of experience into themes or categories reflects the positivist, masculine concern, to order, predict and control life. And yet, in our ordered lives, for others to feel confident in such research, a compromise may need to be made to see a path through the complexity. People are so used to speaking with received voices that they are unable to unravel their own meanings from such texts, but then perhaps teachers, writers and researchers of nursing have not encouraged or facilitated such personal adventures. Narratives can never tell the whole story but they give glimpses to other dimensions not overtly addressed, the gestalt relationship between foreground and background.

Gergen and Gergen (1991) make a distinction between inward looking reflexivity which seeks feedback to reinforce and sustain a particular worldview and outward looking reflexivity which draws on multiple perspectives to challenge a worldview. The former is a 'closed' or single loop system whilst the latter is an 'open' or double loop system (Argyris and Schön 1974). Clearly, to realise a vision always require intense scrutiny of the vision itself, not just the words used but what the words actually mean as lived. And here, I might add, what the words really mean rather than any surface interpretation. This is the nature of reflection. Realising one's vision is the narrative plot and is always problematic.

Pattern

'Narrative fit' is significantly enhanced by the discovery of a pattern match (Spence 1982). Robinson and Hawpe (1986:113–114) note that:

> In order to perceive order and recognise repetition and similarity we must go beyond the surface features in dealing with the world of concrete objects and human social interactions.

A story provides the right balance between uniqueness and universality. Because stories are contextualised accounts they can convey the particularity of any episode. But because they are built upon a generic set of categories and relationships each story resembles other stories to varying degrees. A sense of familiarity is the result of this underlying similarity.

Narrative is persuasive because it *can* accommodate contradictory experience and the complexity of experience. Its structure cannot be static or immutable, it is organic, literally lived, growing, cultivated, responding to new interpretations that emerge from the constant dialectical process of deconstructing lived experience and constructing coherent narrative within the hermeneutic spiral of being and becoming (Giorgi 1985; van Manen 1990). Fay (1987:171–172) writes:

> It ought to be obvious that a narrative cannot consist of a portrayal of *all* the acts people perform and the causal outcomes of these actions ... there must be a principle of selection in terms of which some acts and outcomes are included and some excluded ... the principle most generally employed for this purpose is one which says that events ought to be included which, when related together, for a recognizable pattern by which the nature of the person's lives, or an important feature of them, is depicted. *Such a pattern* is the plot of a narrative.

Narrative resonates with chaos theory in the sense that the practice is complex in its wholeness and yet within that apparent chaos there is order or pattern recognition. Narrative is *movement*; like a stream gathering pace, rhythm, deepening, widening, being shaped by the landscape as it flows towards the sea. I can tune into and flow with the inherent order rather than resists the flow of energy by forcing ideas into boxes. This is a vital understanding in constructing narrative.

Narrative demands liberation from oppressive forms of censorship and expression (Cixous 1996). As I construct the narrative I am conscious of tensions playing themselves out within me, the tensions between finding an adequate expression for my voice in relationship with those I work with and finding an adequate expression to engage readers in ways that might be meaningful. So I resist (even as I feel the demand) reducing the narrative into some explanatory scheme, what Clandinin and Connelly (2000) describe as the formulaic and reductionist boundaries with narrative inquiry. In a world largely governed by professional texts in a formulaic and reductionist vein it is a difficult pull to resist. Elaborate concept identification and analysis obscures rather than illuminates possible meanings when the narrative needs to be open for the reader for potential dialogue.

Between the lines of my narrative description I plant signs that point direction to the significance and meaning of my practice; in a touch, a glance, a pause, a plaintiff smile, a simple action of holding someone's hand. As I wrote elsewhere 'the profound buried in the mundane yet when watched, lifts it into immense significance, valued in its unfolding moment, a light across the reader's soul' (Johns 2002:42). Planting seeds to explode in the reader's mind over time (Okri 1997).

Due to its reflexive nature, the narrative might seem repetitive; yet a new twist is always present for the discerning reader. Reflection helps me to reveal the complexity and uncertainty of easing suffering for people who are dying and their families, pulling out for deeper reflection significant issues such as: What is a 'good death'? What is spiritual care? What is suffering? What is compassion? What is the therapeutic team? Narrative holds these ideas together as a 'whole' in ways that communicate meaning within the particular situation, revealing the common patterns and uniqueness within each situation. It reveals the subtlety and depth of nursing knowledge (Boykin and Schoenhofer 1991) lifting apparently mundane acts into significance. Hence narrative illuminates the complexity of practice as a 'whole' and, as such, is the natural expression for holistic theory and practice.

The reflexive spiral of being and becoming is sometimes a dramatic moment of revelation or it is a gradual almost subliminal unfolding moment by moment.

The narrative is on-going. It is never finished yet as at certain points, the narrator pauses to summarise the journey so far and present an account, notably for academic purposes. The process of understanding ourselves can never achieve finality but is always unfolding and always being revised. There is no genuine narrative that will definitely reveal our true identity (Fay 1987).

The following ideas of writing emanated from the March 2009 PhD school:[1]

- Writing to enable people to be present within the narrative (both those referred to within the narrative and readers);
- Do not close down the interpretative space (with over-explanation – leave the reader space for his or her own interpretation);
- Have a pattern yet without trying to impose order;
- Writing about the point (show but not tell);
- Greater emphasis on reconstructing conversations (sense of drama and being in the present);
- Writing in shorter sentences – creating tension between sentences (in the spaces);
- Using more images and metaphors to hold meaning;
- Making the point – followed by silence.

Of course, many more points can be made. The point of the exercise was considering key issues in scripting the narrative. Writers have love affairs with words. They rejoice that there are so many ways of saying the same thing – or nearly the same thing – because each minute shift in vocabulary will subtly change the meaning and the tone (Manjusvara 2005:20). Every word counts.

Tinkering

I say to the students, tinker around the edges. Open a file and play with your ideas. Play with expression, for who knows how to tell a story, to find the balance between telling the story and being a story analyst. Create images to hold meaning. We can only play and the ideas will take form almost by serendipity. I am reminded of Schuster's qualities of transformational leadership, notably that leaders take risks, experiment and learn and it seems it is just like this. In shaping the narrative they are shaping themselves, finding a way to be the leader they desire to be. It is not easy. I exhort them to take comfort in another of Schuster's qualities of transformational leaders – 'leaders persevere in hard times'.

24 March 2007

As if by serendipity I open Margaret Wheatley and Myron Kellner-Rodger's book *A simpler way* and they write about tinkering – 'this world of exploration is one which tinkers itself into existence' (1999:17).

---

[1] The PhD school is a three-day intensive for supervisors and students studying narrative, held at the University of Bedfordshire. The school is held bi-annually and is open to subscription (www.beds.ac.uk/rpf).

Tinkering resonates with doodling, almost an idle, opportunistic tinkering with the materials yet purposeful towards making something work, as if the words aren't working, or finding new ways to make them work better, to tell the story – 'but life's tinkering has direction. It tinkers towards order' (Wheatley and Kellner-Rodger 1999:17). The writer's search for system is not an orderly linear pattern. It is sensed in moments of revelation by dwelling within the whole messy fabric of words that may randomly be scattered throughout the journal. The relationship between words, events, feelings are not a neat analytic processes but deeply complex that defy simple reduction into orderly systems of thinking and representation – 'but how it gets there violates all of our rules of good process: life is not neat, parsimonious, logical, nor elegant. Life seeks order in a disorderly way. Life uses processes we find hard to tolerate and hard to believe in – mess upon mess until something workable emerges' (Wheatley and Kellner-Rodger 1999:17).

I must believe in this for myself when my aching mind screams for order … perseverance and patience … flowing with the hermeneutic tide as insights emerge of both meaning and form. My students also ache and scream at me when they write and write again, and, slowly form emerges until the sense of creation and beauty astounds them. Creation is a relentless process. It is surrender to deeper intuitive forces beyond the grasping rationale and analytical mind that seeks to impose order. Order is found from within, not from outside. Hence we must create places where we can play, where we can let go of the analytical demand, where we can reveal to ourselves the art of holding creative tension. It is a place where the cubic centimetre of chance becomes a perpetual wide open space, where every moment is a learning opportunity if we are mindful enough. It is about creating our own worlds rather than being confined to a world created by others, as difficult as that may seem in systems governed by dominance and oppression. But it is easy to start with ourselves, with our journals …

I am drunk with reading. I need a walk to let the ideas ripple through and play with them. Reading crowds my mind. At first it excites me and then it overwhelms me. Reading books only for short bursts with a pencil in hand to mark the serendipity. Only then do I *really* listen, open myself to the possibilities of what the text has to say to me, to let the words ripple through me and play with.

In guiding students, I cannot rush them into a creative space. First they must come to realise that their learnt processes are no longer adequate, functional to become who they desire to be. They must realise that learnt processes forged on the Newtonian anvil are constraints to creative becoming. Hence on the surface of things we pull at the order of things, exposing paradoxes, ruffling feathers, making it messy, slowly opening ourselves to the possibilities of other ways. For example: to see the therapeutic encounter between a nurse and a patient as a mystery unfolding and to see caring as an act of love. What possibilities begin to emerge. What tension!

Lou

The following are scratches from my own journal in guiding Lou,[2] notably concerned with finding pattern to her insights about spasticity nursing. It probably won't make entire sense but it does capture something of the rhythm of such work.

---

[2] Used with her permission.

Morning of 27/3/07 – We reflect on the shifting form of her narrative as we endeavour to find a pattern that works. No logic just intuition. It is feeling the flow rather than thinking about it. Lou recognises she is too much in her head. Lou tears at her hair as we take another turn, another twist in search of a better way to represent the work – patterns unfolding, not random although seemingly so, parting the high reeds that obscures any pre-set path but nevertheless creating a path that works. Today we think we have found it based on the recognition of a tension between telling a story and analysing a story ... Lou had rewritten her stories making them more evocative, and taking out the analysing from inside them. Instead she had identified insights from the text and written thousands of words on the insights ... reading it is like ploughing through a heavy field making explicit what the story already says. Where is the balance between story telling and story analysis? A disorientating dilemma yet crucial to find. It is the same as saying what do readers need to be told and what can they discern for themselves. Yet every reader is different. Few are likely to be mindful of their own assumptions as they read. Story *is* theory. Thus it is enough to tell the story in ways the insights shine.

Trimming the experiences, cutting out analysis and suddenly we have so much space in the thesis!

We agree to write a further chapter reflecting on the narrative process (originally in the end chapter) but we can see more clearly that the 'original contribution to knowledge' is not just the spasticity theory but also the narrative construction. This is such a creative process. It shows again that there can be no prescribed narrative theory, that narrative for each student is a unique experiment with self. At first the insights were apparently random and arbitrary. I helped Lou to be more detailed – brainstorming the possibilities of insights in rich detail, but how to organise the insights? Do they need organising?

We play with the idea of using the framing perspectives to open the scope of insights, notably philosophical and role framing insights and then reality framing insights to appreciate the constraints on realising Lou's vision, but for me this didn't work. Too concrete. Developmental framing – using the Being available template as we had envisaged linked to the emerging space theory. Lou responded to these insights – reorganising the insights, and developing them as a consequence but still the analysis is too long. Many of the words she writes repeat what's in the story. They don't really say anything more so scrap the lot! The story is the theory and is the essential ground for the end theory chapter.

Lou is happy for once at the end of the session. We see a strong light filter through and illuminate the text and the way forward ... spontaneous, creative. It now seems so obvious but it needed the steps along the shifting hermeneutic tide to see it. In the process Lou has rewritten the stories as engaging and challenging. She has identified her key insights and framed them. We sketch out the space model ... it is becoming easier to see the emerging pattern by throwing the Being available template over it. In self-organisation, structures emerge. They are not imposed. They spring from the process of doing the work. These structures will be useful but temporary. We can expect them to emerge and recede as needed.

15 June 2007

After our session Lou and I go for a drink. We muse about Chapter 4 – the analysis chapter where she draws to the surface the insights gained through the reflective journey as a model for spasticity nursing. It is not easy. Lou feels tied up in conceptual knots.

She shows me her first draft. She starts with the early formulations and moves towards the latest. It is stodgy, yet we had felt this was the way to go, to make transparent the cognitive process. An alternative would be to start with the latest formulation and work backwards. The intentionality collage Lou did with Rory might be the beginning … she did this in 2005 after finishing the journal (as represented in the narrative). It was from this point the idea of space emerged. Perhaps we should start with that, leading on to her appreciation of Barbara Hepworth and space as an organising metaphor. Unbounded space.

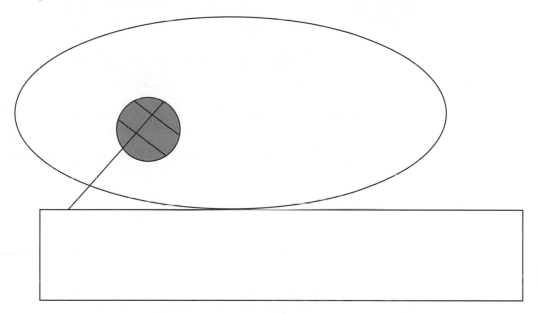

In a way it doesn't matter what the shape looks like. The shape is the artist's creation … the oval is the therapeutic space. The circle represents the mystery of creation itself … the therapeutic process unfolding that is essentially uncertain, unpredictable, and can only be known. The parallel lines represent the family and Lou tuned into each other in precarious harmony reflecting the parallel with the family's own relationship with life.

The space between the parallel lines also represents the balance between connection and separation and mindfulness. The foundation line represents security and tradition, that the relationship does have boundaries of power and tradition that are always being understood and shifted. The bounded oval also represents the team and society, that this relationships takes place within spaces. The position of the circle within the oval reflects the way the relationship is positioned and how that relationship and space itself needs always to be mediated. The foundation stone is the Being available template. This is the adopted interpretative framework Lou used to help shape and mark the stories as representative of her therapeutic quest. We test out if the core therapeutic works. We revise it – 'being available is tuning into the other's wavelength to understand, connect with and flow with towards maintaining and improving the balance of their precarious harmony'. The vision is the foundation. The factors that influence Lou's ability to being availability are randomly patterned around this strange attractor, always shifting in dynamic relationship within the whole:

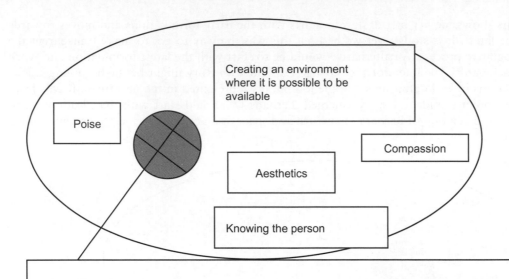

We bombard the space with key insights related to each of the influencing factors:

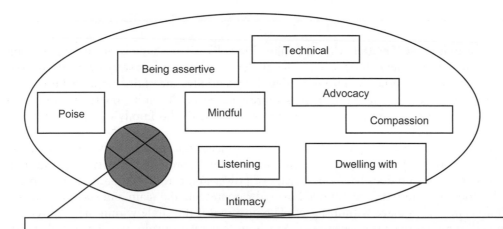

Now these ideas can be discussed, linked back to the narratives where they lie thick on the surface or buried between the lines … washed out with the hermeneutic tide.

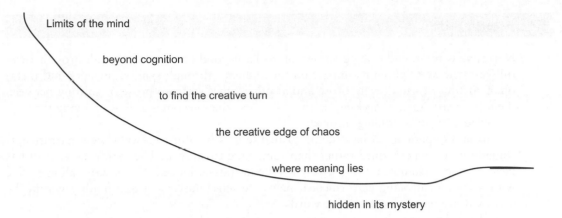

Limits of the mind

    beyond cognition

        to find the creative turn

           the creative edge of chaos

              where meaning lies

                hidden in its mystery

Sitting with Lou
contemplating the final chapter
how to present the work
drawing out the insights
into a coherent pattern
around a strange attractor
… what might that be
that adequately captures the essence
the nature of dwelling with others with spasticity in precarious harmony
in a line.

Inspired by 'space'
dwelling in space
mediating self within self
feeling the edge of creative space
expanding space
shaping therapeutic space
not bounded by space boundaries
created by expectations socially arranged ignorant of the therapeutic demand
how the demand screams
beyond broken dreams
you are the dream catcher.

Sitting in this space
Smithfield market across the road
Sipping a San Miguel in the quiet afternoon
co-creating
dwelling with the ideas
moving beyond the concept
and suddenly a rose blooms!
Theorising
scratching the surface
going deeper
touching the spirit
dwelling with.

Lou eventually developed these ideas further for inclusion in her final thesis (Jarrett 2009).

Representation

Narrative is presented using a variety of media beyond prose, even though prose is carefully crafted to heighten its impact on the audience through syntax, imagery and metaphor. At times I use flowing prose and at other times staccato prose or shifting between them to create impact. Seeking rhythm. The text then becomes a dance moving through its mystery as an unfolding drama.

Through experience, I have come to realise it is helpful to always view narrative as something to be performed rather than something to be read. The performance turn has been extremely significant in the way I write narrative. Indeed, I now write all narrative with a view to it being performed. It helps me sense movement and fluidity within the text as if my hands are sculpting words.

It also helps me to be more parsimonious with words, leaving pauses, spaces, silences, for the reader or listener to dwell in and consider the point being made ... not filling the space with explanation that would close down the potential for dialogue. Less is more (Manjusvara 2005:53).

The use of conversation within narrative is another experiment to find form. Using actual or reconstructed words is helpful to draw the reader into drama as something happening at that moment, as something lived in the unfolding moment.

Picking up the point of reconstructing conversation. The judicious use of conversation gives the narrative a certain *face value* authenticity and sense of drama. Of course, the narrative is no more authentic than a narrative written without conversation, yet it does seem more believable. Paget (1983) led me to recognise the need to use adequate conversation or 'talk' to support 'proof' of practitioner development *and* to portray the subtlety, complexity, context and subjectivity of experience. Looking back through my PhD narratives (Johns 1998) I recognise my increasing use of conversation taken from guided reflection sessions, until approximately 60% of the narrative was constructed through conversations. I believe that conversation best captures the spirit of the work rather than the language of interpretation 'that flattens rather than deepens our understanding of human life' (van Manen 1990:17). Because much of the conversation was led by the practitioner, it seemed natural to use it as the primary source of description (Agar and Hobbs 1982).

Using conversation as central to the narrative construction inevitably incorporates the feelings, goals, needs, and values of the people who created it (Robinson and Hawpe 1986) because these are always implicit within dialogue. The narrative writer(s) make explicit the significant issues within the conversation and fashions these fragments into a whole whose integrity is in its presentation in narrative form (Gergen and Gergen 1986).

Consider these two versions taken from *RAW*:

Tears run in small streams down each side of her face. A proud woman brought to her knees. At every turn something else emerges to taunt her.

'How is Phil coping?'

'He's coping fairly well but finds it difficult to talk about what has happened.'

Coping fairly well – I have a stereotyped image of a man unable to express his feelings. I want to press her about her husband's feelings when she blurts out, 'I won't have any treatment if this comes back. I want to live for my children. I have doted on them, they are everything to me ... but this is too painful. There is no way I can go through this again.'

I ask how she felt me coming today?

Wiping away her tears she says, 'I wasn't worried either way. ...'

Tears run in small streams down each side of her face. A proud woman brought to her knees. At every turn something else emerges to taunt her. I asked her how was Phil coping? She said he's coping fairly well but that he found it difficult to talk about what had happened. *Coping fairly well* – I have a stereotyped image of a man unable to express his feelings. I wanted to press her about her husband's feelings when she blurted out that she wouldn't have any treatment if this came back. She wanted to live for her children she has doted on, they mean everything to her. She said that the things are too painful; that there is no way she could go through this again.

I asked how she felt me coming today? Wiping away her tears she said she hadn't been worried either way. ...

Which version reads better?

RAW was initially written as a narrative reflecting my journeying as a complementary therapist with Gill, a woman experiencing breast cancer treatment spanning over five years and 70 sessions. I then adapted *RAW* to be performed by a single voice and subsequently for four voices. Reading *RAW* as a single voice, the issue of dialogue between myself (as a complementary therapist) and Gill, the woman experiencing breast cancer treatment, was not problematic. However, when another voice read Gill's words it became problematic. It just didn't sound right. The reader could not get the gist of Gill's voice, its intonations and inflexions.

When *RAW* was first performed[3] I did not realise the problem. It was only after working with my dance and drama colleagues at the university on the *Climbing walls* performance did I come to appreciate the *naturalistic problem*. Next time we performed *RAW*,[4] I knew the reading of 'Gill's' voice was wrong. I subsequently rewrote the performance text to reduce the dialogue between Gill and myself, only using 'her voice' to make statements (Johns 2009).[5] The retained dialogue between myself Gill and myself was read by myself.

My performance text for *Climbing walls* (Chapter 10) also contained considerable dialogue between Ann, another woman with breast cancer, and myself (again as complementary therapist). We did permit two brief scenes to be dramatically included with voices representing Ann. It may seem a small point yet such subtlety makes such a huge difference in the performance, as if performance amplifies narrative form. The skill of narrative writing as performance is revealed. It can only be experiential and not prescribed, although the need to avoid the 'naturalistic pull' must be avoided – or else the performance should be written as a play and given over to actors and expert direction.

Prose broken down into single lines becomes a type of prose poetry, or prose that has a particularly timbre that opens up the text and invites the reader to explore between the lines. The first lines of *Jane's rap* are an example of this expression (Chapter 14):

---

[3] Performed at the 14th International Reflective Conference, Aalborg, Denmark, June 2007.
[4] Performed as my inaugural professorial lecture at the University of Bedfordshire November 2007.
[5] RAW performance text is published in Johns C (2009) *Becoming a reflective practitioner* (third edition). Wiley-Blackwell, Oxford. The narrative itself has yet to be published.

I tell Chris a story
A reflection on my practice
Night shift
Around 3 in the morning
He's deliberately cut his arm
Deliberate self-harm
Needing sutures
I recoil
Try to hide my feelings
But feel empty
No compassion
He asks if it will hurt
My irritation
Bubbling to the surface
'Must have hurt when you did it'
I spit
Such a waste of time
Stitching him up

Contrast this text with the narrative (Chapter 13). The performance text is 6000 words shorter than the narrative, reminding me of the maxim – 'less is more'– how meaning can be buried in words. However, the narrative was initially written to satisfy academic scrutiny. It was never written with performance in mind.

Art

I briefly mentioned art as reflective space in Chapter 2. Besides prose, narrative is constructed from diverse art form; imagery, poetry, film, painting, photography, play, movement and dance, etc., whatever the narrator feels suits her in finding adequate representation for holding meaning and unfolding the reflexive narrative. Again, there is no prescription to such work, no theory to guide it beyond the claims of coherence and reflexivity. And again it is not easy.

In constructing the movement within *Climbing walls* we rehearsed for many days to find and explore a form that we felt 'worked'. Working alongside dance and drama teachers made the work less naïve, in the sense it was informed by dance and performance theory, and yet, as April, Amanda and Antje reveal (Chapter 10) there is no performance theory for this type of text. All the more creative.

In *Jane's rap* I position eight chairs in a reflective spiral, each chair represents each of the eight self-harm people spoken about in the text. Positioning the chairs in this way was first rehearsed in my presentation to the Nursing Faculty at Barnes-Jewish Medical Centre in St Louis. It worked. The chairs gave the self-harm patients presence in the performance space. I realised I needed to give them voice. I approached Colleen Marlin, Professor of English at Centennial College, Toronto, to write a series of empathic poems – to give voice to the self-harm patients. When I performed *Jane's rap* at the University of Bedfordshire these poems were read by April Nunes-Tucker, as she sat in turn, in each chair. She had studied the poems carefully to interpret the experience of being a self-harm patient through her posture and voice inflection. As we read the text we moved along the eight chairs. As she read each poem I placed my hand on her left shoulder and looked away. The feedback was very affirming. The random chairs on stage gave a desolate impression of an accident and emergency department, the physical desolation reflecting the inner desolation the self-harm patients must have felt. Asking someone outside health care felt significant in writing the poems, almost as an advocate for the self-harm people. As you can read for yourself, the poems are sensational (see Chapter 13).

Imagery

Images hold and communicate the complexity of experience and meaning. They hold together the whole, adding richness and substance to text, adding layers of texture to meaning, symbolising meaning and complementing language.

In designing my single voice performance of *Climbing walls* (Chapter 10) I researched and constructed a background of images that reflected literally what was happening in the written text – images of women with one breast, bald women, women with wigs, cancer cells, mammography photography. I thought by doing this I would synchronise the words spoken. Most narrative I have seen performed uses a similar approach and I have wondered why I had sometimes felt irritated by this approach. I felt that the images were an embellishment and emotional seduction of the audience. Certainly images can be very emotional in reflecting feelings being portrayed within the text. But images can also be distracting from the text.

So I discarded the whole PowerPoint. Instead I attended an art workshop[6] and let my imagination flow using inks, using the images to open the viewer's own imagination. It was such a revelation to explore this new reflective medium to open a space to explore experience and use painting to represent meaning, rather than impose literal images on the audience, as good as they were.

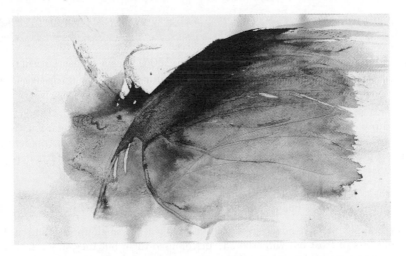

In *Jane's rap* (Chapter 13) I designed a PowerPoint background that consisted of photographs I took whilst walking on Franz-Joseph Glacier in New Zealand – using ice images to symbolise coldness, starkness, desolation, taint, and cutting. I also painted a series of *ensos*, Zen circles of enlightenment (Seo 2007). Each *enso* is painted with one

---

[6]The art workshop was led by Lin Rose and Cindy (ottersqaw@yahoo.com).

brush stroke in a single breath and expresses the totality of our being. Each *enso* is painted a different colour to reflect my sense of feeling within the reflection. Within each *enso*[7] I wrote a six-word narrative[8] to capture the essence of the self-harm person's experience as reflected through Colleen's empathic poems.

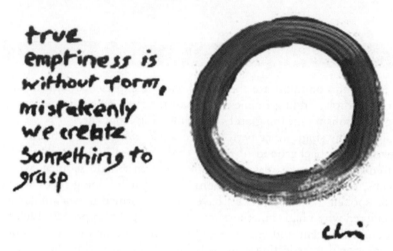

Painting the *ensos* became an extension of my spiritual practice, enabling me to find deeper meaning within the text, opening the performance as sacred space, and lifting the performance into a spiritual dimension. By doing this, April and I were deeply moved by the performance as were the audience, facilitating the primary point of the performance to confront negative attitudes to self-harm patients with a professional audience.

Metaphor

In her leadership narrative, Philomena James (2006) uses a consistent theme of observing crab apples from her office window as a metaphor to link the narrative through a series of experiences.

> I joined my new organisation today. My window looks over a wild garden. The crab apple trees are covered in small yellow apples the size of large marbles. Apparently there is a lunar eclipse followed by a full moon, a time of new beginnings, and that is how it feels. (2006:35)

> The birds are pecking at the small yellow apples on the tree outside my window, taking full advantage of autumn's bounty … it is the fourth week in my new post. (2006:38)

> The crab apple trees are now bereft of leaves. Only a few small apples cling to the branches. The cold kiss of frost has withered and discoloured them but they stay attached to the tree defying both birds and weather. (2006:43)

> I look out of my window and imagine the crab apple trees decked with lights as Christmas approaches. (2006:44)

---

[7] The *ensos* and six-word narratives are set out in Chapter 14 in association with the poems they represent.
[8] The idea of six-word narratives was inspired by conversations with Colleen Marlin.

The trees outside my window have never looked so forlorn, and only the grey mists and short days shroud their vulnerability. it is as if they are suspended waiting, waiting for the signal to emerge again. This is how I am feeling. (2006:47)

The cold winter wind has finally changed direction and eased. I can see tight buds on the crab apple trees ready to unfurl and bring fresh growth. (2006:59)

The garden outside my window is transformed. The crab apples are green and the long grass revived. (2006:59)

Phil uses the imagery of the crab apples to reflect her transformation as a leader, moving through a sense of desolation to new growth and abundance that marked her own leadership emergence after a seemingly long winter, as if guided reflection was the soil that nourished her in the knowing that her leadership would emerge, remaining positive through the harsh climate when it seemed that nothing would grow, or that all might perish.

Narrative thread

Time – the unlimited continued progress of existence and events in the past, present, and future, regarded as a whole. (*Compact Oxford English Dictionary* (COED) 2005:1084)

Constructing narrative is always experiential within the hermeneutic spiral of being and becoming. Within the seemingly chaotic pattern of experience, order is shaped through meaning. As noted, frameworks are utilised to pattern the reflexive development of self-realisation, perhaps creating the illusion that things are more orderly than they really are. The risk with imposing too much order is that meaning gets flattened. It is a fine balance between *showing* the insights within the text and *telling* the reader what the insights are. Yet either way insights are the key to organising organisational structure.

Reviewing my own and others' published narratives, time within narrative has been structured in various ways:

- Chronologically, as a series of (linear) experiences unfolding day by day.
- Chronologically, organised through a series of case studies that may overlap with other case studies.
- Chronologically, organised through a series of guided reflection sessions.
- Chaotically, i.e. apparently random experiences without reference to chronological time.

Between 2000–2002 I kept a reflective journal as a complementary therapist working with palliative care and cancer patients in hospice and community settings. This narrative was organised chronologically as a series of experiences unfolding day by day (*Being mindful, easing suffering* (Johns 2004) published by Jessica Kingsley).

My narrative between 2002–2004 was organised chronologically through a series of case studies (*Engaging reflection in practice* (Johns 2006) published by Blackwell Publishing).

Contrasting the two approaches, I prefer the chronological unfolding of experiences day by day simply for its sense of drama. It feels more spontaneous and creative than the case study approach.

In his narrative (Chapter 11), John-Marc breaks up chronological time by commencing his narrative with the end experience as if setting out the climax, and then retraces his steps from early student days until he catches up with and continues the point of drama he commenced with. This stylistic turn is very effective in heightening the drama, reminiscent of the film 'Crash', which uses this technique to great effect. I have now used this technique myself to structure my autoethnography *Reflection on my mother dying: a story of caring shame* (Johns 2009). In their respective narratives, Latchford (Chapter 7) and Groom (Chapter 12) structure through guided reflection sessions rather than experiences.

Even though I have yet to explore the potential of 'chaotic' narratives, I feel a creative pull in that direction.

Narrative style

I have been influenced by many authors and ideas in shaping narrative, perhaps no more than Ben Okri. In his book *A way of being free* he writes (1997:47):

> Even when it is tragic, storytelling is always beautiful. It tells us that all fates can be ours. It wraps up our lives with the magic which we only see long afterwards. Storytelling reconnects us to the great sea of human destiny. Human suffering, and human transcendence.

Nothing is more important in writing narrative to tune into this idea of beauty – that writing should be beautiful and enchanting. Such beauty is affront to a broken age. Just as science decries the use of story, so health care has diminished caring. Health care without caring is a contradiction. Story is the reconnection. That in writing beauty the spirit can only soar and self can become empowered. The idea that story reconnects is a vital understanding, that in writing I reconnect myself not only to human life and suffering, but also to myself as suffering, particularly if I myself feel dispirited, or alienated. As Arthur Frank (2002) notes, story is remoralising in environments that are demoralising. Narrative refocuses the self at the centre in ways that honour and mend the fractured nature of reality yet in ways whereby a temporal unity or plot is established not just in a written form but within life itself. The art of storytelling challenges the narrative writer to write accounts that capture the imagination.

Yet within the stories lies the truth of the nursing, or any other tradition. The stories shed a light on everyday practice in ways the very roots of the tradition are revealed. The stories are beacons of the effort to realise self as caring. In this sense they are poignant, enchanting and horrific, enchanting through the beauty of caring in responding to the suffering of others and horrific in revealing the suffering of illness and the ways caring is thwarted because of ignorance. Okri (1997:64–65) writes:

> giving truth direct narrative expression is to give it public explosion. the truth –Truth – SHRIEKS: it wakes up all the hidden bullies, the hidden policemen, and the incipient dictators and tyrants of the land. The truth could simply be something that everyone sees and knows already, something that we all live with, sleep with, and wake up to, and die as a result of – the truth could be something so obvious and familiar, but which no-one has uttered … and while it lives, uncried out, it devours, this unacceptable truth we accept in silence.

Through such words, Okri firmly places narrative within the scope of critical social science, without doubt reflecting the oppression he felt especially towards artists within his own country. To speak your truth is integrity. Saunders, in her leadership narrative writes (2006:94):

> Ben Okri inspired me throughout writing this narrative. At the beginning of this two year course, I viewed his work as 'flowery poems' and a clever structure of words. As time moved on I became more aware of my spirituality and as such his words mean more for me now than type on paper. As Okri (1997) illuminated, there is, as I understand, a spiritual level of writing which is in harmony with the forgotten self.

Stories are truthful renditions of experience. They may not be historically accurate in terms of detail. They may be distorted in the self's need to perceive self in certain sorts of ways. Yet, it is still a valid story because people need to distort things for reasons which themselves becomes a focus for understanding and revealing the true self beneath the layers of distortion that mask the therapeutic self. The purpose of narrative is to reveal self and the layers that obscure self because if we cannot reveal the true self then the self cannot be available to achieve desirable and effective work.

I have for many years read narratives at conferences and within my teaching, but is only since the reflective practice conference in Denmark in June 2007, with my first performance of *RAW*, that I consciously embraced the idea of performance as something beyond reading the narrative as written. As I became more mindful of performance, so I began to shape the text as performance. This performance turn led me to connect with drama and dance teachers at the University of Bedfordshire, inviting them to work with me on performance and to co-supervise my PhD students. Working with these inspiring women, I felt as if I had come in from the cold and found a home conducive to the nurturance of narrative.

In Chapter 5, I reflect deeper on narrative style from a feminist slant.

References

Agar M and Hobbs J (1982) Interpreting discourse: coherence and the analysis of ethnographic interviews. *Discourse Processes* 5:1–32.

Argyris C and Schön D (1974) *Theory in practice: increasing professional effectiveness.* Jossey-Bass, San Francisco.

Boykin A and Schoenhofer S (1991) Story as link between nursing practice, ontology, epistemology. *Image: Journal of Nursing Scholarship* 23:245–248.

Cixous H (1996) Sorties: out and out: attacks/ ways out/ forays. In: H Cixous and C Clément (eds.) *The newly born woman.* Tauris, London.

Clandinin D and Connelly F (2000) *Narrative inquiry: experience and story in qualitative research.* Jossey-Bass, San Francisco.

Compact Oxford English Dictionary (third edition) (2005) Oxford University Press, Oxford.

Dewey J (1933) *How we think.* JC Heath, Boston.

Fay B (1987) *Critical social science.* Polity Press, Cambridge.

Frank, A (2002) Relations of caring: demoralization and remoralization in the clinic. *International Journal of Human Caring* 6:13–19.

Gergen K and Gergen M (1986) Narrative form and the construction of psychological science. In: T Sarbin (ed.) *Narrative psychology: the storied nature of human conduct.* Praeger, New York.

Gergen K and Gergen M (1991) Toward reflexive methodologies. In: F Steier (ed.) *Research and reflexivity*. Sage Publications, London.

Giorgi A (1985) Phemenological psychology of learning and the verbal learning tradition. In: A Giorgi (ed.) *Phemenology and psychological research*. Duquesne University Press, Pittsburgh.

Kieffer C (1984) Citizen empowerment: a developmental perspective. *Prevention in Human Services* 84:9–36.

James P (2006) *Being and becoming an effective clinical leader*. Unpublished Master in Clinical Leadership dissertation. University of Bedfordshire.

Jarrett L (2009) *Being and becoming a nurse specialist in spasticity management*. Unpublished PhD thesis. City University, London.

Johns C (1998) Becoming a reflective practitioner through guided reflection. PhD thesis. The Open University, Milton Keynes.

Johns C (2002) *Guided reflection: advancing practice*. Blackwell Publishing, Oxford.

Johns C (2004) *Being mindful, easing suffering*. Jessica Kingsley Publishing, London.

Johns C (2006) *Engaging reflection in practice*. Blackwell Publishing, Oxford.

Johns C (2009) Reflection on my mother dying: a story of caring shame. *Journal of Holistic Nursing* 27:136–140.

Manjusvara (2005) *Writing your way*. Windhorse, Birmingham.

Mattingly (1994) The concept of therapeutic 'employment'. *Social Sciences and Medicine* 38:811–822.

Okri B (1997) *A way of being free*. Phoenix, London. Text extracts used with permission of The Marsh Agency Ltd.

Paget M (1983) Experience and knowledge. *Human Studies* 6:67–90.

Robinson J and Hawpe L (1986) Narrative thinking as a heuristic process. In: T Sarbin (ed.) *Narrative psychology: the storied nature of human conduct*. Praeger, New York, pp. 111–125.

Saunders A (2006) *Transforming self through transformational leadership*. Unpublished masters in clinical leadership dissertation. University of Bedfordshire.

Schuster JP (1994) Transforming your leadership style. *Association Management* 46:39–42.

Seo AY (2007) *Enso: Zen circles of enlightenment*. Weatherhill, Boston.

Spence DP (1982) *Narrative truth and historical truth: meaning and interpretation in psychoanalysis*. WW Norton & Co., New York.

Van Manen M (1990) *Researching lived experience*. State University of New York Press, New York.

Wheatley M and Kellner-Rogers M (1999) *A simpler way*. Berrett-Koehler Publishers, San Francisco.

Chapter 5

A feminist slant

Christopher Johns and Colleen Marlin

This chapter is in two parts. The first part is written by myself, extending the brief essay 'A feminist slant' included in the first edition. The second part is written by Colleen Marlin, responding to the challenge of writing from a woman's body – in terms of how she writes this piece rather than as an intellectual consideration.

Christopher Johns

Virginia Woolf, in her lecture 'A room of one's own', given at Girton College, Cambridge, in 1928, had been asked to speak about women and fiction. Woolf presented 'A room of one's own' as a metaphor for creating space to write a story; a space that had been foreclosed within a society that had not valued women in terms of the way women view the world. Indeed, the dominant stories of nursing tend to reflect the way medicine and organisation value nursing; stories of the nurse valiantly assisting the intrepid doctor in his [sic] technological battle against disease and death drama. As a way of viewing this dissonance of values, Virginia Woolf posited a dichotomy between the masculine and feminine. Woolf (1945:74) reflected the way women's fiction reflects social values as to what counts as significant:

> This is an important book, the critic assumes, because it deals with war. This is an insignificant book because it deals with the feelings of women in the drawing room. A scene in a battlefield is more important than a scene in a shop. ...

Woolf suggests that, throughout history, masculine values have tended to be viewed as more significant. The triumph of the masculine rational mind and reason over the female emotional body. By drawing a contemporary comparison, her words can be construed to reflect professional values and draw a distinction between *feminine* nursing values and *masculine* nursing values. So I can rewrite Woolf's words:

> This is an important book, the critic assumes, because it deals with the high technology of nursing practice. This is an insignificant book because it deals with the feelings of patients and families in the health care setting.

The challenge through story is not to de-emphasise the drama and technology of nursing practice *qua* medical practice, but to emphasise the exquisite nature of caring and the profound significance caring has on the lives of patients and families, and to value the mundane that takes place between women as if in the drawing room or as if a scene within a shop. So mundane that it can be so easily dismissed with the raging war all around to save lives. It is through story that the mundane and the profane can become sacred. It is through story that nurses can make visible, find meaning in, and value this quintessential essence of nursing. And as if to prove the point, it is rarely the high technology that practitioners reflect on. Yet a shadow dims the light to thwart this enterprise. Within the masculine dominated world, some practitioners aspire to have masculine values, whilst others do not assert their values of caring, their voices silenced under the weight of dominant values and the organisation of health care; whereby the dominant values attain priority, making little allowance for what might be construed as caring. Such tensions ripple through the narratives in this book. Tensions born out of the struggle to assert the feminine perspective within a masculine world – the most ironic and most significant contradiction that face nurses – the continual denial of self, the continual suppression of voice even within nursing itself. I felt strangely uncomfortable when I read – 'When a woman speaks to woman she should have something very unpleasant up her sleeve. Women are hard on women. Women dislike women.' (Woolf 1945:109)

But why should I feel strangely uncomfortable about this? That women purport to care for each other, yet fail? Indeed worse, project their frustration into each other – unable to project it into the 'masculine' of those who oppress. The sense of horizontal violence that spills over the top of the water-butt, that leaks along the seams of teamwork. Is it the desire to become masculine that women sacrifice each other and in doing so lose touch with their feminine and alienate themselves from who they are? Visions of caring spiralling down the plughole. It is this tension and struggle that sets up contradiction and plots the stories that nurses share. Stories that highlight the possibility of caring yet shipwrecked against the reef of masculinity. Woolf puts it like this:

> Everywhere and much more subtly the difference of values persist. The whole structure, therefore, of the early nineteenth century novel was raised, if one was a woman, by a mind which was slightly pulled from the straight, and made to alter its clear vision in deference to external authority … she had altered her values in deference to the opinion of others. … Moreover, a book is not made of sentences laid end to end, but of sentences built, if an image helps, into arcades and domes. And this shape too has been made by men of their own needs for their own uses. (1945:75–77)

Woolf suggests that the shape of narrative has been determined by man, built upon a masculine tradition of the way a narrative should be fashioned. As such women (nurses) struggle to find an adequate form to shape their stories because there is no tradition for doing this. When I first ask practitioners to write about an experience using 'I' they stumble, for it is often the first time they have tried to express 'I'. It is as if they try to position themselves outside their experience, to turn themselves into objects to gaze at. When they are enabled to focus on self, the self is often deprecated, diminished, reflecting the way these practitioners tend not to value their experience. And in not valuing their experiences they do not value themselves. In shrugging aside their values they alienate themselves from self as reflected in the struggle to know how to adequately express their experiences or stories.

In her lecture Woolf drew on the novel by Mary Carmichael, *Life's Adventure*, to reflect on the development of women's fiction from the early nineteenth-century pioneering work of Charlotte Brontë and Jane Austen, to contemporary twentieth-century work.

From the novel Woolf cites: 'Chloe liked Olivia … let's admit in the privacy of our own society that these things sometimes happen. Sometimes women like women' (1945:81).

Wolf urged her listeners not to blush and goes on to reflect – for if Chloe likes Olivia and Mary Carmichael knows how to express it, she will light a torch in that vast chamber where nobody has yet been. It is all half lights and profound shadows like those serpentine caves where one goes with a candle peering up and down, not knowing where one is stepping. And I read the book again, and read how Chloe watched Olivia put a jar on a shelf and say how it was time to go home to her children (Woolf 1945:83–84).

Knowing how to express it is the key to narrative, to light a torch in that vast chamber of practice where nobody has yet been. Each experience, each human to human encounter is unique. It has never been enacted before and yet readers will identify with the experience because they are familiar with the vast chamber where they have had similar experiences. The narrative is itself a torch to help the reader shine a light on self and these experiences, and written in such a way the reader can trigger and relate to her own experiences. To adequately do this the reader needs to be able to grasp the pattern of the writer's experience so she can interpret it in her own terms.

Woolfe (1945:104) notes the *pressure of dumbness* caused by the accumulation of unrecorded experience that denies voice to life's vital lessons. She demands that we reach below mundane events to explore the depths of our own hearts. She writes (p. 89):

> I said to Mary Carmichael, holding a torch firm in your hand. Above all, you must illumine your own soul with its profundities and its shallows, and its vanities and its generosities, and say what your beauty means to you or your plainness, and what is your relation to the ever-changing and turning world … of gloves and shoes and stuff swaying up and down among the faint scents that come through chemists' bottles down arcades of dress material over a floor of pseudo-marble.

The writer's pattern contains the threads of her own interpretation yet without imposing this meaning on the reader as the way the narrative should be read – 'how Chloe watched Olivia put the jar upon the shelf' – the profound buried within the mundane yet when watched, lifts it into immense significance, valued in its unfolding moment, a light across the reader's soul. The word profound is used by Woolf:

> One has a profound, if irrational instinct in favour of a theory that the union of man and woman makes for the greatest satisfaction. … And I went on amateurishly to sketch a plan of the soul so that in each of us two powers preside, one male and one female; and in the man's brain the man predominates over the woman, and in the woman's brain, the woman predominates over the man. The normal and comfortable state of being is that when the two live in harmony together, spiritually co-operating. … It is when this fusion takes place that the mind is fully fertilised and uses all of its facilities. (1945:96–97)

Of course what is profound is rarely rational within the unique human–human encounter of nursing practice. It follows from Woolf's reflection that texts written from a masculine-type brain fall upon the woman's deaf ears and vice versa. To this I would add blind eyes. Indeed all the senses are depressed and even denying the feminine's fundamental intuitive and empathic sense. Perhaps this is why so many nurses struggle with theory? They simply cannot relate to it, written as it is from this masculinity with such depressed senses clinging to an illusion that they need only be rational. It is not an appeal to reason that counts but an appeal to sensitivity. Women may need permission and empowerment to listen to their own senses and souls in order to listen to the sense and souls of others. The empathic sense that is vital to connect with and know the experience of the other (Belenky *et al.* 1986).

My fear is that women/nurses have been disempowered through being encouraged to listen with the ears of men denying the sensitivity of their senses. This may be difficult if such sensitivity has become crusted and buried along the edge of rationality where the description and significance of the everyday subtlety of the emotions may not be recognised or valued by nurses. Woolf writes:

> It is fatal for anyone who writes to think of their sex. It is fatal to be a man or woman pure and simple; one must be womanly-manly or man-womanly. It is fatal for a woman to lay the least stress on any grievance; to plead even with justice any cause; in any way to speak consciously as a woman. And fatal is no figure of speech; for anything written with that conscious bias is doomed to death. It ceases to be fertilised. Brilliant and effective, powerful and masterly, as it may appear for a day or two, it must wither at nightfall; it cannot grow in the mind of others Some collaboration has to take place in the mind between the woman and the man before the art of creation can be accomplished. Some marriage of opposites has to be consummated. (1945:102–103)

To return to the metaphor of *a room of one's own*, Woolf suggests the room will need a lock on the door. She throws down a challenge to nurses (and women everywhere) to throw of their cloaks that wrap their feminism and to synthesise the feminine with the masculine. A marriage of souls that finds its fullest expression. Perhaps before such marriage can be consummated to give rein to the feminine simply that the feminine can be known. As Woolf puts it:

> So long as you write what you wish to write that is all that matters; and whether it matters for ages or only for hours, nobody can say. But to sacrifice a hair of the head of your vision, a shade of its colour, in deference to some … professor with a measuring rod up his sleeve is the most abject treachery. (1945:105)

I am not certain that gender of the narrator is so significant. What seems more significant is the value given to ideas such as caring, and how can the subtlety of caring is expressed in ways that honour both what is done and who does it. Bella Madden (2001:25–26) wrote in her dissertation:

> In a simple way, my feminism finds expression in my dissatisfactions and frustrations as a practising midwife. This research is an exploration of those frustrations – teasing out the elements of constraint upon me to practise in ways congruent with my beliefs and ideals. I have already said that the writing of this project is its creation, but I am concerned that I find it so difficult to mould this dissertation into a compact, recognisable, academic piece of work. I search for the freedom to let it develop devoid of predetermined chapters and sections, finding it difficult to think in terms of self-contained, clearly demarcated issues and arguments. I tell myself this is laziness, that what results must be logical, progressive and complete: beginning, middle, end. I worry about assessment, and the need to gain accreditation. But Cixous (1996) challenges me to write my femininity, 'it is the whole that makes sense', and for a while I worry less about the format of the fragmentation. Cixous objects to what she sees as masculine writing, because it is cast in oppositions – it relies on reason and logic for its validity. She identifies women's writing as much more fluid, 'marking, scratching, scribbling, jotting down,' and argues that it is this flexibility that makes feminine writing potentially subversive and transformative. I am after all writing a story about myself here, surely that is not too

difficult? But I am ever worried about the validity of the exercise, how can I make this academic? How can I turn this into knowledge that is 'worth something'? Just as I seek the discourse of resistance in women's narratives, so I resist the patriarchal, rational discourse of academic writing at the same time as attempting to gain by it. How can I reconcile these tensions, or live with them?

Bella can feel the professor's measuring rod prodding her like some cattle prod. Cixous' work legitimises (as if the narrator needs permission) to write from the body, unwrapping self from a logocentrism and phallocentrism that has dominated everyday life, reflected through language. Cixous (1996:97) writes:

> Woman, writing herself, will go back to this body that has been more than confiscated, a body replaced with a disturbing stranger, sick or dead, who so often is a bad influence, the cause and location of inhibitions. By censoring the body, breath and speech are censored at the same time. To write – giving her back access to her own forces; that will return her goods, her pleasures, her organs, her immense bodily territories which have been kept under seal; it will tear her out of the superegoed, where the same position of guilt is always reserved for her. Write yourself: your body must make itself heard. Then the huge resources of the unconscious will burst out.

Deep breath. Vaporised trail that mark such journeys into the unknown. Yet such words are one thing, realising the feminine is quite another. How might this be known if the body has been confiscated? Do I, as a man, disadvantage women as narrators of their bodies? Important questions within a narrative tradition grounded in caring. MY answer – it cares not a joy whether I am man or woman. Being mindful of the tension, we can explore it and seek appropriate expression of the body as I do within my own narratives.

Woolf and Cixous help to balance the feminine and masculine perspectives, in particular to unwrap the more masculine perspectives that have dominated patterns of thinking and writing. Yet, as Mayeroff (1971) says of the nature of caring, it takes courage to step into the unknown. Only by stepping into the unknown with pen poised over paper, can the unknown be revealed. Cixous' words inspire the journey and give courage.

The real drama lies not in heroic acts but in the fabric of relationship, the transparency of my humanness, my vulnerability. Perhaps in an ironic way, such small moments of caring are the understated heroics. Living and dying of cancer *is* heroic. My narrative simply tries to illuminate that. In my experience these moments of caring are often invisible yet make a profound difference to the experience of being cared for and for practitioners who care. Narrative endeavours to capture caring in its wholeness characterised by discrete caring events, each caring moment unfolding into the next. Writing makes such moments visible and reveals their significance. To give an example (p. 213)

> Rachel visibly relaxes seeing Callum so still. She says, 'It's like magic.' I take her hand and say, 'It must seem like that.'
> We pause and still holding her hand I say, 'Your hands are dry.'
> She says 'They are always like that.'
> 'Let me massage them for you.'
> Her subdued smile radiates through the gloom.
> Holding her hand is an invitation to intimacy, a gateway to opening a healing space.
> Like a prop to ease the burden of her suffering.
> Like an olive branch of peace.

Such moments often pass unnoticed in the heroic din. Words come alive in ways that the reader can relate to; feel, engage with, engendering personal reflection and imagination in ways that theory or conventional texts fail to open up the mystery of human existence. Jeannette Winterson in her book *The Passion* (1987/2004:155) eloquently expresses this mystery:

> Words like passion and extasy [*sic*], we learn them but they stay flat on the page. Sometimes we try and turn them over, find out what's on the other side, and everyone has a story to tell ... We fear it. We fear passion and laugh at too much love and those we love too much. And still we long to feel.

Passion words to inspire passion: passion for my practice, passion for my writing, (com)passion for others. Can you love enough? Has the world become so sterile that we fear passion? If so, my narrative is a public exclamation that passion is vital that I want the reader to feel and *flow* with. The rewards are vast for those who come to live their passion.

Bella Madden (2001) further considers the moral positioning of women's voices within her narrative. She writes:

> Our lives are given continuity through narrative construction and reconstruction. Without the opportunity to consolidate and build our own narratives, women, particularly new mothers, literally run the risk of 'losing the plot' of their own life history. As clinical researchers, we have unique access to this interface between the public and private spheres of life, and therefore have a duty if we research it at all, to do so with respect and sensitivity. May and Fleming (1997) argue that there is a moral imperative within nursing research, that demands that we not only look at what is, but also at what ought to be, and that narratives offer such an opportunity, as they are reflections of both ourselves as practitioners and the occupation of nursing/midwifery in general.

De Francisco (1997) feels that to attempt liberating research, we must place the non-dominant group at the centre of our study, and we must force ourselves as researchers out of 'ethical objectivity', which only serves to deny the real affective aspects of our lives and oppression. Our methodology must think globally, that is, it must be rooted in ideas of social structure and the wider forces of society; but act locally by looking at what is happening within the smaller picture of peoples' lives. The point is to make acts of resistance visible, and facilitate their spread. In this way, the concept of power at a societal or interpersonal level is also a positive one – it is not inevitably about oppression. There are echoes of Fay's (1987) warning here as to the danger of replacing one dogma with another – De Francisco argues that we must move away from tendencies to over-generalise behaviour, as well as studying the power differentials between researcher and researched. This is very self-conscious research she is proposing, and it is interesting to note that other feminists see our modern task connected to that of reconstructing our sense of self and identity.

Weir (1995) sees the problem of self-identity as the capacity to sustain and resolve, often conflicting, identities, and that to do this we need high degrees of self-awareness and self-direction. However, the downside to this is that we are burdened by our own insights, as every act becomes one of self-definition, and every meaning problematic. This is balanced by the knowledge that we are, through the process of self-realisation, affecting our world and our place in it. We are awake to the buzz at the intersection of the individual and social forces, and feel the powers exerted on us, our acquiescence and resistance.

But nurses and midwives have traditionally been wary both of feminist thought (Doran and Cameron 1998) and reflexive research. Stereotypes of feminists abound, and are usually negative in the minds of many women. However, as De Francisco (1997) argues, when we stop concentrating on gender differences and look instead to the exercise and expression of power as both a negative and positive force, then our feminism takes a less dogmatic form than many expect.

> It brought buried things to light and made on wonder what need there had been to bury them.
> Woolf (1945:108)

The idea of a feminist slant intends to balance a more dominant masculine perspective that values the heroic, outcome and order more than the subtle and nebulous. The attention to the apparently mundane reveals the essence of care and the deepest insights. Belenky *et al.*'s study on developing woman's voice offers a way of viewing and synthesising the tension between the masculine and feminine within narrative. At the procedural level of developing voice they identified two types of knowing/voice – the connected and separate voices:

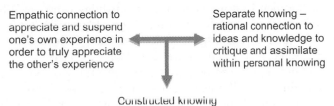

Both types of knowing are significant yet when synthesised within constructed knowing they enable the practitioner to fully utilise the whole mind. The connected 'voice' is the feminine or yin; hidden, dark sensed, intuitive, subjective, whereas the separate voice is masculine or yang; observed, light, rational, objective. As Wilber indicated (Chapter 1) the rational has dominated the intuitive and as such the feminine or yin side has been suppressed.

Colleen Marlin

Writing as woman

It starts with a train trip from Toronto to London, Ontario, Canada. I sit at Union Station, one of my city's oldest landmarks, awed by the beauty of the marble, the columns, the design. The monumental building stands tired, worn, but with its original majesty and intention still intact. I ponder the builders, appreciate the power of legacy, and wonder what it is I will be leaving my children after my time here is up.

As a young woman, I thought it would be books: lovely hard-covered things with my name prominent across its spine. But the publishing I've done has been minimal, accidental, even.

A friend posed the question, 'Why don't you publish more?', to which I had a rush of so many lines of parallel and paradoxical inner explanations, the music in my head morphed to jazz then dissonant noise. The same friend, sometime after the first question, asked, 'Do you write as woman?', and pushed me further with 'How do you know?'.

My reflection starts at the great hall of Union Station. I am here stupidly early in the morning, stupidly long before the train ride I've booked is departing. As woman, I've learned to be mindful of inevitabilities, taking into account all that could go wrong. I've spent decades scanning my environment for snags, dangers, and my earliness attests to my attempt to stay the unforeseen, run interference. I'm on my way to perform at a reflective practice conference two hours west, and in my solitude, in the early hours of morning in this ancient and magnificent building, my contemplation on my friend's questions begins.

At the other end of the great hall, I hear the electronic notes of a machine announcing '*gagne*', 'winner', in two languages, wonder whether those purchasing and cashing in lottery tickets on the edge of sunrise are male or female, and what pushed them to the kiosk so early. I've had years of consistently making the same wish on birthday candles, and knowing I couldn't speak my wish, or it wouldn't come true: to be happy. I kept silent on that solitary, solid wish for years, and still my silence didn't bring happiness any closer to me. And my quiet search for happiness and the roadblocks I've encountered in my pursuit of it have been foundational to why I write. I learned early that things are not as they seem, and that had me turning over logs and rocks, to see what wriggled there. What did the men I know wish on their birthday candles? What motivations do we share? Why have they not felt my compulsion to write? Why haven't the men I've shared space with filled dozens of notebooks with their pains and joys? How have mine paralleled theirs? What is distinctly mine, a woman's experience?

I lug my purse and books and bag and water into the women's washroom. Someone watching me wouldn't guess I'm leaving town for only over one night. I can barely turn around in the stall, with all the stuff I have crammed in there with me. In the relative privacy of my cubicle, I continue my wonderings, turn to read the graffiti on the walls enclosing me. The scratched entry to my right catches me.

'I'm in love with a boy who's too scared to love me too.'
'Then he doesn't.'

The rebuttal etched by another's hand.

As I walk past the men's washroom, I wonder what's written in the stalls there, and have a sense that the entries won't match the ones my sisters have documented. Many years ago, I took a writing course from Isabelle Huggan, a creative writer living in France and teaching in Canada. I lamented to her that all my poems, stories, novellas and scripts seemed to be written about relationship. Her answer: 'What else is there?' I suspect for men there is something more, or at the very least, something else, but for me, matters of the heart pull, haunt, fascinate. That's where I venture, in my alone time.

I moved houses relatively recently. When exhaustion hit, I stopped unpacking for a while, and when the task resumed several months later, I surprised myself with the contents of a couple of boxes I'd lost track of. One spilled forth old love letters, in my hand, returned to me by my ex-husband, with his laden retort, 'This is how you used to feel about me.' Another had cards and letters and photos from lovers past, memories unearthed loosening a torrent of tears. I sobbed, reading of friends, men, sentiments I'd held passionately, now somewhat forgotten, or more to the point in the case of some, trying to be forgotten. I wondered, with the quantity and intensity of the communication received, what it was I must have penned in their direction. I was too emotional to read anything but fleeting words from the tight script in the Hilroy notebooks, full of heartache in my young woman's printing. My handwritten printing is larger now, my comments more bold, but still, the majority of writing I do reaches no ears, eyes, hearts beyond my own, still deals with matters of swollen hearts, mine and others'. Contemplations on love continue to consume my imagination.

My swift flip through the archives of my disappointing past reveal reams of material related to the topic of love. I ponder at its opposite. Not hate, perhaps indifference, or something verging on fear, and it freezes my heart altogether.

And so on this dark spring morning, arms achy with the awkwardness of my bags, I set them down, stare at the word 'Men' on this other washroom door, and wonder more deeply what's scrawled on the walls of the men's washroom, wonder how it's turned out for the young woman who's shared my stall, and experience with love and lack of love.

I make my way to stand in line behind the grizzled man with a tired, stickered guitar case. I'm curious what music he chooses to sing, I feel he sings the blues. I write them. I rarely share them.

Something in the ageing musician's countenance is reminiscent of my ex-husband, perhaps what appears to be self-containment. Many incidents contributed to the demise of my marriage, its final death knoll inspired by our distinct responses to a Tom Stoppard play, *The Real Thing*. In the summer before our parting, my then husband and I attended a Granville Island theatre to see a production that got us talking about love, monogamy and the pursuit of individual pleasure. We didn't see eye to eye.

I realise, inching my way forward in the line of passengers heading to London, that Stoppard's words were the catalyst for our first real talk about our attitude to love, 15 years after we'd been together. It strikes me as an odd thing not to have talked about earlier in our sharing of time. Close to the end of our marriage, the particulars of my unhappiness found their way into a highly autobiographical story my husband found accidentally in our shared office. The state of our marriage got discussed through discourse about the characters in the story, at a safer distance than talking about ourselves, I suppose. My ex wanted me to rewrite the character of the male to make him more sympathetic. I wanted him to see the plight of the female character. Writing had been dangerous. Writing my pain through the heartache of my protagonist had us face-to-face talking of our own dysfunction, discord, irreparable disappointment.

The two young women in line behind me talk excitedly, apparently second guessing the words and actions of a man one of them is trying to have some kind of relationship with. I doubt he knows he is the object of so much discussion, and doubt if she is aware that so much of her creative energy is spent trying to create a relationship that doesn't pain her. I wonder if the young woman keeps a journal, and writes her heart out, as I have done and do. I suspect the reason I write is because of all the speaking I felt I couldn't do, and all I needed to say. I push my red bag forward with the press of my functional red shoe.

I'm the second girl in a family of three, the youngest a male, a match for my Leo father in both sun sign and size of character. I knew at five, hearing the thrill in my father's voice announcing the arrival of my sibling, 'A boy!' – that I, as female, was somehow a disappointment from birth. The males in our house, father and son, were outgoing, gregarious, storytellers, charmers. The other two females, both Cancers, were gifted as nurturers, the hospitable, capable ones, offering audience and sustenance. I think back to what I learned in technical class while studying broadcasting at university. I caught on swiftly. The male plug is pronged, out there, obvious, its phallus looking for something to penetrate, the 'doer' or hero. The female plug doesn't protrude; instead, it's receptive; it receives. I knew my role as woman; it was both modelled and taught, though it didn't come naturally. In a household with two women so suited to both 'receiving' and giving, there was me, my gifts not so functional. Being the second female, and a different kind of daughter, I didn't catch on to cooking or cleaning, or feeling good about only listening to the conversations going on around me. I wanted a more active role than nurturer or audience. I wanted to act, and to 'do', too.

I had the nosey qualities that can make for a good writer, and cause a lot of grief. I eavesdropped, wondered, asked. I sat under tables and behind closed doors, listening hard, in hopes a secret would fall or fly to me. I pretended to sleep from the back seat of our family car, while my ears extended to draw in the conversation of my parents. I knew from very young that in order to learn more, I had to be very still and silent, to have them think I wasn't listening, so the adults would speak their secrets within my earshot. I heard things I shouldn't have heard. I knew of suicides, brutal car accidents, pregnancies outside of marriage, mental illness. I knew of money troubles. I knew of cancer. I knew my uncle died in a transport accident in thick fog, his truck crashing in to a rolled truck fallen over in the centre of the road, and exploding, flames consuming everything on impact. 'All that was left was his belt buckle.' I knew his wife had declined his invitation to join him on that particular trip. I knew my uncle's death caused my father to cry, not something I'd witnessed before. I knew that, from eavesdropping and watching. And I watched closely. What was going on there? What did that gesture mean, that shift in facial expression, that reaction to what was said?

The young woman in line behind me becomes quite agitated. There's that perennial frustration … 'Why doesn't he get it?' I turn to steal a glance at her, her face the shape of a moon, smooth, yet already, the lines between the brows beginning to form. I've seen that, the furrows on my female friends' faces, the hurt and confusion etched deep in ageing foreheads. The young woman interests me: her end of the conversation, her youth, her pleas spoken to a female friend, not the male she's wanting something else from.

I'm affected by her. I imagine I'll remember something of this moment on some future day. Without my being conscious of the 'what' of it, something of this scene will catch and take hold in me: how her frustration makes two parallel lines on her forehead, how her shoe is worn down more on one foot than the other, how she fingers and twists a silver band on her thumb, how a bit of hair attaches itself to the hint of moisture on the inside edge of her lip. Some of the particulars of this woman, this scene, will enter me, and will embed themselves in the porous cubicles of my undiscerning memory tissue. Sometime future, for no apparent reason, I'll have a flash of an image from this particular moment in time, as if caught in a painting. And this flash will cause me to think back on this young woman, and all the splendid, concerning, concrete details of witnessing and eavesdropping on her conversation on this singular day waiting in this particular line for a train in Toronto. I'll review the scene, and it will shift, no longer so much a painting, stilled and inanimate, but more a moving picture, vibrating with life and possibility, energetic. No doubt I'll be hit by it, wondering what that scene holds in way of truths, if I scratch there for a while, and follow the liquid lines taking shape before me. What will be revealed to me, if I pen the scene, and see what emerges? If I remember, I'll wonder about why I've remembered what I have. I'll wonder what it means. What is secret, invisible, stirs the story, until, like an image in a dark room's vat of magic chemicals, something comes into being, now visible, now meaningful.

I'm aware on my wait for the train, that the setting here, the people in this scene, hold something of interest for me: the man in front of me, serene and solitary, the young woman behind, agitated and full of longing, the contrast between the two. And so it has been with my experience of writing. Something catches me, I call it a cause for pause, and my glance lingers there, my mind turns, my heart engages, and I wonder, either in the moment, or when the image reappears for contemplation.

I've been interested in story from young, listening to it, and imagining it. I spent hours as a child engaged with department store catalogues, not picking out clothes to order, our household finances wouldn't allow for that, but instead, picking up threads of story, inventing lives for the models whose faces I saw repeated page after page. I could learn something, through the stories told to me, and I could also discover my own truths, through the stories I made for myself. I've brought along Virginia Woolf's thin and poignant text *A room of one's own* on my voyage. She spots the fundamental quality of fiction that manages to survive, and names as significant the notion of integrity. 'What one means by integrity, in the case of the novelist, is the conviction that he gives one that this is the truth. Yes, one feels, I should never have thought that this could be so; I have never known people behaving like that. But you have convinced me that so it is, so it happens.' (Woolf 1989:72)

There are moments, scenes, that won't let me go, sit pulling at me for possibly decades before I have the courage or need to step there. As a child of seven or so, sitting silently on the other side of a closed door, small ear pressed to the wood, I heard that my father, a good man as I knew him, a humble construction worker, was responsible for the death of another man. I heard my father's voice tighten in his whispered conversation over tea with my mother. I learned that the bucket of my father's crane had swung around and knocked down a man who shouldn't have been at that place on the job site, that my father jumped from his crane and ran to the man's side, that my father bent to him to ask what he could do, that the coffee truck came in at that moment alerting the men of its presence with its characteristic bell, that the dying man requested a cup of coffee, that my father sprang to get him the coffee, that before my father ran back with the weak coffee, the man died. I knew that I could not tell my parents I knew any of this, for it was a secret, something unspoken, that I should not have heard. I knew I one day would need to write of this, and so far, this 'knowing' has remained silent fodder in me. I've stepped close to the heart of the story, with a postcard story called 'Caffeine', but this version stays safe, compared with the story I continue to sit on.

Caffeine

My da's a bit of a tightrope walker, surefooted as a coon approaching dinner. He walks steel beams, joining struts of downtown high rises. He's sure, of foot and ability.

'No building I've worked on is ever going to fall,' he said, watching over and over the slow tumble of the tower of New York City. My mother refused to watch the news with us. She just kept swiping madly at the kitchen counter, the way she does when he goes on about stuff she doesn't like to hear, her head turned away from where we were sitting.

My da's muscles are like the steroid users I've seen in my brother's wrestling magazines. He can lift the pair of us, one under each arm, and spin us until we want to puke, and he's not even panting.

Since moving to the city, he takes us to each new job site, tells us what the building's going to look like, how many stories, what they'll use it for. He takes photos of us against the backdrop of his latest project. You can barely see us against the massive girders behind.

We know the dangers; he's told us that, too, though Mom shushes him. A fall from the third storey, there's a chance of survival. A fall from the fourth, you'll be looking into the light.

'Aren't you afraid?' I ask him often, partially because I think he likes to answer that, and partially because I like to hear his answer.

'No need to be afraid.'

'But aren't you afraid of heights?

'No need of that. Don't look down, and you don't know how high you are.'

My Uncle Clay works with Da, only he is afraid.

'Jesus Christy, kids, drop a penny from your pocket up there, and the steel underneath ya trembles like a trampoline after a high jump.'

Mom shushes Uncle Clay too.

Then there's this day. A wicked wind churns up from the lake, out of nowhere, unless you can read the sky the way my da and Uncle Clay can.

'Best be getting ourselves down.' They begin the process, cautious as can be, doing what they know to do, so said Da after.

Only this time Da says Uncle Clay looks down, for just a second.

'I've always told him, don't. You just don't. Can't.' Something happens, and gravity gives a mighty haul on Uncle Clay and yanks him to the sidewalk at the foot of the building they are so especially proud of.

He falls from the third storey, I'm guessing. And whatever it is in place to save him, doesn't.

My da is flying down the stairs, flights of stair, to the ground, crouching there beside his brother, and asking, pleading, 'Clay, what can I do? What can I do?' Just then, the coffee truck comes by, rings its bell.

'Get me a coffee, would ya?' my uncle says.

My father does, but Uncle Clay dies before the coffee has a chance to get cold. My da's quit the coffee, says it's not good for his adrenaline.

This 'knowing', and other tight holdings of secrets, and the eventual, inevitable unearthing and blurting of secrets, the need to speak, hurdle me sooner or later into creating story.

I pat my pocket for my train ticket, take a sip of water, watch in the distance, two women embrace, a long embrace. I doubt that straight men would embrace in this way. I'm curious about the relationship between these two. I know these women have a story that would interest me. I wonder about it, wonder where it overlaps with my own.

There is a wonderful Canadian anthology of 34 reflective pieces written by women, collected in *Dropped threads: what we aren't told*. As its editor, Marjorie Anderson, notes in her thought-provoking foreword, the authors, in choosing what to write about,

identified gaps in their communal talk and named life-altering surprises in their individual lives. Most spoke of serious issues, of surprise bruisings or blessings, private moments of intense connection or bewilderment ... to identify the areas of surprise and silence in their lives ... more than one respondent commented on the courage it would take to write on personal issues that had long been beyond the limits of acceptable expression. A few women identified experiences which they could not write on because the pain was too new or the fear of judgment still too strong ... Others approach distinctly personal moments with caution and then veer away, as though the walls around the silences they've been keeping are impenetrable'

They tell us that once life slows down enough for reflection, women uncover truths several beats away from the expected and the promised. (Anderson and Shields 2001:viii, ix)

As a young woman, I rarely, barely allowed myself space for deep reflection. My various roles and my approach to them called for my time and attention. I hadn't yet learned about being a 'good enough' student, friend, employee, wife, mother. Margaret Atwood, one of Canada's more prolific and innovative writers, understands the dilemma I faced and shared with other women with a predisposition towards writing. 'Any woman who began writing when I did, and managed to continue, did so by ignoring, as a writer, all her socialization about pleasing other people by being nice, and every theory then available about how she wrote or ought to write. The alternative was silence' (Atwood

2001:139). Early, I fell into the trap of thinking I needed to earn and win the love and attention of others in order to grow my own self-esteem, and in so doing, set myself up for sharing characteristics of both stress-prone personality types, types A and E, the driven one, and the one who does everything for everybody, else. I learned to be super-woman. I knew the drill. Like Atwood, I knew:

> Women are socialized to please, to assuage pain, give blood till they drop, to conciliate, to be selfless, to be helpful, to be Jesus Christ since men have given up on that role, to be perfect, and that load of luggage is still with us. This kind of insatiability is particularly damaging for women writers, who, like other writers, need private space and as women, have a hard time getting any, and who are called by inner voices that may not coincide with the strictures of prevailing policy-formulators. (Atwood 2001: 144)

Atwood understands Woolf's premise no doubt, has lived it. I look up at the clock. We'll be boarding soon. I'm eager to return to the words of Virginia Woolf. I believe Woolf would understand what my approach to writing has been – haphazard at best, what's propelled me to write – the pains of my own experience and what I've witnessed of others', what's kept me from publishing what was written – a mix of 'Who do I think I am?' and 'Don't say that', not that or that.

I couldn't grant myself the time or focus to write seriously, but still I kept my journals, and in them, documented moments that wouldn't please others to read about. My journals didn't involve much contemplation or mindfulness. I didn't intend them to matter. Instead, they were the valve on the pressure cooker of my life, the safe way to let off little blasts of steam, whatever sudden hits of emotion I could no longer lid and contain. When I look at the stories I have managed to write and share, I know their beginnings came from bursts of scene and emotion scribbled in my journals. I share Margaret Shaw-MacKinnon's sentiment of what can come, through expressions in solitude. 'So often in women's lives, our thoughts fall like seeds into the rich loam of privacy. It is here that they blossom, exotic hybrids never to be viewed by the public eye. And yet, it is in these private musings that we can potentially find the quick of our personal, countercultural truths' (Shaw-MacKinnon 2001:221).

My journal has been an incubator for the wild seeds I have collected in my pockets and scattered on white blank pages. I appreciate Woolf's impression of how fiction comes to be. 'What were the conditions in which women lived, I asked myself; for fiction, imaginative work that is, is not dropped like a pebble upon the ground, as science may be; fiction is like a spider's web, attached ever so lightly perhaps, but still attached to life by all four corners.' (Woolf 1989: 41)

I find this a compelling image. Whatever tales I weave spin from a real place. And so often, the fiction I have a powerful response to has its roots deep into the author's unique life and perceptions. Tillie Olsen, in her powerful, highly autobiographical short story *I stand here ironing*, has her narrator unravelling a stream of consciousness monologue while standing at an ironing board and contemplating, with no shortage of guilt, why her first-born is so troubled. My heart somersaulted with the hit of the words, the narrator hoping upon hope for her daughter to know she has greater significance to the mother than the inanimate dress the mother so diligently presses. I want my own two to know this as well. The domestic and professional tasks that can so consume me don't matter to me as they do. They are much more than any of that.

Now that my children have their own adult lives and roles, reflection is something I allow myself, time is more my own, and the truths of un-mined memory leap and lunge at me. I allow myself the time for contemplation. My journalling today allows space for insights and analysis about the spills and blurts of thoughts and emotions. I'm part of two writers' groups ... one, a group of women who gather the first Saturday each month to write spontaneously on topics gently, lovingly tossed into the centre of the circle, what was written to be read back, without criticism; the other, a mixed group bent on constructive criticism, who read and re-read one another's work in advance of meeting, then gather, intent on offering astute and detailed feedback on how the work can be improved. In the latter group, I've been reprimanded for writing things my fellow writers can't believe. Regularly, they buy my fiction as truth, and resist what I've written that most closely represents what I've actually lived. 'That wouldn't happen,' they say. 'But it did,' I say. And I recognise the veracity of author Anna Quindlen's words I heard quoted at a workshop on self-reflection: 'Facts sometimes need fiction to be told truly.'

I recently wrote a story about a woman in labour, wondering at her husband's temporary but lengthy absence from the delivery room, wondering if he had returned the short distance to the family home to sleep with her best friend, there keeping vigil over their first born while the protagonist laboured. My group didn't believe my tale, yet I know what thoughts distracted me as my belly convulsed agonisingly with the approach of our second child. I know what I was wondering during my husband's absence. I also know it's quite possible he just left to make phone calls, to check on our daughter as he said he was about to do, to arrange things for his anticipated absence from his work day. I know he may have been gone only a short time, too short to realistically be engaged in what I'd wondered about, yet still I know I wondered.

Things not remembered
I remember the pain. Sharp. Unnecessarily unbearable, surely. Telling myself 'You're not going to die ... you thought that last time, you didn't ... buck up, buck up, f ...!' Looking over my shoulder to locate my husband, his green eyes barely catching mine, before looking away, patting his clumsy paw on my quaking shoulder. His breath on my ear, a whisper, 'I'm just going to check on ...' Our first born, asleep in his bed, our friend pulled from hers to come and watch him. Then upside down faces of nurses, noticing my doctor wasn't yet there. Time passing. Their saying, 'Not yet, don't push yet,' and my really wanting to. The purple dot, somehow seen from inside my own forehead. Quiet washing over me. Body splitting in two. Bottom half writhing, pulsing with life eager to see light. Upper body stilled. Serene. Attention focused on that purple circle, mesmerised, a kid of inner hum, a bee inside a flower's heart. Mirror being adjusted. Flash of rumpled green. Familiar smiling eyes of my doctor. Awareness of my husband's hand again on my shoulder. The smell of soap. Wicked yank of pain. No breath. Then new baby's breath exhaled in a cry, already alert to the world's cruelty.
I don't remember how long he was gone. Don't know if it was long enough to go the short distance home, undo his pants, do his thing, zip himself up again.
I don't remember if I even want to know.

Recently, another story sprang from me, a woman gone a bit mad, temporarily, at the incessant photographic images of a broad mouthed, smiling woman promoting herself on political placards stuck in neighbours' lawns, the smiler being the former lover of her love. 'Wouldn't happen.' 'But it did.'

Sprayed
I don't really know what got into me. She hadn't done anything personally, not really. But there she was, Mary Veinot, face bigger than the moon, airbrushed and smiling forcibly from political

posters on study sticks stuck into neighbours' pristine lawns. The Liberals had me surrounded. I've got nothing against them. Some friends are Liberals, not that they've been by lately. Guess I've been a little sad. Another break-up. Nothing like that to have the scaredy cats scurry. They've been through this with me before, granted; it's never pretty. I can carry on. Perhaps I do cry more vehemently than seems necessary, but heh, it takes what it takes. I read that in a self-help book.

It had something to do with Ms. Veinot's smile in that doctored photo, that look of 'I've got something you want,' or 'I'm getting something you're not'. She sports more than the standard allotment of teeth, more than most have the DNA to produce. She could do damage with that wide mouth of hers. And I knew where it had been. I knew plenty about Mary.

Hers was a signature giving authorisation for elevators to ride up and down, and carry a prescribed maximum number each trip. That's the kind of power she's had. And now, her cunning lips turned up at me, she wanted more.

She's had her way with Maurice, my ex. She'd grabbed him, literally, at a fund-raiser wine and cheese that maybe could have done with more cheese and a little less wine, at least in Mary's glass. Maurice, impressed by her forwardness, jumped her, fast and frequently, over a twisted summer of gluttonous fore, during, and after play. Seems she had a thing for shoes, accessories and elevators. I wish he hadn't told me that. To be honest, I had asked.

Guess I'd had too many repetitions of Mary's mouth on the walk between the Canadian Tire and home. Walking is supposed to be good for you. My therapist suggested more of it, but maybe not such a good idea this day. I'm not big on smug, yet there, ... Mary, Mary, another Mary, reminding me of her importance, that she was worthy of my vote, reminding me of my own failed relationship. The spray paint was destined to camouflage the decay of my backyard furniture. 'Be constructive, re-create your world.' My therapist thought artistic expression would do me good. Rather suddenly, and without premeditation, trust me, I blasted several swirls of Night-star Silver on Mary signs. The therapist's suggestion was a good one; I did feel better.

I'm not keen on a man in a uniform. The visiting official didn't think marring Mary's face had been such an inspired idea. He wanted an explanation, looked puzzled when it was revealed Maurice wasn't even my most recent ex, and Mary happened long before he and I had our time. 'Why?' The officer pressed.

My recent ex liked Mary's face, her big, wide, open mouth. He would have jumped her, too.

'She's got more than her share of teeth,' I said, as good an answer as any.

My writing group didn't think I'd ever have the opportunity to look at my ex's face on political signs on lawns to the left or right of me. I had. They didn't believe a sex scene I'd lived, didn't buy what had gone on at a nude beach in Vancouver, didn't accept my description of a bathroom door hacked at by firefighters in their attempt to save my friend, his wrists spilling red into his wife's white tub.

A Toronto writer and musician, Paul Quarrington, in giving instruction to aspiring writers one Saturday winter's morning at Humber College in Toronto, advised them to write about the things in their lives they don't want to admit, the 'thing that bothers you the most'. I believe my strongest work has that at its heart, yet that very fact is what has kept so many of my manuscripts in my file cabinet drawers, and so many concept, unexpressed, still contained in me. It's a rebellious act to wave in others' faces one's own dirty laundry.

I read a poem at Humbers' School for Writers, a brave act, considering the narrator confessed my own wants and fears.

> Careful
> 'Be careful what you wish for'
> I've been told more than once

That doesn't stop me
From wanting what I don't have

I wanted her beauty

I ask too many questions of boyfriends
I knew where his ex worked
I knew
She had huge round breasts
And wore tight low cut topes
To show them off
To win better tips
To have the men licking
Wing juice from their fingers
Wishing to lick her
I knew he'd been jealous
At a work Christmas party
When she openly flirted with
The admiring, hard-cocked males
Desperate for a taste of her
Knew it was hard for him
Knowing she had liked the thought
Of all those men wanting her

I wanted to be wanted like that

I knew where she lived
I saw her outside her house one day
Waiting for the bus
Traffic-stopping beauty
And my heart lurched
As I saw first hand
What kind of beauty makes a man
Unable to forget
What he's had
What he wants still

I knew where he wet
That less-than-perfect new years
While I was puking
Wishing he was there to hold my hair out of the way
To hold my hand
To hold my gaze
But he answered her call
Came in sheepish at five in the morning
Scared to see me awake and waiting for him
Unhappy I quizzed him on where and why
Less surprised that I was hurt
That he'd gone to her
Pumped her full of himself
Let his large hands get tangled in her mess
Of long thick black dream hair

He found it hard to shake his want of her
I, my image of them

And he went away
Resisted her appeals
She'd had another child
No doubt wanted him to raise his one
As he had done with the one before

And with time
I stopped thinking of it
Followed a new man
Who took me to the very bar where she was known
Lusted after
And this new man
Spoke of her beauty
Ad I wondered why again
Through another man's eyes
I had to see her again
And I felt badly
At the sight of
My own thin hair
My modest breasts
My cellulite

And then this other woman
Who knows I know
About the woman men want
Been intimate with men
Who have left large tips
Gone home with big fantasies
She tells me
About the woman I wanted to be
About the third baby
About her not having a place to live
About her going down with her baby
Into the valley
With the other homeless
And setting up a kind of camp
Not a kind enough camp
To keep away the cold
And how it got her
Bit her leg off
And now

This woman of great beauty
With her baby
Without her mind
Without one of her long beautiful legs
Is more than little down on her luck

I doubt that my ex will go back to lay with her again

And I am in my home
Owned
Warm
Looking out on thick white snow
Not frightened for my life

My hands rest
On both my legs
I will attempt to be
More careful
With what I wish for

I'm not proud of my jealousy, my wish for that kind of head-turning beauty. It's hard to look at myself this way. It's hard to be this kind of honest.

Martha Brooks, in her essay 'One woman's experience with the ecstatic', writes, 'Memory is the force that links all life. It makes us pay attention even when it is painful to do so, marking us in way that can sometimes leave us mute or howling' (Brooks 2001:206). Sad memories of secrets not shared have silenced me, then so needed expression, as to be messily, organically released. Sometimes the words multiply in my journal. Sometimes, what presses to be told finds its way into fictionalised story, where it nervously grows without expectation of an audience, where sometimes it even fears what would happen if the story were to be read. Then the story stops itself. So many of my stories have stopped themselves. 'Go fearwards. Go where the energy is' is the mantra of the writing teacher Barbara Turner-Vesselago. Fear can stop me.

The most vocal of the women behind me in line is on her cell phone, her voice exasperated. I wonder if she has called the man she's been preoccupied by. I wonder what he's said. The musician in front of me inches his luggage forward. I echo his moves, slide my bags ahead two feet. I check my watch. It's close to time.

In my early thirties, one of Toronto's dailies published a short story of mine, 'My favorite uncle', based on a pivotal moment in my preteen life, when an uncle on a hot summer's night, a storm brewing, came upon me in my makeshift bed on a sofa in the far off, lonely corner of the house, his words apparently intended as comfort against the storm, 'Don't be afraid of the thunder', the heat of his breath and hands with their exploration, terrifying. I can remember only to a point that night, remember the fear I'd become pregnant, being too young to yet know the mechanics of how that happened; however, his inappropriateness, and my not knowing all that happened, has haunted me since, sent me to therapy. To this day, I have an ambivalent relationship to potato chips, the token he offered me the next morning, either as a gesture of 'thanks' or a bribe to 'keep quiet'.

I'd sat on that story for over two decades, and only felt the irrepressible need to write it when my own girl child grew. The fear of not telling my tale was now greater than the fear of telling it. I needed to do something to stop the cycle, to keep my own daughter protected from the likes of my sick uncle. When the story was published, my sister called, to offer a thin compliment … 'It is believable.' She, too, had been approached by this uncle, only she had the benefit of three further years of living and the capable, confident attitude of the first born. She'd told him to take a hike. She reported that our mother, upon reading my story, had said, 'It wasn't that bad,' my own mother having been touched by the same man, at the same age, yet making a limiting judgement on my experience. She'd dropped a few words about her preteen night, but her truth was revealed less through her off-handed reference to a night she passed off as inconsequential, and more through her adult woman's avoidance of my uncle, her brother-in-law, her body language wary and keeping a distance. At so many events, I'd watched her watching him, keeping her back to the wall, never turned on him.

Sharon Butala, in her essay 'Seeing', writes, 'I think of my mother, who knew so much she never said, but whose wisdom darkened and deepened her eyes as she gazed at me'

(2001: 218). There are so many women whose eyes have seen more than they are willing to share. A woman working at the college where I teach read my story, whispered, 'It happened to me, too.' She then confessed that she, at sixty-five, hadn't ever told anyone until my story nudged her to share her truth with me.

The story was published while I, as a newly divorced adult, was on a camping trip with my parents and children. I watched my father while he sat in the driver's seat of his immobile mobile home, silently reading the fictionalised version of my harrowing, irreversible moment in time. He put down the paper, left the camper, and never spoke of my story or the incident that prompted its writing. He remained friends with my uncle.

When I received word that my story won the contest I'd entered and was to be published, the first adult person in my path was my ex-husband, come to pick up our children. I greeted him with the welcome news. Then I had also been met with silence. I wondered if there was a conspiracy among men. And I knew the women of my family were embarrassed by my forwardness in speaking the unspeakable. The year after the *Toronto Star* published that story, my mother asked nervously, 'Are you entering the contest this year?' I took it that she'd prefer if I didn't. I relate to Lorna Crozier's (2001) description of family in her essay 'What stays in the family.' My parents' beliefs, values and behaviours were rural, small-town. I learned early to bite my tongue and stay silent about any dirty little secrets – no one else needed to know. And I learned I was to lid my resultant pain and sadness, or better yet, try to forget the secret and accompanying emotion ever existed.

Some time when I was a young-married, my mother happened on a collection of poems I'd written called 'Down home', based on childhood memories of times on my grandparents' dairy farms. On our overnights at the Marlin's, I slept with my elderly grandmother, Verlie, who each night peed in a chamber pot under our shared bed. The stench sickened me, the sound disturbed me, the brilliant colour in the china basin the next morning repulsed me. The experience had a memorable effect on my senses. I had ignored a big lesson of my upbringing by choosing language to express that, and other lived moments on the farm. I grew up in a family where it was modelled and made perfectly clear what could be talked about, and the bad stuff wasn't on the song sheet. 'We were told: If you can't say something nice, don't say anything at all' (Atwood 2001:135). My mother's reaction to my poetry was adamant, judgemental. 'That's not very nice.' My reply to her was one of frustration: 'You've raised me to be "nice". That's why I need to write.' 'Collyanna', as many have called me, needed to express her shadow side as well as the good. My writing embarrassed my family. I could only persist when feeling bold, or being in a zone where I could forget, for a moment, the family creed.

I watch, as people getting off a train are greeted by those who have come so early to fetch them: the open arms, the waiting greeters who rush forward, the ones who hang back. The words exchanged and the silences. Several people ahead, one woman with short, cropped hair offers another a drink from her water bottle, a nice, loving gesture. The second woman drinks. Do men share water bottles? I've had more than one ex tell me they won't share beds with other men, even when sleeping arrangements are tight. They'd rather sleep on a bare cottage floor than climb into a big bed with another sleeping male, even if he is a close friend. Perhaps wondering about this will one day prompt story.

Several years back, I wrote a play called 'Nice', a comic and highly autobiographical piece about a young woman who was ill-treated by men, mainly because of her seeming inability to say 'No'. Its inception was prompted by something as simple as my doctor at the time asking me advice about love. I'd been intrigued with that reversal of roles: the healer asking the patient for wisdom. I remember my horror on opening night, to see a bluish-white haired octogenarian take the seat in front of me, front row. I thought ahead to all the bawdy bits, the racy, off-colour, rude and risky things I'd written, about to be delivered by the actors on stage. I was hellishly nervous at what would be the old woman's judgement and dismissal. I was hugely relieved and surprised when she laughed uproariously at what I'd intended as funny. I knew it was dangerous to write what I'd lived, because as my mother observed, it 'wasn't very nice'. I had a scare more recently, to see the woman who had been my doctor and inspiration for the play in the very theatre where the play was performed. Was she there years before, for my play? Would she have recognised herself, in my comic reinvention of her? It takes courage not only to write, but to publish and produce. I've had this dilemma – speak my truth and risk being alienated by those who share my gender and those who don't, or make light of my experience and seek to incite laughter not serious contemplation.

Margaret Atwood hit on this in her essay, 'If you can't say anything nice, don't say anything at all': 'The double bind: if women said nice things, they were being female, therefore weak, and therefore bad writers. If they didn't say nice things they weren't proper women. Much better not to say anything at all' (Atwood 2001:139). And so the judgements sent me, as Atwood predicted, into bouts of silence, until the containment of secrets and memories again filled me to bursting, blasting, and blurting. Much of what I've written jumped from me first in unconscious 'leaks', things expressed, despite myself.

The man in front of me shoulders his guitar case, lifts his computer case, and shows his ticket to the VIA Rail employee. I show mine. Once on the train, I choose a window seat, facing the direction we're headed. As is my habit, I want to see what is happening outside my window. I press my face to the glass, and let images play on me. Remembering the purpose of this voyage, I retrieve and open the folder of poems I will be reading at the conference, but instead, return my gaze to the grey urban morning. My own city looks different from train tracks than roadways. A young woman the age of my own child chooses the seat beside me, stretches out, falls asleep. I suddenly have low-grade anxiety, recognising now the 'what if's' … what if she's hung over, what if I need the washroom, want to get up to stretch my legs? Know I won't want to disturb her. I'm amused at my own absurdity. I'm aware that it's this line of inquiry, my child's mind toying with the 'what if's' that gives me something to write about. I'm also aware that it's the 'what if's' that have stilled my pen, and silenced me. What if's have kept my writing in drawers. What if I embarrass those I love? So it went when I was a young guest accompanying my parents to their friends' apartment for dinner. I was tossed paper and pencil to keep me entertained while the adults enjoyed pre-dinner talk. I drew like a mad thing, and proudly showed my artwork to the assembled. 'This is my mom. Naked.' Even though my child's hand's life-drawing was primitive, generic, not recognisably my mother, this image did embarrass her. I knew in creating the picture, I had done something wrong. I knew to still my pencil. I stopped drawing for over a decade.

And so why haven't I published more? Alice Walker, author of the much respected novel *The Colour Purple*, in her essay, 'Beauty: when the other dancer is the self', confessed to being nervous when an article was about to be published about her and her work, that her people, family, would find out her books were 'scandalous'.

When I forget myself and dare to write, I write about things that would embarrass my mother. And while I've been inspired by what if's in terms of seeing the possibility of story, I've also been distracted and stopped by them. As a daughter, then a wife, then a mother, I was conditioned to be watchful, vigilant, attentive, to anticipate and think about consequence. I was raised to scan my environment, to attend to, nurture, protect.

I was raised to have a sharpened awareness of lurking dangers, of what needed doing in the moment.

The train whistle sounds as we approach a crossing. I twist to see washed clothes dancing on the line, all the clothes dark in colour. The young woman beside me turns softly in her slumber. True to form, I hope my movement hasn't disturbed her. And what I've been thinking flies away from me for a moment. So many important epiphanies have evaporated or scampered off, with the jolt of demands near to me.

I relate to Betty Jane Wylie's (2001) observations in her essay 'The imaginary woman'. I know the role of woman has been focused on raising the babies and making the home, taking care of people and place, all the while grounded, steady, unruffled. We've needed to be mindful, watchful, anticipating what needs our attention, and ready to deal on a moment to moment basis with whatever comes our way. We're to solve, soldier on. It's been the rare bold or lucky woman who could afford to stop and stare at the sky, to contemplate the abstractions of life. We've been busy taking care of immediate demands, and that's the polar opposite to the luxuriating in concepts that precedes the creation of art.

Atwood thinks that a large motivation for women to read writing by other women isn't just to learn about craft; our interest in our sisters' work was 'in something much more basic: we were curious about the lives of these women. How had they managed it? We knew about the problems; we wanted to know if there were solutions. For instance, could you be a woman writer and happily married, with children, as well? It did not seem likely. (Emily Dickinson, recluse. George Eliot, childless. The Brontës, dead early. Jane Austen, spinster. Christina Rosetti, her wormholes, her shroud.)' (Atwood 2001:137)

Watching the passing backyards, I consider my lifelong quest for happiness. Perhaps as one drawn to write, it wasn't my destiny. Virginia Woolf speculates:

> That woman, then, who was born with a gift of poetry in the sixteenth century, was an unhappy woman, a woman at strife against herself. All the conditions of her life, all her own instincts, were hostile to the state of mind which is needed to set free whatever is in the brain. (Woolf 1989:51)

I know the conflict between an ache to express and explore, and a hyperawareness about the wants and needs of those I care about. Two and a half decades ago, after a party my husband and I attended, I was surprised when he was headed for home, forgetting our children were at the babysitter's and needed picking up. I wondered at the liberty in being able to forget for an evening, the whereabouts of his children. My children have been amazed at how I could spot them blocks off, when they should have been at school, but instead, were taking their freedom; amazed at how hearing young strangers on a bus name the address of a house Halloween party they were bedecked to attend, had me somehow knowing my own child would be there too; how the squeal of tyres outside our closed front door would have me leaping up, pulling the door wide open, knowing that screech somehow had to do with one of my offspring. My instincts are strong, in matters affecting my children.

Before motherhood, as a young creator, I'd had fantasies of writing a novel. Why not? I had ideas, energy, previous expanses of time dedicated to running and catching up with my own imagination. Even a month before the birth of my daughter, I had the idea I would write splendid prose after her birth, while my young one slept, played, entertained herself. I had seriously overestimated a child's capacity for sleep and self-sufficiency, and underestimated the number and degree of essential responsibilities requiring my attention and energy. Outside of motherhood, I had no idea about the depth of a new mother's fatigue. From inside of it, writing morphed from a real possibility to a vague and nagging wish: what I would do, once everything else was done. At my annual physical sometime after the birth of my second child, I complained of being tired, deeply, wearingly tired, tired beyond belief, tired beyond hope of recuperation. The doctor, also a family friend, said 'Colleen, you've complained of being tired since Eva was born.' He wasn't wrong. I remember when my son was a few weeks old, standing with him in my arms in the dark in the middle of a sleepless night, and looking through his window at the hospital where he'd be born, but a block away. I wanted to secret him back into the nursery, just for one small night, to have the nurses attend to him along with the newborns, while I slept without worry. Since becoming a mother, my sleeps had been less restful, a consequence of a mother's vigilance, keeping an ear open to the nocturnal needs of my children. It's safe to say that once I became a mother, I was more than a little distracted. The realities and demands of motherhood burst the bubble on my novel writing fantasy. I had to find another way to feed my hunger for self-expression. Certainly my children's prominence in my world influenced not only what I chose to write about, but also how I wrote and what I wrote. The reality of motherhood nudged me in the direction of supreme realism: I didn't have the time or energy or attention to develop something as time-consuming or complicated as a novel: long, uninterrupted spans of time were just not available. I found my way to the short story. I needed to write smaller pieces that I could stick to for a short period of time. I wrote in bursts and spurts, with the kind of urgency that comes with necessity. There was pleasure in that, grabbing a stolen moment from my complicated life to visit the life of an imagined character.

Like so many women, I started writing furiously, clandestinely, in stolen moments. I snatched titbits of time while the children were sleeping or away visiting, while dinner was cooking and laundry was spinning. I spoke story aloud while driving, partially an attempt to entertain the two tempted to fight in the back seat of our car, partially to help me keep my sanity by giving me a chance to continue to generate story, however short. I have countless postcard stories, and beginnings to longer pieces. I have filing cabinet drawers full of pieces begun, but not finished, as the calls of motherhood pulled me back to the there and then. But they were started, and even just beginning a story, that mattered to me.

Inventing story does interest me. I've been creating story before I could write. My father would frequently attempt to bond with a new suitor by bringing out the 'She's so weird' tales. Amongst the nuggets was the standby: 'When Colleen was little, you'd walk by the room she was playing in, and hear a whole mess of different voices coming from there. You'd think there were a dozen kids in with her … and there she was, playing all by herself.'

Do I write because there weren't children my age on our street to play with? Do I write because I needed to make imaginary friends for myself? Do I write because I'm confused, and writing brings me explanations? As a college professor, I've often sent my students to read Joan Didion's (1993) essay 'Why I write'. I wanted my students to appreciate what I had learned through my own motivation to write: I write in order to reveal to myself, my thoughts, my observations, my desires, my fears. Discoveries come.

This habit of mine to invent, to step into the lives of imagined people, got me in trouble with my family. So much of my experience was rejected with their automatic response: 'That didn't happen. You made it up.' And how it sends story scrambling, scattering, to have it accused of fabrication, my story and my history, apparently figments of my over-zealous imagination.

My parents didn't believe my impression that another uncle's uncle was, in fact, mean, didn't like children, was worthy of my fear. My parents didn't believe I had heard of a woman who, somewhere close to my grandparents, ran naked under the summer's sky behind high walls, in an attempt to have the sun heal the boils and other skin ailments plaguing her. My parents didn't believe my uncle had done something 'that bad', didn't believe that my marriage was worth leaving when my husband 'hadn't beat me and was a good provider'.

Even with the soft sleeping breath of the woman beside me, I feel liberated, being on this train. This freedom echoes that I've experienced on the ferry rides to and from Vancouver and Nanaimo on Vancouver Island. When my children were small, I saw so few rented movies from start to finish. To this day, I far prefer to go out to the movies, where the pull of my life's demands can't find me. And so it is on this train. There is nothing for me to do, other than not disturb the sleeping woman at my side, watch the passing scenery, the scenes in the train with me, and the scenes playing from my own memory bank. There isn't anything for me to resist doing, in order to take time to reflect and imagine.

And so I look out the window to my right, at the lush landscape. I like seeing life from the backyards. This view matches with my own writing process. Backyards contain what is ordinarily hidden from view. Backyards contain the organic mess of life. Backyards have the secrets. At one crossing, there is a flap of yellow caution tape, the kind used by police to show where the public is not welcome. Years ago, when I complained to my therapist that it was hard to write with my children at home, he gave me some metres of police tape, suggesting I put it across the portal to my bedroom which doubled as my writing chamber, to alert them they were not welcome at that time, that I was busy, that they would have to fend for themselves for awhile. Yellow plastic tape with black letters: 'Caution – do not cross'.

I pull '*A room of one's own*' from my bag, wanting to read more of Woolf's reflections on women writing … and not writing. This somehow feels good preparation for the reflective practice conference I am barrelling towards.

I'd heard the title of Woolf's book as a young woman, thought I knew Woolf's premise. I'd spent the years since my divorce being hard on myself. There's nothing like self-flagellation to scare away concepts and language. After my marriage ended, I had a room of my own, yet still couldn't produce pieces ready for publishing. I wondered what my problem was. In reading Woolf's text, I know now, it's not just the space, but also independent money, and even more powerful for me, a certain freedom, since 'freedom and fullness of expression are of the essence of the art' (Woolf 1989:77).

Like so many women, from necessity, I wrote with a kind of feverish desperation. Tiny stories flew out of me, fast, ridiculously fast. Giving writing a larger space in my life would have felt irresponsible and self-indulgent. In my filing cabinet, I have ten novellas, written one a year for ten years running, each on a Labour Day weekend when my children would be away and happily occupied with their dad for three days, and I could claim the time as a writing marathon without guilt. Writing short pieces in one sitting, without any concern my children would need me, worked better than the yellow tape, 'Caution. Do not cross'. The therapist was male, gay, childless. His suggestion as a concept was brilliant. I, female, single, a mother, couldn't make practical use of it. Instead of its being a beneficial strategy, it became a family joke.

The train picks up speed. A couple across the way order tea from the man in uniform. I'd like tea as well, but know if I do, I will be disturbing my neighbour's slumber. I take another sip of water, and turn again to the window. A gold cupola sits on top of an ornate church in a reserved Ontario town, looking like a gold dipped Dairy Queen ice cream cone. The grass, this May, is neon green from extensive rains, yet there and there and there, parched patches, dry, golden, burnt – incongruous. From its backyard, I see a mansion, now housing funeral proceedings. I wonder why it is that small town Ontario funeral homes occupy the best architecture. I'm intrigued with this view of the world, the view that isn't normally seen, the backyard view, ordinarily hidden from others. The backyards aren't the place of pretence. The backyards let me in on secrets. I see two dogs in a muddy field, one, shiny black, asleep, the other, golden and long haired, keeping vigil. I wonder which, if either, is female. I see an ancient tree, fallen, uprooted, lodged in the river, changing the course of the water. I see a house trailer parked at such a steep angle. I know there'd be no comfortable, horizontal sleep possible on any of its beds. I see a split in the earth, a giant slice into a ravine, an easy place to tumble. I think of the film *Thelma and Louise*, and their flight in the convertible off a cliff's edge, choosing certain death rather than risking capture. I discontentedly ponder why so many women found the film empowering instead of depressing. And how is it that the skinniest, sloppiest of fences separate rambling backyards from the railway tracks we're flying on? I fear for the grand-children I imagine visiting their elders in these old houses, fear their curiosity will take them to the far end of the lawn, fear they'll push through the hole in the fence, to play tag on the tracks in our path. I'm a woman who turns when I hear a child in a grocery store call 'Mom'. My heart lurches when I see a stranger trip on the sidewalk. My skin vibrates with near-misses of people I don't even know.

The woman beside me crosses her left ankle over her right. This I notice. I notice and I notice and I notice. And noticing is what causes me to write. And noticing is what causes me to stay silent.

The rivers and streams are brown with the mud of spring run-off. I recognise that often stories come to me only after the waters have risen so high, they overshoot the banks, and all hell breaks loose. I get, absolutely, how the present is coloured by the past, how the muck I've lived adds grainy texture to the muck I'm in. And so it is for my sisters.

Once again, I open the folder on my lap. Within its covers, eight poems for me to know intimately, in preparation for the conference, written by me from the perspective of eight different self-harm patients admitted to an emergency department in England under one nurse's care. How did these poems get written? What do I know of self-harm?

When I was very young, my cousins had an aunt who was the most beautiful woman I'd seen to date. Unlike my pale hair and eyes, her hair was dark and rich, her eyes the colour of chocolate or garden earth at night. She wore a red velvet dress to her wedding, or perhaps I made that up. Perhaps it was to her funeral. She, when 11 or so in 1953, was selected as Ontario's representative to board a train travelling from the west coast to the east coast, picking up one special girl child per province, to go across the big water and attend the Queen's coronation. A few years back, these girls-now-women gathered, to celebrate the fiftieth anniversary of their shared honour. All were in attendance, save the beautiful woman I'd looked up to. None knew the reason for my cousins' aunt's absence. Suicide. After her marriage. After the birth of her first child in wedlock. Long after she'd given an illegitimate child up for adoption. 'Post-partum,' my mother shared when I'd asked her, as an adult, why she had turned her husband's hunting rifle on herself. Sometimes the answers I get to my questions have too few words to be of much use. Another friend of my parents and role model in my childhood, Edith, told me when I was eight she had to get a second copy of a gospel record another cousin sang on, *The revelations*. She'd worn out the first copy. I'd never known anyone to wear out a record, couldn't guess how many times she'd played it. She told me when my mother was out of the room that God was calling to her. That he needed her. Shortly after, she set fire to herself in her husband's workshop. As a young woman, but long after it happened, longer after it had been a safely guarded secret, I learned accidentally that a dear cousin had tried to take his own young life. His size alone saved him. A smaller man would have been poisoned beyond resuscitation with the amount of intense pharmaceuticals he'd spilled in his system.

Over a decade ago, my best friend Susan invited me to her and her second husband's home in the country. She wanted to write a screenplay with me, inspired by the drama and humour of her life's story, centred on women gathering in a hot tub. I drove out to her farm house with my pad of blank paper, my suitcase, my eagerness. My kids were at their dad's. Her child was with his. We had the concept. We had writing experience. We had love of language. We had rich and tumultuous lives to draw from. We had the place to ourselves. We had in a big supply of coffee, evaporated milk, and frozen pizzas. We had her hot tub to sit in while brainstorming where to take the tale. I stayed for three days. Nothing got written. Cigarettes got smoked, ashtrays emptied, dishes washed, dogs and cats and birds fed, phone calls answered and made, pain shared, floors swept, photos pointed to, stories begun, and stories begun, and stories begun, but Susan's distractedness, the demands of her present and perhaps fear of what would be encountered to enter story deeply, had her doing something else the whole time I was there. Honest writing is somehow an act of rebellion. It would be risky. Despite my having overnighted there innumerable times before, that stay was the first I'd seen Susan appear at the breakfast table without her make up on. I had wanted to cry, it was so poignant, seeing her paper-ish white, pocked face, open and vulnerable and exposed like that. Susan had a scar on her hand that looked to me like a peace sign. In few words one day she revealed the mar had been the consequence of the lit end of a cigarette pressed on her one hand, by the other, self-inflicted. She didn't eat much during the visit intended as our writing retreat, but had the coffee pot in action all day and night long. She drank black coffee in a mug, then Pepsi then coffee then Pepsi … black liquid … hot and flat, cold and bubbled … white mugs full of black liquid. Unbearably hungry, I made myself a sandwich. While it was raised to my mouth, Susan took my plate away to wash it. I thought back to a painting I longed to own, one by a northern Ontario artist, where a woman intent on her task is out putting up her laundry against a black sky, as the storm waters circle and rise, threateningly, around her waist. Images I can't shake push me to write.

Susan killed herself shortly after that visit. She, former on-air TV news reporter, college teacher of Film Noir, wife of a news cameraman, woke from their marital bed, tiptoed through the dark house, climbed up on her roof, and suspended herself from the television antennae, the source of her and her husband's livelihood, and the source of her disappointments. She dangled there by a rope until her husband woke, looked through the house for her, went outside and stomped the acreage searching for her, then looked up. She hadn't managed to write her screenplay. She had left in longhand a series of instructions for her husband to carry out, after her death. Susan inspired one of the ten novellas, *Strays*. In its writing, an imagined history appeared for the Susan-like character inspired by my dear friend. It gave me a jolt, wondering if my fiction was in fact, the real story of her life. Had I inadvertently, through fiction, stumbled on the truth of Susan's unspoken past? Ask the questions, and answers come, though not always ones easy to face.

There is my friend whose fingers are chewed by the cruel workings of her own teeth. When we brunch, I can tell how anxious she's been in her week, by the rippings and scabs. The young daughter of another friend who, suffering post-traumatic stress, has kept away nightmarish images by cutting herself awake. The student who wrote a suicide note on the back of her final exam for my course. The other students who have cried in my office, vibrating with too much pain to want to stick here. The woman who lost her only child to a strange disease in the schoolyard one lunch hour, and now desperately wanted to leave the world to join with her daughter: 'She needs me.' There is my close friend who knows it's a miracle of science and medications that she is still here, with all she's contemplated over her decades of darkness. There's the memory of my having stood too close to the edge at the subway station, wondering how it would be to pick a moment and leap to the tracks, not a suicidal thought exactly, but certainly a thought borne of familiarity with severe sadness, as I would call it then, depression, as I know it now. I write, because of what I don't know, and what I need to know.

There's been much in my particular life that's caught my attention, the world glimpsed from the corner of my eye. So much has turned my head, and urged me to wonder, ask the 'What ifs'. Margaret Atwood gets that it is an act of courage to say the unsaid:

> Those who pledge their first loyalties to isms often hate and fear artists and their perverse loyalty to their art, because art is uncontrollable and has a habit of exploring the shadow side, the unspoken, the unthought. From the point of view of those who want a neatly ordered universe, writers are messy and undependable. They often see life as complex and mysterious, with ironies and loose ends, not as a tidy system of goodies and baddies usefully labeled ... Plato excluded poets from the ideal republic. Modern dictators shoot them. (Atwood 2001:143)

It's no wonder my parents preferred me not to write, not to call attention to myself. What I choose to write, or what chooses me, isn't always pretty. Writing is a bit of an archaeological dig. I put the shovel in the earth, without knowing what the spade will turn up. My messing about with memories, imaginings, concepts and language has had unpredictable finds along the way. But as I age, containment of what I have to say is less possible, less desirable.

The whistle blasts again. The backyards are more closely spaced. We're on the edge of London, Ontario. I've lost time, as happens when I contemplate. The young woman beside me sits up, yawns, rubs at her eyes, and looks past me, out the window. The sun hides today; the moon is a few days past full.

Art is the great leveller. Art making is universal. There is no culture that doesn't engage in making art. Yet I know, writing for me is not what writing is for others.

Why do I write? I suspect it's because in my household of gifted male storytellers, I learned to appreciate story, learned its arc and shape from what I heard, but as female, didn't have space to speak. The men's voices filled the rooms. I suspect it's because I was a weird little kid who got sun burnt and car sick and with no kids my age on the street, preferred to stay indoors, to save pain and loneliness. And in my alone time, I got used to invention in order to entertain myself and understand others. I suspect it's because I have always been keen to know more, to learn, and that motivated an insatiable curiosity. I was nosey. I paid attention. I clued in to some things, with the information I had available. And I was left to imagine what I didn't know, and that was plenty. I write because I catch movement out of the corner of my eye, and I want to know what goes there. I'll shine a light there, see what's hiding just beyond view, in the shadows. My eyes adjust to the darkness after I'm there for awhile, and then, I can see more. Virginia Woolf appreciates that if a strong writer 'knows how to express it she will light a torch in that vast chamber where nobody has yet been. It is all half lights and profound shadows like those serpentine caves where one goes with a candle peering up and down, not knowing where one is stepping.' (1989:84) When I write, I do not always know where I am stepping.

Why don't I publish more? As Virginia Woolf knows, 'interruptions there will always be' (1989:78). For years, my not publishing related to shortage of time and my own inability to name writing and editing as worthy priorities. It seemed not to have a function as significant as what I'd been conditioned to put first. Now, my not taking more work further relates to fear. I have no wish to embarrass my mother. I've learned I'm not to call undue attention to myself. And I need to feel strong, have all my ducks in a row to suspend self-criticism, and trust the process.

Do I write as woman? That question has me wondering if I write as a Canadian. A few years back, a friend with a successful photo archive business offered a placement position to a student from France hoping to learn the ropes. In her stay in Canada, Veronique did lots with the group I spend time with. I laughed, thinking she'd return home to France with a misunderstanding about Canadians if she took us somehow to be representative of our nation. My personal quirks, my idiosyncrasies contribute to the particular woman I am and the specific writing I do. A few years back, I was in an ancient-for-Canada movie theatre, seeing a French film, *Amélie*. I found it charming, amusing, quirky. I was there with my French boyfriend. Prior to choosing our seats, I bumped into my ex, Fred, the man in my life before the French man. I laughed uproariously through the film. Alain, beside me, remained silent. Seven rows down and five seats over, Fred's gales of laughter bubbled up simpatico with mine. Ours were the only belly laughs in the whole place. We, alone, found the same moments funny. There weren't other female voices expressing amusement. I often attend film with two of my closest female friends. One laughs when I do. The other is unmoved by what I find hilarious. I have lived long enough to appreciate that my reactions are idiosyncratically mine alone.

My experience is not synonymous with that of all other women. I have had a particular life. I am the middle child, and second girl, in a family of three. I was afraid of being pushed down the wishing well next door, afraid of the shadowy neighbour to the south. I skipped grade four and was forced to leave my first best friend behind. I had a bold and gorgeous and adventuresome penpal who lived in Illinois, USA. My skin was pale, my eyesight bad, I would practise walking through my house with my eyes shut to prepare myself against future blindness, my athletic abilities, nil, my curiosity, large. I was molested by my favourite uncle. I knew about things often kept a comfortable distance from children. I married young. I divorced young. I've had over a dozen significant relationships since, with writers and actors and drug dealers and a chef and educators. I've suffered chronic fatigue and fibromyalgia. I've lost my niece, my dad, four close friends to death – numerous others to change of circumstance or difference and indifference of opinion. I've been affected by what I've lived, what I've lost, what I've wanted, and that informs what I choose to write about.

I write as woman, because I am interested in the subtle and the unspoken, what goes on in the backyards. I write what the moon sees, not from the perspective of the sun. But to be more clear, I write as 'a' woman, 'this' woman, not all women. Yet what I see through these blue-grey eyes, what I feel from this pulsing heart, what I express through my muddled thoughts, can be understood by others, men and women alike. Literature's great gift enables us to go from the particular to the general, one woman's story to a more universal story.

The train slows and stops. Fellow travellers are already standing in the aisle, bag in hand, ready to descend. The woman beside me isn't getting off in London. I have to climb over her to exit. I drag my luggage in the direction of the women's washroom. These cubicles are pristine, no messages written here.

I think about love and happiness, and want of both, as I get in a taxi. I feel a hit my heart, and know I will soon be writing of a woman reading graffiti in a train station washroom. I think about Virginia Woolf and wonder if freer at 55, I am now ready 'to use writing as an art, and not as a method of self-expression.' (1989:79–80) Whatever is ahead for me, I know, like Alice Walker and so many others who have pushed past fear to create, I have used writing to heal, used writing to 'write myself into the light'.

References

Anderson M and Shields C (2001) *Dropped threads: what we aren't told*. Vintage Canada, Toronto. Text extracts reprinted with permission of the author.

Atwood M (2001) If you can't say something nice, don't say anything at all. In: *Dropped threads: what we aren't told*. Vintage Canada, Toronto. Text extracts reprinted with permission from the author.

Belenky M, Clinchy B, Goldberger N and Tarule J (1986) *Women's ways of knowing: the development of self, voice and mind*. Basic Books, New York.

Brooks M (2001) One woman's experience with the ecstatic. In: *Dropped threads: what we aren't told*. Vintage Canada, Toronto. Text extracts reprinted with permission from the author.

Butala S (2001) Seeing. In: *Dropped threads: what we aren't told*. Vintage Canada, Toronto. Text extracts used with permission of the author.

Cixous H (1996) Sorties: out and out: attacks/ways out/forays. In: H Cixous and C Clément (eds.) *The newly born woman*. Tauris, London.

Crozier L (2001) What stays in the family. In: *Dropped threads: what we aren't told*. Vintage Canada, Toronto.

De Francisco V (1997) Gender, power and practice: or putting your money (and your research) where your mouth is. In R Wodak (ed.) *Gender and discourse*. Sage, California.

Didion J (1993) Why I write. In: *In depth: essayists for our time* (second edition). Compiled by CH Klaus, C Anderson and RB Faery. Harcourt Brace, Fort Worth, TX, p. 173.

Doran F and Cameron C (1998) Hearing nurse's voices through reflection in women's studies. *Nurse Education Today* 18:64–71.

Fay B (1987) *Critical social science*. Polity Press, Cambridge.

Madden B (2001) *Working with women following traumatic child birth*. MSc dissertation, University of Luton, Luton.

May C and Fleming C (1997) The professional imagination: narrative and symbolic boundaries between medicine and nursing. *Journal of Advanced Nursing* 25:1094–1100.

Mayeroff M (1971) *On caring*. Harper, New York.

Olsen T (2001) I stand here ironing. In: C Shrodes, H Finestone and MF Shugrue (eds.) *The conscious reader* (eighth edition). Longman Press, Needham Heights, Massachusetts, pp. 180–186.

Shaw-MacKinnon M (2001) Birth, death, and the Eleusinian mysteries. In: *Dropped threads: what we aren't told*. Vintage Canada, Toronto.

Walker A (2001) Beauty: when the other dancer is the self. In: C Shrodes, H Finestone and M Shugrue (eds.) *The conscious reader* (eighth edition). Longman Press, Needham Heights, Massachusetts, pp. 28–34.

Weir A (1995) Toward a model of self-identity: Habermas and Kristeva. In: J Meehan (ed.) *Feminists read Habermas: gendering the subject of discourse*. Routledge, London.

Winterson J (1987/2004) *The passion*. Vantage Books, London.

Woolf V (1945) *A room of one's own*. Penguin Books, London. Text extracts reprinted with permission from The Society of Authors as the Literary Representative of the Estate of Virginia Woolf (UK).

Woolf V (1989) *A room of one's own*. Harcourt Brace, Orlando. Excerpts from A Room of One's Own by Virginia Woolf, copyright © 1929 by Houghton Mifflin Harcourt Publishing Company and renewed 1957 by Leonard Woolf, reprinted by permission of the publisher (US).

Wylie BJ (2001) The imaginary woman. In: *Dropped threads: what we aren't told*. Vintage Canada, Toronto.

Chapter 6
Awakenings

Aileen Joiner and Christopher Johns

Aileen Joiner is a psychiatric nurse. Her narrative unfolds the 'reality shock' of reflection as she came to confront and work towards resolving the forces that diminished her. It is a powerful drama that reveals the way intelligent nurses can become disempowered within health care systems. Aileen's narrative is constructed from the three assignments she wrote while undertaking the English National Board for Nursing, Health Visiting and Midwifery (ENB) course A29 course – 'Becoming a reflective and effective practitioner'. This four-module course is offered (at level 3) within a BA in Health Care Studies degree for post-registered health care practitioners. On this course, students work in small guided reflection groups (maximum eight) to reflexively learn through their stories of everyday practice that they bring to the group. Aileen was guided by myself and by Cheryl Watson, my colleague at the then University of Luton, who worked with me as co-supervisor on this course. The students' first assignment asks them to write up a reflection they have shared within their guided reflection group. The second assignment asks them to construct a personal theory of reflection. For their third assignment they construct a reflexive account of personal development around an area of practice. Each assignment has been designed to plot the practitioner's development through the course. This narrative has been pieced together and edited by Christopher Johns from the first and third assignments I wrote during the course.

My first assignment

People live in a crisis that ripples across their beings, rippling below the surface of conscious thought. Such crises can be observed by paying attention to the signs, yet most people live in a state of partial visibility as if wrapped up in themselves perhaps to keep self from exploding. Reflection is a trigger to release this tension.

Johns and Freshwater (1998) state that reflection 'gives us wings to soar as we emerge from our cocoons' (p. x). I certainly feel that I am at the stage of wanting to burst from my own cocoon and I want to use my fledgling attempts to ensure that I do soar professionally and personally. Reflection is the personal opportunity for me to look through my own window, which Johns (1998) describes as 'a window to look inside, to know who I am as I strive towards understanding and realising the meaning of desirable work in my everyday practice' (p. 9). This definition seems useful to me as it provides the image of a personal space … . I am beginning to associate reflection with personal time out …

permission to break from 'performing' in order to consider the 'performance' and the need to plan future 'performances'.

I have always kept a diary and have been encouraged to reflect in my journal through the course. Much of the course is delivered in small guided reflection groups. After our first session I wrote in my journal:

> I sat in a room full of strangers stating I had left nursing in the '70s because I didn't like it. With that came the realisation that after all the studying, all the work, I still felt the same way! It washed over me, a strange experience, a flooding sensation from foot to finer tips. Physical but deeply emotional. I tried to explain in a later session of clinical supervision with my ward manager ... 'but you're good nurse Aileen, very professional, everyone says so, etc.' ... Yes, but is the professionalism the armour I use to keep self together through a multitude of experiences I find exhausting, stressful, distasteful and frustrating. Nursing is far from my expectation, my personal practice is not what I want, it is confined by so many limitations. All my idealism forced to the recesses of my mind, never perhaps to be realised. To change the face of something so massive at what cost to myself? At what worth to others? Chris Johns has spoken of people being marginalised. I have always have the capacity to marginalise myself, never good at conforming to satisfy others. What am I doing? Onwards with studying. Why? Will this provide some key to unlock disappointment, or will it be a balm to bring about acceptance of what is, and where I'm at? Reflection so far seems to raise more questions, but can I answer some? I am unable to separate myself from my practice. So much of nursing is personal, the professional may separate the personal side, but the personal fragility provides much of the human touch. There is not much opportunity to personalise the rigid practices of the ward routine. Much verbal encouragement is given, but little happens. The routine continues, the relentless routine. Probably there is safety in the routine, and a workforce of long serving nursing assistants who pride themselves on maintaining the routine, continue the past and reduce the future; although I work with people who would reshape what we do. I need to reshape what I do, because it swallows me like a whale. This all seems negative, but I feel more positive in expressing my doubts. I am aware of my feelings within myself daily. I am always aware of my impact individually, I am not complacent about the issues that affect my feelings about my job, but maybe I am worn down ...'

It seems to me that this piece of reflection has enabled a much needed cathartic therapy for myself. Heron (1975) felt catharsis enabled the dissolving of scars from emotional vulnerability. Valentine (1995) said that nurses, and women were nurturing, caring, loving kinds of people – the antithesis of confrontation. This does not allow for the integration of assertiveness as a personal trait. I believe that many women like myself are skilled at being assertive, but consciously choose to use alternative traits to deal with certain issues, to reduce exposure of vulnerability. By this I mean I can reflect on several ways of dealing with my dislike of my current situation, but know that I will not act alone, or completely independently choosing just for myself, since the consequences affect far more people than myself. Bendelow (1983) found that by avoiding conflict it was turned inwards and experienced as stress, a feeling I relate to, knowing stress and frustration are constantly with me at work.

My reflective account shows a lack of energy throughout. Peers (from the group) described feelings of sadness, hopelessness and profoundness. I reveal some of myself and my conflict within to weigh what I would like to change personally against the reality of what I work with daily.

I felt that this group of people saw me then as helpless and hopeless. Yet this is wrong! People who know me well would laugh at that suggestion. Yet honesty causes me to acknowledge my restrictive upbringing, strong on conforming (though I do not always do this), doing what is right, not challenging, with little meaningful communication. All this leads me to feel I have long fought to be different and yet fundamentally remain the same.

Graham (1998, cited in Johns and Freshwater (1998)) talks about a sense of humanness and personal identity belonging to the patient. I would argue that the nurse too, has that right of personal identity, especially during reflection and essentially during practice. Social groups (such as our reflective group) are very important in maintaining a sense of humanness. I think this ties in well with the fragility I talked about. I know I am fragile; that makes me sensitive to myself and others. Humanness allows us to remember that fragility is part of being human.

My second assignment

It occurs to me that at the point of narrating my journal I had viewed my professional manner as armour to hold myself together, but with reflection I review my original feelings and now wonder if this was also a valuable tool to prove to others my sense of capability, sense of responsibility etc. With the unfolding of my reflection, I can begin to see how my own notes illuminate and transmit meaning to theory. My personal learning curve is increased as I start to see beyond myself and understand, liberating the tight reign on my emotions.

On reflection, clearly I am incongruent in my beliefs and have been guilty of holding back, to my own cost, to my own cost. Although I hold strong beliefs related to equality of opportunity, personal rights, etc., I have been confused by the complex world of the struggling nurse where there is no automatic right and I lost sight in my attempts to be submissive, in order to conform and be accepted. This perception I now feel, is distorted and I struggle to make sense of my feelings.

Miller (1977) cited in Oakley (1984) identified characteristics that develop from belonging to a dominant or subordinate group which helps me underpin my difficulty in changing my situation, while nurses continue in the subordinate group of submissiveness, and the culture in my own environment is managed, based on submissiveness and ever coping!

My recent experience would have been less stressful had I been myself from the onset and unafraid, but I was brought up to practise self-sacrifice – 'You can't always have what you want …', and I have transferred my upbringing to my career, fearing I could not make wrong right and I should sacrifice my own values to be employed. There is now within me a recognition to change. I have highlighted fundamental problems and surfaced my tension. I can see how important my need I to bring to the surface the underlying value systems from my past which are valued as crucial importance to change. Johns was so right (1998) about being unable to cleanse ourselves from our histories.

Even within my own reflective group where I am the junior grade listening to others' reflections, I am reminded that I am merely an 'E' grade! Especially when I listen to reflections by others that highlight attempts for managerial grades to rule over others with patriarchal supremacy. I do believe Newman (1994) when she says that 'who people are' can be read as a pattern rippling across the surface of their being, and just as I read my own ripple (guided by my supervisor), I can read those patterns in my group and I vary in response. I am ambivalent, frightened and bloody-minded all at once in sharing my thoughts with theirs. I feel I began as a qualified nurse after a difficult training period, where there were definite and known attempts by the college where I trained to make life more difficult when I 'fought' them on several issues that I felt strongly affected my values. In this way I felt first hand their power over me and the effect it wielded over my future, and I currently consider whether that experience so affected me that I lost my autonomy to express my opinion without fear of punishment. This view has been further supported by experience within the team where I work. The reality of the situation means I must work with what is, yet I carry some bitterness, a useless emotion, which always adds to through life's path and saps me of energy to grow. I can see some fluttering that is within me to grow, and this may encourage me to seek a new job in due course. I can relate to Moira's experience and feel in her story my own.

When I shared my reflection within the group I was offered the visual image of a jungle; to cut space in the undergrowth using a machete, to sit in the trees dropping anger into the space below. I am amazed at how effective this visualisation has been. I have added my own pattern – dropping coconuts on people I feel anger towards. It is surprising how many coconuts I have dropped! This has made me aware that I do hold on to anger, not only towards myself, but towards others, especially those I cherish and value. I think I am very self-critical and know I can be caustic and hostile, and so have avoided the confrontation and need to utilise 'pricking the bubble' in order to reduce the anger I hang onto.

I can see that the questions will continue in my reflection because, although one can consider the contradictions and debate ways forward, there is then the need to make choices. I stand in front of a bridge I must cross. That is, making the choice. For me, I think it is essential that I do make the correct one, as much of my personal well-being will depend on it. It seems I must repair some confidence along the way.

Johns (1995) found that reflective practitioners always interpreted extant knowledge for its relevance to their practice. Watson (1998) states that it is necessary to use theory as a lens for reflective seeing which helps bring the mountain and the marsh together, the mountain being Schön's (1987) high hard ground of technical rationality, whereas the marsh is Schön's enduring metaphor for the messy indeterminate nature of professional practice. I feel I have inhabited the depths of the marsh and can now see and find meaning in the mountains and their relationship with the marsh in the wider landscape and in doing so, I am understanding more of how my feelings are impacting so strongly on my practice. But this is not an automatic process, rather an extremely complicated one, a long therapeutic journey where I will look back on this analysis as crude and unskilled as I become more proficient. I have acknowledged my own discomfort but surfaced some strengths in my abilities too. I have shown a pattern in my life. There is much truth that learning through experience is arduous work (Johns 1995).

My third assignment

I pick up my journey through the third assignment some four months later. During this course a lecturer commented on her awareness while reading my work, of tentative steps occurring in becoming more positive and affirmative of myself as both a person and practitioner. This is true – I am aware of subtle and real changes taking place within myself and my work. One major change has been the acquisition of a new role with promotion. This was a result of exposing and surfacing tension in (my previous role) where I began to realise I was totally frustrated, unable to meet my practice potential or any personal satisfaction.

Guided reflection gave me the opportunity to allow myself time and space to 'spring clean' emotions long held onto, deep within emotional depths. The theme of these emotions has been ever present in my reflective work. Now my reflective practice feels like a new dawn, a new horizon of opportunity towards realising nursing therapeutic potential (Johns 1998).

> Reflect the actions and the words
> The good times soar on wings of birds
> The sad times tear my soul apart
> And cause my heart, my life to chart I look within myself so deep
> My thoughts remain within my sleep
> They stay aside my waking day
> Over and over, in encased depths they lay.
>
> Reflect the care, the love, the act
> The need to show an emotional pact
> Between what I am, what I do, why I care
> Was it just, was it right, was it fair?
>
> And if I can reflect who I am
> Will you challenge me if you can?
> And if I reflect that I care
> Will things change? Do they dare!

I wrote this poem when I began to reflect on the meaning reflective practice had for me. In the poem I express some inspiration for improvement in my life as a whole. I now realise how central the many emotions I carried within me were to the nurse I was becoming. I was inspired by Johns' comment (1998) that reflection gives us wings to soar, as we emerge from our cocoons but this was balanced alongside many arduous years of being many things to many people where I arrived exhausted from the emotional labour of dealing with other peoples' feelings and regulating my own emotions, what James (1989) has termed emotional labour.

Over time I have been able to create the time and space to recover from emotional entanglement, having come to recognise that nursing is almost parasitic in the way it takes psychological reservoirs of one's personality and that one needs a strong sense of self to recharge our batteries. When evaluating emotional work, what we say depends on who we are talking to, what shared knowledge maybe assumed, and what kinds of reaction are anticipated (Frith and Kitzinger 1998). My own emotional work has been influenced by many complicated personal and practice events. Initially, as a newly qualified nurse, I found the stress of coping with adults attempting such behaviours as self-mutilation and attempted suicide draining and isolating since there was little opportunity to explore feeling, especially in a unit where such behaviours were an almost daily occurrence. One positive aspect of listening to others reflecting is to realise my stresses are shared by others. At the same time I was nursing my mother who died of cancer, my son left home to go to university, and I changed jobs and my batteries went flat. Emotions are fruitfully seen as embodied existential modes of being. Work commitments and a busy lifestyle contributed to me carrying them as baggage – picking them up and dumping them as time allowed, but not exploring them, letting them go or renewing them. Work spent considering this now is charging my batteries. I have come to recognise how dangerous my lack of self-interest in sorting them may have been, and if I am honest, I can see how I reduced myself as a practitioner by 'capping' my true feelings as this extract from my journal illustrates:

> Don't hold my hand, please don't hold my hand. I cannot hold yours. You are dying and you know it. I know it too – I see it in your eyes. I know you are frightened. Your fear is not within the layers where most people hold onto theirs, when they are well. No, it is on the surface, covering you. It is beyond your skin all around you in the room. I feel it. I know it and I must cope with it.

> I do everything to make Margaret comfortable. The position, the pillows, the light, the warmth. All are considered. A sip of water, a fumble with the charts, take the blood pressure, keep the oxygen nearby. Soothe the relatives, say the right things.

> Are you watching me? I'm good, you can tell I've done this before. They think I'm an expert and unaffected. There are no experts in this and the effects mix with my own bereavement.

> Her hand is so fragile, small and like a bird's shaking as life flows away. How large my hand seems. Ugly next to Margaret's. Every time I approach the bed she attempts to grab my hand – she is seeking reassurance. I know I must hold her hand and show reassurance in my eyes. I say something soothing but I'm not there. I think now as I write of all the hands I've held and wonder if anyone will be there to hold mine. When you think about how many people we love in our lives that hold onto our hands, parents, partners, children, no wonder Margaret wants hers held now as she dies …

As a nurse I have held many people's hands during times of pain and stress. It is never easy to do. To me it connects you so physically with them. I think I am exposing more of my shadow self but I'm cautious since there isn't enough guided reflection space to deal with it all, and like others, this year I worry about the impact of coping with newly surfaced emotions. Zerwekh (1995) wrote that it is always a turning point when nurses can find and celebrate humanity and competence that at first may be hidden by suffering and degradation. She says nurses search for ways to validate people who have lost faith in themselves or no longer believe in their own power. I'm searching in my practice for their humanity and mine. If I must find it to be considered an effective practitioner I may fail, but if I work amongst people who can see elusive this achievement is, I can relax in being human and frail. … my recurring theme. Possibly I am becoming more effective practitioner because I accept fragility. I have learnt that while I can create a therapeutic environment for others to release their emotions, I am not a machine and must therefore find appropriate expression of my own, in order to be available to others. I use the Being available template (Johns 1998) as a mirror to see myself. Do I like the reflection? I like it more. I recognise now that I am very strong, have coped with much and those aspects of me that show fragility are warm, human and okay. Life experiences force me to be more honest about who I am and what and why I contribute towards others as I do. Having previously looked in some depth at the gender issues and prevailing attitudes between doctor and nurses, I concur there is a definite set of constraints as to what nurses are able to do for patients and themselves.

It seems realistic to say some of my reflective patterns have been painful and I have had to think about managing myself during reflection. If I am hard on myself does that follow I am hard on my patients? I have discussed being less hard on myself and know the kindness I extend to others can be extended within, but the barrier is not altogether down. Chapman (1983) concluded from Menzies-Lyth's work (1988) on the ritualistic practices utilised by nurses to protect them from anxieties, that individual behaviour attempts to defend one from the primitive anxieties evoked by death, dirty tasks and intimacy. I have found myself attempting that protection, yet overtly steering myself from ritualistic practice in the hope of achieving more holistic care; being much more comfortable with a strong belief that patients are people with minds and soul and feelings, and not object bodies given up to medical domination.

However, my delivery of effective care is variable since my reflection about Margaret shows a gap between the performance to meet the need as I interpret it and the deeper levels of myself as I reveal them. Cultural patterns of avoidance, the forbidden topic of death govern interactions around dying patients in hospitals (Glasser and Strauss 1965, cited in Chapman 1983). This must surely contribute little support for the nurse who cares for these patients, attempting somehow to support patients, relatives and others, while managing their own emotions throughout. Fortunately, I find myself thinking about many issues in a different way, attempting to step free of ingrained cultural and socialisation limitations. Now I am beginning to see how restricted I have been in myself.

Watson (1998) said that reflective caring practice helps us to stop and think, to pause in the midst of action. I have certainly done much of that. Watson felt this resulted in us being more aware, more mindful, authentically present, allowing a redirection. She likened it to being a simple shifting of one's consciousness from being harried, hurried or rushed, to being still, to find one's quiet centre. When I think of this I am inspired to be calm yet the days are often so hectic. I was known to say to those who knew me well I want peace in my life, but the reflection I have *laboured at* this year makes me think that the peace I seek is here in the quiet centre of myself; and if I had the courage to exorcise my shadow self I would find more peace. In response Chris said, 'The shadow self does not need exorcising, it needs embracing because it tells us important things about ourselves.' Through reflection I come to acknowledge and value my shadow self and integrating my shadow self with myself. Perhaps on this level we most need the challenge and support of guidance.

During my first assignment I realised I was at a bridge that I must cross successfully to maintain my own mental health. Now I view myself crossing that bridge and reflect on Johns' words: 'Assure your bridge is strong with a well defined plan' (1998). *Truthful* reflection has helped me focus my plan and I begin to see what the future could hold and more importantly, there is now a time for me to be kinder to myself.

I have changed my job. I was not prepared to continue in a restrictive routine that didn't recognise individual patients' needs. I've grown by becoming more self-determining, by choosing my own values and ideals, grounded in my own experience (Mayeroff 1971, cited in Johns 1996). This shows a personal right to become whole (if that is fully achievable) through choice and based on experience. It fills me with confidence that the person I am, while unique, is okay and in that I feel less isolated from other practitioners and also some independence, which shows progress in itself since I previously commented on feelings of isolation and lack of harmony.

I have explored relationships amongst work colleagues and I am finally realising some of the effects these relationships have had on my well-being. I was seen as a confidant and lent on for support, yet needed much support myself … more than I admitted to openly, whereas now I look for support. I was seen as capable, yet often questioned that of myself, feeling my integrity and logic opposed others. While I am guilty of using others in the workplace I too was used and exploited by friends and superiors and when it was overt at times I tolerated it even when I recognised it, but that perspective is changing. Johns (1992) states that nurses must develop new ways to effectively support each other in their mutual roles.

I wrote in my journal:

that my time on the unit has been fraught with frustration and I have seen myself wanting to be more involved, often part of a routine I disliked, of events that I wanted to challenge and part of a team whose support varied ... yet again nothing is certain, I cannot be sure my choice of job will be better ... I often ask myself why do I put myself through so much?

Already I see events repeating themselves, yet I do see them and work towards responding differently even as the less than welcoming reception has left me guarded and confused, wondering about the psychological cost. My sensitivity re-emerging, depleting my batteries again, yet the opportunity to reshape something is not lost on me and I am able to utilise new reflective coping strategies, ensuring not to absorb too much. Let them keep their problems and prejudices which are not mine.

Reflection has equipped me with so many intrapersonal and interpersonal skills, but it is there for the reader to see that there is great turmoil between what I am and what I do:

> Its not that I am black or blue
> Nor any shade that's blurred from view
> Its just that when I want to care
> to show for you that I am there
> The nurse I am just doesn't dare!
>
> But there is a new and changing me
> A person grown who now can see
> the callous cruelty of what was done,
> The right to care, but live, have fun.
> And in doing that change the job for which I trained
> So there's more of me and less that's drained.
>
> I'm not where I want to be
> I want more, I want to be free
> To give to others better choice to start
> To practice life and work from their heart
> A sense of self in all they do,
> That's not dependent on hierarchy such as you!

The ghosts I have carried from my experiences as a student nurse are not laid to rest – I am trying but still they are not exorcised – 'the callous cruelty of what was done'. 'The right to care, but live and have fun', is my hope that nurses will drop this need for devotion and sacrifice and come to understand the best ones have a life as well and all have the right to one. The final verse shows a desire to have a role in shaping the experience of other beginners in nursing so that ultimately more will be able to challenge the hierarchical structures and professional dominance that restrict us from realising our therapeutic potential and destiny. Then the mountain and the marsh may well come together.

From old end chapter: Aileen's narrative

Aileen's narrative reflects the way reflection gives her permission to let go of containing a self that had become constrained, conformed, afraid, exhausted, frustrated and helpless.

In this respect, reflection is reclaiming control of the self. The reader may ask 'What theory lies here?' Perhaps theory is a misleading word. Perhaps insight of the relationship between things would be a better descriptor.

At the core of Aileen's narrative is the idea that reflection facilitates the expression of her voice as cathartic expression. Finding a voice that sheds light on the shadows within, a voice that is accepted and honoured, a voice nurtured and allowed to soar, a voice that reconnects the authentic self. Aileen notes 'Zerwekh (1995) wrote that it is always a turning point when nurses can find and celebrate humanity and competence that at first may be hidden by suffering and degradation.' Zerwekh's insight is confirmed.

As Aileen noted 'one positive aspect of listening to others reflecting is to realise my stresses are shared by others.' Aileen recognised herself in the words of others, both the spoken word of the group, and the literary word of Zerweck, confirming Belenky *et al.*'s (1986) observation that women need to be reconnected to communities of caring. Then recovery is possible and possibilities emerge.

References

Belenky MF, Clinchy BM, Goldberger NR and Tarule JM (1986) *Women's ways of knowing: the development of self, voice, and mind.* Basic Books, New York.

Bendelow M (1983) *Managerial women's approaches to organisational conflict: a qualitative study.* Unpublished doctoral dissertation. University of Colorado, Denver.

Chapman G (1983) Ritual and rational action in hospitals. *Journal of Advanced Nursing* 8:13–20.

Frith H and Kitzinger C (1998) 'Emotional work' as a participant recourse: A feminist analysis of young women's talk-in-interaction. *Sociology* 32:299–320.

Glasser B and Strauss A (1965) *Awareness of dying.* Aldine, Chicago.

Graham I (1998) Understanding the nature of nursing through reflection. In: C Johns and D Freshwater (eds.) *Transforming nursing through reflective practice.* Blackwell Science, Oxford, pp. 119–133.

Heron J (1975) *Six category intervention analysis.* Human potential research project. University of Surrey.

James N (1989) Emotional labour: skill and work in the social regulation of feelings. *The Sociological Review* 37:15–42.

Johns C (1992) Ownership and the harmonious team: barriers to developing the therapeutic team in primary nursing. *Journal of Clinical Nursing* 1:89–94.

Johns C (1995) Time to care? Time for reflection. *International Journal of Nursing Practice* 1:37–42.

Johns C (1996) Visualising and realising caring in practice through guided reflection. *Journal of Advanced Nursing* 24:1135–1143.

Johns C (1998) Opening the doors of perception. In: C Johns and D Freshwater (eds.) *Transforming nursing through reflective practice.* Blackwell Science, Oxford, pp. 1–20.

Johns C and Freshwater D (1998) Preface. In: C Johns and D Freshwater (eds.) *Transforming nursing through reflective practice.* Blackwell Science, Oxford.

Mayeroff M (1971) *On caring.* Harper, New York.

Menzies-Lyth I (1988) A case study in the functioning of social systems as a defence against anxiety. In: *Containing anxiety in institutions: selected essays.* Free Association Books, London, pp. 43–85.

Miller J (1977) *Towards a new psychology of women.* Beacon Press, Boston.

Newman M (1994) *Health as expanded consciousness.* National League for Nursing, New York.

Oakley A (1984) The importance of being a nurse. *Nursing Times* 83:24–27.

Schön D (1987) *Educating the reflective practitioner*. Jossey-Bass, San Francisco.

Valentine P (1995) Management of conflict: do nurses/women handle it differently? *Journal of Advanced Nursing* 22:142–149.

Watson J (1998) A meta-reflection on reflective practice and caring theory. In: C Johns and D Freshwater (eds.) *Transforming nursing through reflective practice*. Blackwell Science, Oxford, pp. 214–220.

Zerwekh J (1995) Making the connection during home visits; narratives of expert nurses. *The Hospice Journal* 10:27–44.

Chapter 7

Finding a new way in health visiting

Yvonne Latchford

Background

Before embarking on my dissertation, I had studied with Chris in guided reflection[1] during which time I had reflected on about my work with two families with child protection concerns. I became increasingly aware of contradiction and conflict within my role, which became the driving force behind my determination to find a better way for health visiting in child protection work at a time of turbulence within health visiting.

The government consultation document *Supporting families* launched in November 1998, *urges* health visitors to rise to the challenges of developing a modern approach and a 'high quality early investment', shifting the focus of health visiting from dealing with failure towards prevention. This involves questioning traditional roles and working styles in order to find new ways of working that involve 'new partnerships and inter-agency and multi-disciplinary working to deliver high quality and effective services to address the challenges of inequalities, parenting and family policy'. This renewed government commitment to expansion of family support services is an extension of the underpinning philosophy of the Children Act 1989 that placed a new emphasis on family support and formalised the notion of working in partnership with parents. These government initiatives have placed early family support interventions firmly at the heart of the challenge for health visitors to find a new way.

Historically this has not been the first major government challenge to change health visiting practice. Welshman (1997) suggested that health visiting remains 'a prisoner of its history' due to its inability to extend its scope of practice. Welshman charted the course of resistance by health visitors to expand their role that eventually resulted in expansion of social services provision to the detriment of health visiting during the 1950–1960s. Despite increased opportunity due to 'wider economic, social and medical changes' and, despite government encouragement to expand the 'traditional field of work with mothers and infants', health visitors on the whole did not expand their work into the newer arenas of preventative work. If resistance to change has become woven into the fabric of health visiting history, then it is essential that positive, enlightened

---

[1] ENBA29.

responses to new challenges are developed to ensure the future survival of the profession. Health visitors must choose to proactively meet these challenges or passively accept that nothing can be done. Reactions to the new government proposals provide some early indication of the current professional mood. Initial response to the *Supporting families* consultation document support the need for an expanded role of health visitors whilst recommending that there needs to be a substantial increase in health visitors to achieve this goal. This article also outlines government recognition that in order to expand its role, health visiting needs a fundamental change. The article entitled 'Family policy doomed without increase in health visitors' chooses, however, to de-emphasise change, and focuses instead on the need to increase health visitor numbers. Although such increase may be relevant, it could nurture a passive response in health visitors. Accepting that nothing can be done without more health visitors will deter an alternative positive debate on change and action. Although disguised, the more disturbing suggestion is that health visitors who do not change will fail to become involved in new policies. As these policies are gong to determine the nature of future provision of family support in the community, a passive stance may affect the way the government considers the future role of the health visitor. In the light of the wider acceptance that work with young families remains a priority and still dominates the workload, how can health visitors afford to sit back and ignore these new initiatives in primary care? We know through past experience that if health visitors do not rise to the challenge of change then others will. These are important issues for the future of our profession.

There are also strong influences within health visiting that traditionally nurture a sense of passivity, so it becomes even more crucial to find a way to create the conditions of empowerment within the ranks. There is a need to find a way to challenge resistance that will potentially 'act as a counterweight to the desire for change and will induce people to accommodate themselves to the discontent they are suffering' (Fay 1987:29). Within this research I have taken up the challenge to find a new way. I will illuminate the way I have become empowered to change my everyday practice, and question and actively participate in changing an entire working culture through the medium of guided reflection through my on-going relationship with Helen and her family.

Helen

Helen is separated from her profoundly handicapped husband and lives with her two children, Natasha, aged four years, and Robert, aged six years. Helen has manic depression, which is presently controlled by lithium. Helen is a devoted and loving mother and when she is not ill she copes with the children very well. Acute bouts of illness have occurred twice in the two years I have known her. The first time was just before I met her. At this time the children had been placed on the Child Protection Register and Helen had been taken into hospital. Soon after her recovery the children were taken off the register and were returned home to their mother.

My early experiences were set against a background of Helen's mistrust and anger stemming from her sense of not being heard, a metaphor for her powerlessness. Belenky *et al.* (1986) suggest that women's sense of voice can be used as a metaphor for their experience and that the 'development of voice, mind and self are intricately intertwined' (p. 18). At this stage, Helen's sense of self and inner voice was struggling to emerge and was being denied. I found it necessary to find a way to peel back these layers of anger in order to connect with her and to build a relationship with her. Her anger at this time was preventing any significant access to the family by social services or health visitors. Helen viewed any access as an intrusion and was immediately resented. At this time she was taking steps to sue her previous health visitor and social worker. Her anger was due to her feelings that she had been misrepresented, misquoted and misunderstood during the child protection process. My early aims with her were to find a way of regaining trust and building a caring relationship that could empower her to move forward in her life.

Guided reflection provided me with a safe clearing so I could see around me. I realised that I had been frightened of Helen and I wondered why this should be so. I began to question the way she had been labelled, noting in my journal that 'it would have been difficult for anyone to see the real Helen under such a dense fog of negative labels'. This inner questioning represented my first determined steps towards coming to know my true self in context of my work with clients. I pondered over her words, 'I don't mind you, it's health visitors I don't care for'. I asked myself why this should be, and in doing so I began to scrutinise the role of the health visitor in child protection work. I gradually became aware of feelings of tension and contradiction between my sense of self and my sense of role.

One example of an issue I explored at this time was the increasing emphasis on risk assessment and assessment of vulnerability including the use of clinical guidelines and checklists in health visiting child protection work. Although this was accepted practice, I saw that according to research, this was at odds with more tacit, intuitive ways of knowing which health visitors would rather pay attention to. I also looked at the ways that child protection work encourages health visitors to act in covert ways (Dingwall 1982; Taylor and Tilley 1989), and how this was at odds with the need for health visitors to develop 'open and honest' relationships (Department of Health 1995). Through guided reflection I had begun to expose contradictory ways of working within my practice. It was a time of sudden clarity, a time of enlightenment 'marked by the emergence of a disposition which is intent on subjecting social arrangements to rational inspection, and which is bent on breaking with the done thing when examination shows it to be unwarranted' (Fay 1987:67). It became clearer that I needed to break with the old order to find a better way for health visiting in child protection work, a way that enabled me to realise personal and professional beliefs and values in actual practice.

Research process

'It has been said that it is possible only on the page, in stories, that we can be so tender to one another, so free, so humane, so brave and so pure' (Okri 1997:43). For all these reasons, in my early days as a reflective practitioner, it was a profound experience to give expression to my personal feelings and perceptions within the pages of my journal. With the benefit of guided reflection however, the true significance of Okri's words in terms of my health visiting practice soon became much clearer to me. I became aware of the limitations of reflection without guidance, as I gradually realised that becoming 'true' and 'free' were not as straightforward as I had first perceived.

I did not journey alone. Sharing my stories with Chris I found that my practice began to change in ways congruent with my ideals of desirable practice. In choosing to write about and sharing certain experiences I opened myself to the possibility of gaining new insights and understanding opening the possibility to show 'the lived quality and significance of the experience in a fuller and deeper manner' (Van Manen 1990:10). Engaging in a free and open dialogue with Chris enabled me to peel back the layers of interpretation even further as he introduced his own perspectives and understandings. Through discussion and by drawing on literature I came to understand why things were as they are and what they might become. Together we are able to co-construct new meanings and new possibilities, the 'dialectical play which Gadamer calls the fusion of horizons' (Weinsheimer 1985:210).

My motivation became focused and I became increasingly empowered and knowing to act on new insights. I became liberated. Within education the conditions of liberation can only be achieved when the educator's efforts 'coincide with those of the student to engage in critical thinking and the quest for mutual humanisation' (Freire 1972:49). Freire believed that the relationship must be primarily one of partnership based upon a profound sense of trust in the student's ability to act as a conscious and creative being. As such my journey became our journey. We contracted to meet for one hour every month. In total we met seven times between August 1998 and April 1999. Between these sessions I used a journal to reflect on my visits to Helen which became the basis for our dialogue within guided reflection. I took notes of our dialogue, which I wrote up immediately after each session to capture the essence of what took place and which I used to unfold my journey.

First guided reflection session

I talked about my visit to see Helen at her home. She was warm and friendly and readily talked about how she was coping. I asked whether she had heard anything from social services regarding obtaining access to her conference notes. She said she hadn't and became angry. She talked about going to see her solicitor again. I remember thinking how sad it was that we were still having the same conversation after all this time.

Although Helen knew I shared her frustration it was not enough. I tried to talk to her but she became even angrier. I wasn't afraid although I felt concerned for Natasha who was playing nearby. She said, 'Mummy is angry with you', and I said, 'Yes mummy is very angry, but I don't think she's angry at me.' She then went to play upstairs. Helen said, 'You always make me feel so angry' and asked me not to visit anymore. Then she lifted a large plastic box over her head and slammed it down on the floor next to me. I didn't feel frightened but was unsure what to do next. The force had split the box in half. I remember wondering if this was taking catharsis too far. Then it happened. She began to talk to me between copious tears. She talked to me about feelings of despair and hopelessness. I asked her how she now felt. She said that she had only ever broken out like that once before in her life and then apologised, asking me how I felt. I said I was glad she had been able to release some of her anger but that perhaps it was a bit too threatening for me. I said it was also a shame about the box. She smiled at this comment and seemed much calmer.

Chris and I discussed the value of catharsis and humour as therapeutic responses to the other's anger. Chris pointed out that an intervention could only truly be cathartic if it was followed through to the end as had happened during my visit. He challenged me to consider whether or not I had been in danger or had placed myself at risk. Although I had not felt frightened, I felt there had been an element of risk due to intensity of Helen's anger. Chris encouraged me to reflect deeper on this anger.

I thought it might only take is a letter from social services or some demonstration of concern to neutralise this anger. Instead they chose to ignore her and this compounds her feelings of helplessness. It's not access to the notes she really needs, it's recognition.

She said she would write another letter to them and I said I would write to support her if she felt that would help.

Chris expanded, 'It may be that Helen can't have access to her notes in which case all you can do is clarify that. It would be better to have this in writing so Helen can see action has been taken. This raises another issue though – why can't she have access to the notes? What is there to hide?'

I said 'It seems that social services are just paying lip service to their espoused philosophy of empowerment. If they wish to be empowering why not allow her to see the notes – what harm would it do? She would be able to have her say, and respond to their comments and move on. They have not even replied to my letter. It seems nobody is listening to either of us.'

I felt the pattern of Helen and my own mutual powerlessness. I felt the powerful and controlling influences of social services on us. I wondered why I have never before considered my relationship with social services in terms of power? Reflecting on the significance of the session I felt I better understood Helen's anger and felt more connected to her. I need to reflect on the lack of response by social services and the nature of relationships between health visitors and social services.

I had reached a turning point with Helen. Her smashed box is a metaphor for my inner cathartic feelings of release. It jolted something deep within me as I became aware of a deep frustration and anger that after all this time the causes of Helen's anger had not been resolved. With Chris, I have endeavoured to peel back the layer of Helen's and my own anger so I could better know and connect with Helen, to be more available to enable her to realise her best interests. It is only as I began to look at myself and to realign my values in tune with Helen that she started to trust me. Being clear about my values and purpose as a health visitor is paramount. It is at the root of guided reflection, working towards resolving contradiction between my values and my actual practice. Although Helen still had nothing good to say about health visitors or social workers, her trust gave me access to the family. Now this trust was threatened by her renewed anger.

Chris had drawn attention to Belenky *et al.*'s idea of voice as a metaphor for empowerment. He had challenged me whether I, we, could develop a more powerful voice that is heard?[2] Becoming aware of my *silence* was revealing. Belenky *et al.* (1986) link women's silence with oppression, ways in which silent women 'see blind obedience to authorities as being of utmost importance for keeping out of trouble and ensuring their own survival' (p. 28). Keeping out of trouble and surviving may have become a way of being for myself, and health visitors in general. I need to unmask this spectre of oppression. It's not just Helen who is struggling to emerge and find an authentic voice. In becoming empowered I can better enable Helen to become empowered.

There is a prevailing lack of understanding about the health visitor role and much seems to depend on individual perspective. One study that set out to consider consumer perspective uncovered a lack of knowledge about the health visitor's role (Collinson and Cowley 1998). In this study, health visitors had failed to explain their role and this had created a mismatch of client and health visitor perceptions resulting in a failure to

---

[2]Belenky *et al.* (1986) identify five types of voice: silence, received knowing, subjective voice, procedural knowing – separate and connected, and constructed voice. Each level of voice represents the woman's power ranging from silence where the woman's voice is oppressed, through to constructed voice where the woman speaks with an informed, assertive and passionate voice, although that does not guarantee her voice is heard.

fulfil client expectations. This in turn had generated negativity towards the health visitors. It seems that health visitors themselves are uncertain of their role and therefore experience difficulty in explaining it to others. This uncertainty may be exacerbated due to the increasing pressure for health visitors to make their role explicit within service contracts for purchasers. Health visitors for example are resorting to the use of clinical guidelines despite evidence to suggest that these tend to be unsupported by research, and an increased use of scoring indices based on invalidated material that potentially constrain and erode professional judgement (Appleton and Cowley 1997). In this way, health visitors are denying and disguising the true nature of their work and are therefore contributing to the prevailing lack of understanding of the health visitor role. This is bound to affect the way that health visiting is valued in the community. In terms of understanding power relationships, it is feasible that within this prevailing climate of vulnerability and uncertainty, health visitors may feel less able to assert themselves. These conditions are far more likely to reinforce the feelings of passivity, reactivity and dependency that bear all the hallmarks of oppression (Belenky *et al*. 1986). Freire suggested that self-perception is oppressed is impaired by 'submersion in the reality of oppression' (1972:22). Freire maintains that at this level, the oppressed are more likely to attempt to identify with the oppressor than to recognise or to struggle against contradiction. Perhaps within this climate of vulnerability health visitors have internalised a feeling of subordination in their relationship with social workers whose powerful, statutory role in child protection work has steadily grown as health visitor numbers have steadily fallen. Perhaps we have found it necessary to align ourselves more with social services in order to survive.

Second guided reflection session

I reflected on my conversation with Jo, a social worker who is interested in the way I work with Helen. She agreed that Helen should either be given access to her notes or at least get a response. It was such a relief to speak with someone on my wavelength. I told her that I couldn't understand why social services had blocked Helen's attempts to see her reports if they were genuinely concerned with empowering clients. Jo agreed. She said she wanted to pursue this issue with her manager in her own supervision. At last someone is listening!

Some colleagues asked me about my research. I said it was concerned with finding a new way for health visitors in child protection work. This provoked curiosity. They asked me what I thought was wrong with the way things were now? I explained that over the past 18 months guided reflection had helped me to see and examine things I had never questioned before. I gave example of the ways I had changed my perspectives and in turn my practice, notably shifting from covert ways I felt health visitors worked with families in child protection. Initially they all disputed this. I stood my ground noting that this had become clear to me after I had been guided to expose contradictions between my beliefs and the way I had practised.

When I said I had questioned my beliefs, something in the atmosphere changed. Both Jo and my health visitor colleagues warmed towards me. I think my words were effective because they were honest. They paid attention to me because the purity of striving to realise beliefs was irresistible to them as caring practitioners. I realised that my experience of guided reflection had somehow set me apart from various colleagues. I felt so powerful. I am powerful! I am able to assert myself in convincing ways. Kieffer (1984), in his

Table 7.1 Attainment of participatory competence through four phases of involvement (adapted from Kieffer 1984)

Phase	Development
Era of entry (birth of struggle against conflict)	Birth of emergence of participatory competence Integrity violated provoking and mobilising sense of frustration and powerlessness towards an empowering response
Era of advancement (continuing struggle)	Maturation of empowerment through extension of involvement and deepening understanding through intensive self-refection with the help of an external enabler
Era of incorporation (continuing struggle)	Reconstructs sense of self as author and actor in environment. Learning to confront and contend with barriers to self-determination leads to a sense of mastery and competence in the individual's sense of being
Era of commitment (continuing struggle)	Adulthood of participatory competence – integrates new abilities and insight into reality in meaningful ways

study of the emergence of citizen leader empowerment, described four distinct and progressive phases of skills and insights leading to attainment of a 'real and self-perceived sense of participatory competence' (p. 12) (Table 7.1). At the first phase or 'era of entry', Kieffer believes that empowerment is provoked through a sense of 'outrage' or 'violation of the sense of integrity' and is a time when 'individuals are first discovering their political muscles and potential for external impact' (1984:19). This was my era of entry. it was my emergence from my sense of anger, frustration and helplessness. This session marked my transition from a sense of moral outrage (Pike 1991) intensified by the constraints that were blocking my attempts to empower Helen into a sense of freedom to act in congruent ways. Guided reflection had not only enabled me to become aware of my inner struggle but was now fuelling it in order to sustain my emergence.

Third guided reflection session

Helen had cancelled our appointment to meet at the nursery. She had angrily said to my colleague that she didn't see the point of meeting. I felt so despondent. I called it 'the black hole' in my journal. I couldn't see how I can move forward. She blames health visitors and social workers for her anger. She tars us all with the same brush. On reflection, I know I am being negative but can rationalise her reaction. Her anger has always been bubbling away and this is just another eruption. It' a catch 22 situation though. I can't easily arrange to see her when she's so angry, but I need to see her to help her move through her anger. Her anger is preventing me from gaining access to the children. I ask Chris, 'How can we protect children if we don't have access?'

Chris felt that Helen's inability to have access to her notes is the root of her anger. He proposed using ethical mapping (Johns 1999) to help me clarify my 'right response' within the situation:

Authority to act?		
Patient's/family's perspective: Helen believed she has a right to be heard and wants to be given the opportunity to respond to the accusations on the document	I can't show Helen the notes but I can support her attempts to gain access to them	*Social workers' perspective:* The social workers said Helen would be more upset if she read the report
The situation/dilemma		
Is there conflict and how might it be resolved? Cut through the conflict of interests by suggesting to Helen we go to social services together	Helen's inability to gain access to the reports and to seek redress	*Ethical principles* Autonomy – I feel it is her right to decide whether or not she will be upset. Protecting her from hurt is a perverse form of parentalism
Power relationships?		
Nurses' perspective: My colleagues agree I should support Helen. However, they feel I should not visit her on my own while she is so angry	I wonder to what extent social services management influences my actions as a health visitor in child protection work?	*Organisation's perspective* My line manager has already let Helen see some paragraphs of the report but she was not allowed to take a copy home so she still could not respond. Access has to be permitted by social services

Considering how I have reacted to similar situations in the past, I realise my embodied sense of powerlessness *vis à vis* social services. I would have withdrawn to avoid conflict and my own discomfort. I would have seen resisting social services as futile.

Applying the ethical grid enabled me not only to clarify and understand my position but also to realise that understanding in itself was not enough. I could feel the contradictions, and imagine ways I could confront these people who I perceived to be more powerful than me. Using the grid helped me to sustain and build upon my sense of inner struggle against conflict so essential to sustain my emergence at Kieffer's level of advancement and incorporation (see Table 7.1). This now embodied sense of awareness was enough to propel me out of a 'black hole of passivity towards determined action'. As Fay (1987) said 'it is only when acting on the basis of considered reflection, when one's actions express one's rational judgements as to what is best, that one can be said to be truly free' (p. 76).

Without guided reflection I wondered if I would have even attempted to find a way to maintain any form of intensive, preventive intervention. Still, it would have been professionally acceptable at this point to revert to the recommended core surveillance programme that currently frames health visitor intervention (Hall 1996) and tends to represent the minimum level of health visitor intervention with pre-school children. Yet Helen's children were not on the Child Protection Register and there were currently no concerns about the children's well-being. As Hall pointed out, child surveillance is only part of the recommended child health promotion programme and is secondary prevention. Hall envisaged that there be 'more emphasis on primary prevention' (1996:223).

If I had withdrawn, my ability to continue working with this family in a primary preventive way would have been compromised. In some ways the core programme has made it easier for health visitors to withdraw from primary prevention. I could have simply left a calling card suggesting Helen come to my clinic. I may have chosen to view this as empowering in that it enabled Helen to make up her own mind about whether she needs to see the health visitor. In terms of primary prevention however, how can I expect Helen to anticipate her health needs without any help? Isn't anticipatory guidance my role as a health visitor? The first principle of health visiting is the search for health needs and this 'is based on the outreach nature of health visiting when unacknowledged needs may be identified' (Orr 1990). The new public health White Paper *Supporting families*, together with the Acheson Report, 'Inequalities in Health', have placed primary prevention at the heart of government policy. The clear expectation is that health visitors will move away from a problem-solving approach and move towards intensive, effective primary care support (Turner 1998/9). Health visitor support has now not only been recognised as being an effective primary care intervention, it is now being actively encouraged within health policy.

In her spirited keynote speech to the Health Visitors Association (HVA) Annual Professional Conference in 1988, the HVA General Secretary, Shirley Goodwin, made an impassioned plea for a 'virtual revolution in some of the basic tenets of health visiting' and for health visitors to create the climate for radical change necessary for health visiting to become relevant to the needs of the people (Goodwin 1988). This plea was in anticipation of the recommendations of the pending report of the Third Joint Working Party, commonly known as the Hall Report (1996), which set out to systematically review and to improve child health surveillance. In her speech, Goodwin described health visiting as a 'gloomy picture of a beleaguered even demoralised profession, frustrated about what it would wish to do but cannot'. Recognising the need to move away from directive, secondary prevention child health screening and surveillance approaches, she urged health visitors to become involved in identification of individual parental needs in order to create participatory opportunities for primary care and 'support of parental confidence and competence' in line with the Hall Report's recommendations. Although it has been 11 years since that landmark speech, there is evidence to suggest that health visitors remain trapped in the narrow and restrictive straight-jacket of health visiting practice that she first described. There still remain tensions between participatory and directive styles of practice even though there is now renewed emphasis on primary care and the need for a shift in the relationship between parents, children and health professionals to one of partnership, rather than supervision, in which parents are empowered to make use of services and expertise according to their needs (Hall 1996).

A recent study for exploring ways of determining effectiveness of health visiting interventions unmasked conflicting tensions between participatory and directive styles of practice and suggested that some professionals were still setting their own agendas as opposed to empowering people to set their own agendas (Dolan and Kitson 1997). This study drew attention to recent evidence that suggested that health visitors were still viewing their 'workload' as being a constraining element to developing their role. 'Workload' has traditionally been given as a reason for inability to expand and develop the health visitor role even though there is evidence to suggest that modifications of workload have positive and empowering outcomes. Health visitors in Nottingham's Strelley Nursing Development Unit became the first community-based project to win a substantial King's Fund grant for targeting resources to areas of greatest need and for finding ways to work in partnership with clients (Jackson 1994). An alternative health visiting framework was proposed and developed focusing on family health promotion and child health, high intervention work and public health. These were all primary care health strategies. In order to make any impact within these areas with no extra funding, some health visitors initially decided to reduce and to prioritise and redistribute caseloads. Other health visitors, during a recent 'Sure Start' funding bid, found that they too were able to develop an innovative targeted practice after consciously deciding to reduce routine case work (Bidmead 1999). These projects provide good example of what can be achieved when health visitors decide actively to tackle the problem of workload. These endeavours may become essential as that the very 'bread and butter' of health visiting practice is currently being threatened. Sure Start core services, outreach and home visiting, support for families and parents, primary and community health care and advice about child health and development and family health, and support for people with special needs, including help getting access to specialised services, are remarkably similar to the core services that many health visitors would consider to be their everyday practice.

However, the government has recognised that the nature of intervention varies greatly between health visitors. Whilst recognising that 'some health visitors are already able to provide support for the family' (Dolan and Kitson 1997), the government also recognises that some health visitors do not. Despite this, the government now expects that all health visitors will 'extend and improve what they already do' (Sure Start document p. 12) and will develop innovative proposals to ensure a lasting support to families that is 'long enough to make a real difference' (p. 6). The government also expects that health visitors will develop this support within existing resources and that is why radical and innovative changes are being sought. If health visitors do not change and re-focus their work, new models of support will evolve to usurp the health visitor role. Indeed there is already evidence of this happening. Recently in Hackney, the views of 202 family members were sought as part of some research funded by the Department of Health. It is unsettling, as Cook (1999) noted, that although these families had access to an individual health visitor, many still 'expressed a wish to have open access to a family adviser in general practice who could listen to and discuss concerns and possible responses' (p. 69). In response to the survey, it was felt necessary to develop a new 'Well family service' for the 6800 people within those caseloads. The key elements to this new approach were described as being home visiting, a consistent relationship on the user's terms, parenting education, emotional support and advocacy. Most health visitors would probably list all of these things as being key elements to the 'old' approach of health visiting. The developers of this new approach however, have no such expectations., declaring that 'with larger caseloads, higher levels of statutory child protection work, increased routine tasks and extended development testing, health visitors are not in a position to offer a targeted service to vulnerable families' (Cook 1999:171). Even more worrying, the key target group of 'families with children in need to fall below the current threshold for social service support' (Cook 1999:169) are currently just those families that represent the 'holding work' or 'grey area' that increasingly takes up much health visitor time. More families are being supported in a holding relationship by health visitors, who are finding that social services departments are 'often only accessible if a referral is described as a child protection issue' and that social workers are putting less effort 'into intervening and working preventatively at an early stage with families' (Appleton and Clemerson 1999:134). In reality, the important emotional work that health visitors are involved in with families at best is undervalued and at worst remains invisible, thus contributing to the perceived need to develop 'new' services that mimic and supplement the health visitor role. If such a significant proportion of health visiting work remains invisible then it becomes essential to develop a sense of clarity about what we are actually doing with health visiting practice. Without such clarity, negative assumptions are flourishing and successfully disguising the true therapeutic, primary care nature of health visiting intervention. Without such clarity I would have been unable to move forward out of this self-induced silence of hopelessness towards a sense of inner certainty and confidence linked with empowerment. As Freire (1972) said 'as critical perception is embodied in action, a climate of hope and confidence develops which leads men to attempt to overcome the limit situations' (p. 72). To again cite Freire (1972), in challenging the 'concrete historical reality' (p. 72) of my health visiting practice and within the wider profession, the only real 'black hole' or 'strait-jacket' to practise is likely to be a self-perceived one. Through guided reflection I have moved my perceptual goal posts, have readjusted my sense of reality and am now ready to move forward in my work with Helen with a sense of inner certainty and confidence I have never experienced before.

Fourth guided reflection session

I had acted on my conviction and phoned Helen today. She made it clear early in the conversation that she didn't want to talk to me. She had given up on health visitors! I remind myself that whilst she had never accepted me as a health visitor she had always accepted me as a person. I drew strength from this and staying with her, empathised saying, 'I know how you feel. It's like we're banging our head against a brick wall.' I encouraged her to think about the ways we were slowly making progress. Gradually she opened up and talked to me and eventually decided that she would like me to accompany her to social services. I said I would be away for the next two weeks and we could go when I returned. I'm dismayed at the lack of response by social services. I ask myself, 'Why is it so difficult? Helen *doesn't ask for much at all*. What is it that they are afraid of? It's such a struggle for me, let alone for Helen. We're both battling against the odds … but why!' However, in so far as much as social services are concerned, I now feel resolute and decisive. I know my continuing support will help to strengthen Helen jut as Chris's guidance gives me strength to do it. I feel as if I am entering into battle! Warrior pose, a moral crusade to fight for integrity and liberate from oppression. Trumpets blare.

Chris repeating the words, 'Helen doesn't ask for very much at all', gave me the opportunity to reconsider them not just in terms of my frustration, but also in terms of their true significance. The more I thought about it, the more incomprehensible the situation became. If health visitors and social workers really wish to work in partnership with families, this level of openness and honesty should surely be less difficult. In wishing to challenge the contents of a report written about her, Helen was attempting to take back some control and yet this goal had for the last year been unachievable. I could now see that this was unacceptable and that it was time to question why this should be.

However, health visitors being open and honest with clients has proved to be problematic. Following a pilot study within six primary care teams, a child protection working group decided to conduct a study to develop a tool that would encourage an open and honest relationship with clients (Glew and Heron 1998). As part of the study, health visitors were asked to broach the subject of child abuse with families at the six-week development check. Not only was there a low response rate to the study at 35%, some of the remaining sample admitted that they found raising the subject of child abuse difficult. Although the authors put this down to the stressful and distressing nature of child protection work, it is feasible to make a further assumption that this level of openness and honesty was too difficult to contemplate. Bell (1995) identified the therapeutic benefits of encouraging parents to become involved at the initial child protection conference also highlighted how health visitors 'had greater difficulty than social workers in presenting negative information about parents and children in front of them' (p. 256). It is strange that even within the prevailing climate of partnership building with families, that health visitors are experiencing such incongruence between their espoused beliefs and values and their actual practice in child protection work. This in itself is revealing and so worthy of further critical scrutiny.

Focusing on the ability of health visitors to act in self-determined ways, it is clear that a high degree of structural autonomy (Batey and Lewis 1982) exists within health visiting as health visitors are 'expected in the context of their work to use their judgement in the provision of client services' (p. 15). Although health visitors cannot expect complete autonomy, as they function part of an organisation, freedom to make independent decisions exist in almost all setting where nursing is practised. The more complex the patient's problems and the more persons involved in the patient's care, the greater is the need for independent decisions by nurses related to the practice of nursing (Singleton and Nail 1984). Despite this it is clear that under certain circumstances health visitors feel constrained and unable to realise their caring beliefs in actual practice. Within the child protection arena it seems that health visitor ability to maintain levels of self-determination are significantly reduced. It may be that attitudinal autonomy is being compromised because health visitors do not perceive themselves to be free to use their judgement in decision making (Batey and Lewis 1982). I recognise that I may have been labouring under this type of constraint in my work with Helen. Reflecting on my experiences I can now see the impact of social service interventions on both Helen's life and my practice.

My attempts to help her gain access to her notes have been to no avail. In this disempowered state of silence I can now see how I have unwittingly colluded with social services and how, in doing so, I have compromised my professional integrity. Holden (1990) highlighted that nurses have a tendency to collude with doctors who are practising in unacceptable ways although this in turn 'strikes at the very core of their personal and professional integrity' (p. 402). This becomes intolerable to nurses and causes conflict between the medical and nursing professions. Collusion with social services has encouraged me to give up my sense of autonomy and power and to act in ways that are against my beliefs and values. It seems therefore that increasing child protection work merely serves to contradict the very nature of health visiting practice and that this may be the reason why these interventions have so often seemed intolerable to me and to other health visitors.

In my silence I have also unwittingly reinforced a perception that social services are relatively more powerful than health visiting and that this may be contributing to my feelings of disempowerment. Holden (1990) suggests that to take back the reins of responsibility nurses need to prioritise their desires in order to decrease frustration, employ a critical awareness in order to act on their own convictions and to develop a strength of will in order to maintain a sense of personal integrity. I am now able to prioritise my desire to become more therapeutic and am developing the critical awareness necessary to help me realise these desires in actual practice. Developing an inner strength is my next challenge if I wish to restore a sense of self-integrity. Indeed this is the next major challenge for health visiting if health visitors genuinely wish to embrace the notion of true partnership with clients. However, within child protection work, there seems to be a weakness of professional identity and attitude that has resulted in collusion with the perceived values of social services and this needs to be further explored.

Collusion with social services may have been facilitated due to the increased bureau-cratisation and rigidity of framework for health visitor involvement in child protection work since the publication of the Children Act 1989. This act outlines the duties and responsibilities of health authorities and National Health Service (NHS) trusts in relation to child protection work. Significantly, the Act recommended the 'identifica-tion of the senior nurse with a health visiting qualification as a designated senior profes-sional to become a member of the Area Child Protection Committee' and also the 'identification of a named nurse/midwife for child protection matters' (Department of Health 1998:3). These new posts together with the Act's emphasis on duty to comply with requests for help from a local authority have laid a foundation for increasing links between health visiting and social services in child protection work. This has been to the extent that health visiting is increasingly and mistakenly described as being a statu-tory agency (Browne 1994). Although it is recognised that the Children Act 1989 imposed no statutory duties on health authorities, there has been a strengthening of bureaucratic links with statutory agencies especially those with social service departments and this may account for the misconception of the health visitor role. Increased bureaucratisa-tion may also have contributed to the weakening of professional autonomy in health visiting. Hall (1968) has suggested that there is a tendency for autonomous professions to be less not more bureaucratic and that a 'rigid hierarchy of authority seems more incompatible with a high level of professionalism' (p103). The increasing rigidity of framework to health visitor intervention in child protection work may have contributed to the perception of less autonomy and control. It may be that health visitors who have not been given the space or time to consider these issues have become blinded by the reality of this oppression, and so believe that becoming more like social services is the most effective way to gain power and control (Roberts 1983). Freire's (1972) work suggests, however, that identification with the oppressor results in a loss of sense of individual awareness, self-esteem and confidence. This ensures that a cycle of oppression is set into motion, which, in turn, perpetuates the perception of subordination. It is possible to see that within this cycle a weak sense of professional identity could emerge. Hall (1968) suggested that some 'established professions have rather weakly developed professional attitudes', the strength of which 'appears to be based on the kind of sociali-sation that has taken place both in the profession's training programme and in the work itself' (p. 103). It therefore seems that both in training and practice, health visitors must find a way to unveil, examine, and challenge dominant values in order to break the cycle of oppression and to strengthen professional attitude (Watson 1990). Restoring a sense of professional integrity will enable a caring morality to emerge and to shape future practice congruent with our beliefs and values about the nature of desirable practice.

Guided reflection strikes at the very core of an oppressive cycle by providing the safe place necessary to facilitate awareness and fuel conflict (Johns 1998). I can see the source of oppression at face value so that although my own position is intolerable, it is within my power to change the situation. Within my continuing struggle for self-determination, it is a time of creativity, strength of purpose and strength of will. This developing sense of inner being relates well to the attainment of a sense of self-mastery and self-competence within the 'era of incorporation' (see Table 7.1). I have rejected the misplaced, negative images of health visiting in favour of a truer, clearer understanding of my position in terms of relative power. That in itself is strengthening and in becoming strengthened I know that I am now far more likely to be able to sustain an empowering, therapeutic relationship with Helen.

Fifth guided reflection session

I had talked to Jo again about Helen and had also seen Helen during a visit to the nursery and Jo had telephoned to let me know the outcome of her supervision session. She said she felt disgusted at the response of her manager. She felt there had been no co-operation. Her manager's retort that Helen was definitely not allowed to have access to the records made Jo angry. Yet she was also anxious. She feared she could get the sack for talking like this. She had tried to express her view, which was very similar to mine, but this had been to no avail. She said there was nothing more that she could do and said that unlike me, she would not be able to surface her feelings of disgust about it in supervision. We compared supervision experiences. Jo was supervised by her line manager, who was far more likely to scrutinise her practice than to help her clarify her beliefs and values. I explained that my supervision experience had been empowering and had encouraged me to focus on finding ways to empower my clients. Jo wanted to support me. She said that she had not realised health visitors became involved in advocacy work with clients. We talked about this and other types of therapeutic interventions in health visiting. I told her that Helen had said she had made an official complaint to social services over 18 months ago, and that although the complaint had been acknowledged, there had been no further response. Jo said that she would ask her manager to write to her and that she would telephone Helen to talk about this. She gave me names of the people she thought Helen could contact to make a complaint and said she would send me a copy of the 'complaints' procedure. She wished me luck.

A few days later I met Helen and the children at the nursery. Jo had explained to her that she couldn't have access to the notes because they were officially the children's notes. She seemed pleased she had at last received a letter but said she was still angry and concerned about the possibility of her son gaining access to the notes in the future. She wanted to be given the opportunity to clear her name. She seemed a lot calmer and more receptive to my help. We talked about the possibilities of recommencing counselling sessions in the New Year. She said she found it difficult to focus on counselling when she was feeling so angry but was willing to try when Natasha had settled into the nursery. I suggested that she put her thoughts and complaints down in writing and gave her the list of names Jo had given me. Helen seemed keen to pursue this and so we arrange to meet after Christmas in order to allow time for a response.

I have generated many more questions than answers but I can see the common thread of oppression and empowerment through the sessions. It is clear that I am further along than Jo in my journey or struggle towards self-determination as reflected in our contrasting supervision styles. Jo had indicated that the underlying emphasis of her supervision was concerned with ensuring she responded in normative ways reflected in her sense of being monitored and controlled. It had been a revelation for her to realise the emphasis of supervision could be empowering. Johns (199) has revealed the stark contrast between a controlling and emancipatory style of supervision depending on the intent and emphasis of the supervisor.

My conversation with Jo had fuelled her sense of conflict to the extent that she began to articulate her own sense of powerlessness and this had been a revelation to me. Up until this point it seemed to me that Jo had passively accepted these constraints and they were so powerful that even with an increased awareness, she had still felt unable to support me in an overt way. Her supervision silenced her to the extent she could only speak with her supervisor's words rather than her own. Freire (1972) believes that in doing this the 'oppressor' who has stolen the words of others will begin to develop doubts in the abilities and competence of others and in turn will become 'more accustomed to power and acquire a taste for guiding, ordering and commanding' (p. 104). In contrasting our supervision, Jo felt her position to be intolerable and that she had nowhere to go to explore this dissatisfaction in a critical way. She felt trapped within a cycle of oppression where there was no opportunity to find a way towards emancipation from the conditions of domination. I can now more easily comprehend why Helen and I have often felt it has been an uphill struggle to gain support from social workers. It must be difficult for social workers to become empowering as practitioners under such a regime. In the light of my understanding of the increasing influence of social services on health visiting, it was now important to further consider the impact of Jo's experience on my desire to become an empowering practitioner.

Whilst comparing my supervision with Jo's had been illuminating I knew my experience was by no means universal. Supervision within health visiting child protection work has historically developed in a way that mimics social work supervision (Bond and Holland 1998). Recently, Scott (1999), a health visitor child protection adviser, declared that 'the value of supervision in child protection work is constructively to challenge, guide, and direct the contribution of all practitioners in the multi-disciplinary prevention of abuse' (p. 762). Scott highlighted the way supervision can be linked to the annual individual performance review to help identify weak practice. She clearly demonstrates her support of the notion that supervision in child protection work can be used to monitor and control. There is evidence that this style of supervision in child protection work is being imposed on health visitors in the same way it is currently imposed on social workers. Recently, health visitors in Bedfordshire received a proposal for a mandatory protocol for supervision of child protection work and management of poor practice. The protocol stated that supervision sessions would become mandatory for all professionals who have completed a CP1 (initial child protection referral form) and for those with children on their caseloads who are on the Child Protection Register. It also stated that 'in the event that poor practice is identified during a supervisory session the matter will, in the first instance, be discussed with the individual and then referred on to the child protection advisor for further consideration'. The aim of this style of supervision is obviously to 'police' and to control the workforce, and as such, is disempowering by nature. Braye and Preston-Shoot (1995) note 'for empowerment in social care to have meaning, the organisational culture must move away from that of power (control of expert) and role 'emphasis on given tasks and procedures) to that of community (learning with users). Such a culture would seek to use and enhance the power and authority held by users, while recognising that professional power and authority remain legally mandated, and may have to be exercised' (p. 115). My work with Helen has helped me to understand the ways in which as a health visitor I can unwittingly collude with oppressive forces and so compromise my professional practice. Especially in child protection work where organisational aspects become more complex due to a blending of ideologies' it is essential that we are able to maintain a sense of control over our working culture if we are to succeed in becoming empowering practitioners. In order to achieve this goal an empowering type of supervision would seem essential.

Sixth guided reflection session

Before I met Chris in session six I sent him an e-mail:

Yesterday something wonderful happened. I'm still reeling. When I went into work there were messages from various people who were all very concerned about Helen and her children. From the moment I picked up the messages I tuned into you and I thought of all the things you have taught me in guided reflection. I thought of Helen and began to draw together all the fragmented strands of knowing. I looked into myself becoming more and more in harmony with her. It felt like nothing I've experienced before. I just knew that whatever I did next would be good for Helen and would protect the children. AND IT WORKED! It is a long story that I cannot wait to tell you. After a very long and tiring day with Helen, the children, child care social workers, mental health care social workers, psychiatrists and managers, the children were protected and happy in a foster home and Helen was in hospital receiving the care she desperately needed. None of this would have happened if Helen and I had not been so connected.

This had been an emotional and passionate communication. It had felt like stars were colliding. All our work within supervision had come together in a way that enabled me to intervene in time to prevent harm to the children. This work had become living evidence of a new and effective way to protect children through health visiting and guided reflection.

I described the intervention by reading my last journal entry to Chris:

The messages I received had been from the school nurse and the headmistress (Mrs Johnson) of Robert's school. Luckily the school nurse was in her office and I was able to talk to her. She said that Mrs Johnson had become increasingly concerned about Helen's mental health over the last two weeks. She said Robert was coming into school late, sometimes not arriving until lunchtime. Helen had been striking up strange, inappropriate conversation full of sexual innuendo with members of staff and writing long, confused letters to Mrs Johnson. I telephoned Mrs Johnson who confirmed her anxieties. She said she had contacted the duty child care team at social services. I contacted the duty officer (Lynne) who had taken Mrs Johnson's referral. Lynne said she had received two referrals expressing concerns about the family. The other referral was from a worried neighbour. Despite this, she had decided to pass these referrals on to the mental health care team. I registered my concern by saying that I wished to refer the family back to the child care duty team. I explained that the children had both previously been on the Child Protection Register and that although no longer registered, there were still child protection concerns in relation to mum's mental health. The social worker explained that a visit had been organised for Monday afternoon by a member of the mental health care team. I telephoned Helen. I asked her how she was feeling and she said 'awful'. I asked her if she needed help and she replied 'yes'. I asked her if she would like to go into hospital and again she simply replied 'yes'. She began to cry. I said that I would like to come straight over to see her and bring a social worker with me. She agreed saying 'I'm not coping with the children'. I could hear them laughing and screaming in the background. I immediately telephoned social services and they agreed to visit that (Friday) morning. I took the mental health care social worker (Kay) in my car and we arranged to meet Lynne at the house. When we arrived, Kay said she would rather wait for Lynne to arrive. I said I felt uncomfortable sitting outside Helen's home and I went to knock on the door. I was shocked when I saw her. She looked so tired and drawn. Her hair was greasy and lank and her clothes were dirty and had been put on inside out. As soon as she saw me she started to cry and I still remember the sadness I felt as she led me through the house. Although Robert is six years old, he was running around wearing nothing except a nappy, a T-shirt and a crucifix tied around his neck by a boot lace. Both he and his sister were wild, running and screaming amongst chaotic piles of toys, wet laundry, remains of food and other debris. One minute Helen was crying and the next she was laughing. Robert was eating a biscuit and I asked him if he was hungry. He took my hand to show me 'what Mummy cooked for dinner'. It was a saucepan full of the charcoal remains of a wooden spoon and a newspaper. He said 'we all watched the fire until it went out'. By this time the social workers had come in and Kay had started to assess the state of Helen's mental health. She concluded that it was not necessary to admit her to hospital. In disbelief I showed her the saucepan and said that although I was not trained in mental health nursing, it was obvious to me that she needed help and could not be left alone to cope with the children. Eventually it was agreed that Helen should be admitted on a voluntary basis and that the children should be taken into foster care. However, Helen refused to sign the document. To my amazement, Lynne responded by saying that there was nothing more she could do if that was the case and stood up as if she ready to leave! I offered to read the document to Helen and after some moments she said that she would only sign it if I read it to her. There was so much trust between us. Soon after this there was a flurry of telephone calls and the children left quite happily with Lynne. Robert seemed relieved. He said 'You are taking mummy away to make her better aren't you?' Kay and I took Helen straight to hospital and the consultant later decided that she was suffering from an acute episode of manic depression. I attended a decision-making meeting at social services the other day and was shocked to find out that it had been organised even though Helen was still in hospital and so was unable to attend. I immediately expressed my concern that this meeting should go ahead without her and they agreed to cancel and re-schedule the meeting. It was so easy. The whole feeling of the meeting was somehow different.'

Chris asked me to clarify what I thought was different about this situation. It was because the social worker who chaired the session seemed to know everything about the history of Helen's case. She may well have read my letters to social services and comments I had made at meetings over the last year. They may at last have had an impact. Anyway something had changed and it was more empowering for Helen so I was pleased.

Within those moments my responses had been natural, confident and in harmony with the needs of the family. Helen and I had worked together in true partnership. Yet without the trust and connection that had been nurtured in guided reflection, I could not have intervened in such an effective and preventive way at this acute time of need. The session demonstrates how I have developed a critical awareness within the supervision process that has brought about a sense of maturity and competence as described by Kieffer's fourth phase of involvement (see Table 7.1). At this level, Kieffer considers that it becomes more possible to integrate apply personal knowing in a meaningful and proactive way. He points out, this awareness can be difficult to achieve without the support of an external enabler. In moving as I move, in tune with my needs, my supervisor has been a dynamic and strengthening influence and had mirrored my desire to become empowered in practice. Such is the parallel nature of work within supervision and clinical practice when the underlying commitment is to become more available to work with others in therapeutic ways. Whilst I am aware that the struggle towards emergence will always continue, I also have an overwhelming feeling I have moved on, have chosen a good path and that things will never be quite the same again.

Seventh guided reflection session

Helen has been discharged from hospital. She and the children were well. I have attended two case review meetings at social services. One was a positive experience the other one was very negative. The first review meeting went very well for Helen. She had been allowed to bring her friend into the meeting to act as an advocate because she had said that sometimes she was unable to explain herself clearly and was consequently often misinterpreted. The chairperson encouraged her to talk throughout the meeting and listened attentively to the advocate. In the end, the decisions made were based primarily on Helen's wishes. It was decided that she would continue to have increasing access to the children and they would return home when she had fully recovered. She seemed relaxed and happy. It had been the first time that she had ever truly participated at a meeting in my experience.

Chris perceptibly questions, 'Something has changed?' Indeed. There has been a noticeable shift in perception and attitudes. It has been a gradual shift that has recently gathered momentum. When I think back to my first piece of reflective work with Helen, I recall the ripple effect of my own change of perception. looking at labelling theory helped me to understand the ways Helen had been affected. Labelling had negatively influenced our early relationship. This, and other early reflections helped me to critically question my perceptions and to see the true Helen. Gradually, others began to change their perceptions and became more sensitive and co-operative towards her. I attribute the more recent changes to our joint determination to continue to be seen and heard. We are both emerging with a sense of inner confidence. At the case review meeting, everyone took great care to ensure she had her say. It was wonderful.

Chris challenged me, 'How did it differ during the next meeting?' The next meeting was awful. I was told that the chairperson, Mrs Granite, was a social services child protection team leader. Things started to go wrong from the outset. When Helen explained she had brought an advocate, Mrs Granite said the advocate could support but not talk.

Chris challenged me, 'Did you question this?'

I replied 'Not at that point. I was quite shocked. We were asked to read through the care assessment carried out by Helen' two social workers. As Helen began to read it she became quite agitated. Due to her past experiences she feels very threatened by this kind of document. She didn't agree with some points but was firmly denied the right to comment. Mrs Granite reminded Helen that she had already been given time to read through it. I suggested to Helen that it might help her to write her feelings down on paper. She agreed and so I asked Mrs Granite if it would be possible to include her comments in the report. Mrs Granite's reaction was startling. Reminding me that she was the chairperson and had not asked me to speak, she entirely disregarded the idea. I resolved to have my say in the meeting when it was my turn to speak. During the discussion about Helen, however, I was not asked to contribute at all. Instead I was asked to comment about the children. As it was apparent to me that the discussion regarding Helen had ended, I said I would like to discuss the outcomes of a conversation between Helen and I regarding future support. She had told me of her fears and concerns about the future and we wanted to make sure there was a safety net of support in operation in case she became suddenly ill again. At this point Mrs Granite asked me to clarify my involvement with the family. I explained about the nature of my supportive work with Helen. I must have used the word 'therapeutic' because suddenly she exclaimed, 'You are a health visitor and you do not have a therapeutic role! Your job is to assess children's development. I've been a social worker for 20 years and I should know the role of the health visitor by now!' Although shocked at the inappropriateness of this outburst, I felt confident and talked to Mrs Granite about the nature of health visiting interventions with parents and children. I offered to send her a recent paper that uncovers the therapeutic role of the health visitor (Cody 1999). Suddenly Helen said, 'I have no problem, I understand her role'.

Chris interjected: 'A profound moment?'

I felt very calm. I found myself using the Burford cues (Johns 2009) that I now use so naturally within interactions. I thought of Mrs Granite and asked myself: 'How does this person make me feel?' I visualised the space between us. I was able within those moments to remind myself of our separate roles especially in terms of power. She suddenly seemed far less threatening. I asked myself 'Who is this person?' and thought of her role in child protection. The previous chairperson had not been a child protection social worker and their styles were so different. I wondered whether her oppressive style arose form her beliefs and values about her practice or from the culture she worked within. Perhaps it was a bit of both, but whatever the cause she could have been overwhelmingly powerful.

Chris again interjected: 'But she wasn't?'

No. Both Helen and I were able to respond in a convincing and assertive way. My comments about the safety net were acknowledged and discussed and everyone listened to Helen talking about her fears for the future. I then went on to discuss the children's general development. We had our say despite the odds and actually we were the powerful ones!

Chris asks, 'What is significant?'

The second meeting was not as awful as I thought. I managed to shift the balance of power which enabled a positive outcome for Helen, chipping away at the same old block and it finally paid off. Helen has become increasingly confident, able to assert her own ideas about the future safety of her children, and people are listening! I feel very optimistic that we will be able to protect the children from harm in the future.

Chris affirms, 'Your mutual sense of empowerment shines through your words.'

I respond, 'Its true. I do feel empowered and it has rubbed off on Helen.'

Despite the odds, Helen and I had articulated our wishes and contribute our ideas with a heightened inner clarity and confidence. It was a time of transition into a newer way of knowing. Through the empowering and parallel nature of guided reflection we had both found a way to reclaim our sense of self. Belenky *et al.* (1986) refer to this as speaking with a *constructed voice*, where women have learnt to speak with a unique, authentic, informed and passionate voice. This voice transcends the *subjective voice* whereby women have an increased sense of private authority but lack the 'tools for expressing themselves or persuading others to listen' (p. 134). As my story reveals, there is a 'transition from sense of self as helpless victim to acceptance of self as an assertive and efficacious citizen' (Kieffer 1984:33). Fay (1987) describes this combination of power and will as emancipation, or a 'state of reflective clarity in which people know which of their wants are genuine because they finally know who they really are, and a state of collective autonomy in which they have the power to determine rationally and freely the nature and direction of their collective existence' (p. 205). Helen and I were both developing this sense of self-determination. Our work was now taking the form of cultural action (Freire 1972) witnessed in the transformative change in others' attitudes and shift in the balance of power in our favour.

Conclusion

I have repeatedly referred to my experiences of guided reflection as having been an unfolding journey. It felt as though I was at the foot of a hill that obscured my view but only needed to be climbed to reveal new and exciting pastures. It turned out to be a long and steep climb along a path strewn with boulders that impeded my journey of realisation. With commitment I persevered, dissolving or shifting the boulders through understanding and empowerment.

My understanding became increasingly involved and complex as new insights emerged into my consciousness, peeling back the layers of self-distortion in order to reveal myself to myself, and clear the path to reach my goal. The turning point came just before Christmas between the fifth and sixth sessions when I felt as if I had reached the top of the hill revealing a whole new vista. I had been able to construct a better way for health visitors. My work suggests demonstrates that child protection work often contradicts the espoused philosophy of health visiting and so becomes a source of tension for health visitors. Perhaps health visitors feel uncertain about their role, which leads to a lack of confidence and a passive acceptance of the status quo. This has resulted in an increasing alignment with the secondary preventative 'detection work' that has traditionally been the focus of social work. This alignment is apparent in the way supervision within child protection work is currently being developed and which mimics the style of social work supervision that, through Jo's experience, appears as fundamentally disempowering.

Significantly, examination of current government initiatives reveals that there is an opportunity for health visitors to become proactive and creative and to develop a new way of working based on intensive and effective primary care interventions. It is therefore time for health visitors to take stock of our position within child protection work. My work indicates that in forging blindly ahead and increasing our surveillance role and crisis intervention work, we are increasingly departing from our espoused beliefs about desirable practice.

The experiences I continue to share in guided reflection affirm my new way of health visiting as if I am free falling down the hill. I have become more positive, confident and assertive. In many ways I realise this story is just the beginning. As Belenky *et al.* (1986) note, 'even amongst women who feel they have found their voice, problems with voice abound' (p. 146). The ongoing struggle for constructivist woman is not to find voice but to make others listen. This must mean developing a collective voice that can effectively challenge not only perceived internal constraints but oppressive and disempowering work cultures. It is my assertion that this can be achieved through the empowering and transformative process of guided reflection.

Footnote

Yvonne's narrative has been slightly edited from the original published in the first edition. Whilst the references to the literature may now seem dated, the issues remain fresh today. Health visiting continues to struggle with its identity and role in response to government initiatives.

The narrative is an exemplar of empowerment, the struggle to understand and shift forces of oppression towards leading more satisfactory lives – Yvonne's fundamental insight into the reciprocal relationship between her own empowerment and the empowerment of her client. As Yvonne became empowered through guided reflection (as framed within the narrative by the work of Kieffer and Belenky *et al.*) so did her client – both emerging from a victimic sense of self to an agentic sense of self as they began to take control of their respective lives (Polkingthorne 1996).

References

Appleton J and Clemerson J (1999) Family-based interventions with children in need. *Communnity Practitioner* 72:134–136.

Appleton J and Cowley S (1997) Analysing clinical practice guidelines. A method of documentary analysis. *Journal of Advanced Nursing* 25:1008–1017.

Batey M and Lewis F (1982) Clarifying autonomy and accountability in nursing services: Part 1. *Journal of Nursing Administration* 12:13–18.

Belenky M, Clinch B, Goldberger N and Tarule J (1986) *Women's ways of knowing: the development of self, voice and mind.* Basic Books, New York.

Bell M (1995) A study of the attitudes of nurses to parental involvement in the initial child-protection conference, and their preparation for it. *Journal of Advanced Nursing* 22:250–257.

Bidmead C (1999) Bidding for success: making a sure start application. *Community Practitioner* 72:166–167.

Bond M and Holland S (1998) *Skills of clinical supervision for nurses.* Open University Press, Buckingham.

Braye S and Preston-Shoot M (1995) *Empowering practice in social care.* Open University Press, Buckingham.

Browne K (1994) Preventing child maltreatment through community nursing. *Journal of Advanced Nursing* 21:57–63.

Cody (1999) Health visiting as therapy: a phenomenological perspective. *Journal of Advanced Nursing* 29(1):1–8.

Collinson S and Cowley S (1998) An exploratory study of demand for the health visiting service within a marketing framework. *Journal of Advanced Nursing* 28:499–507.

Cook A (1999) The well family service: a new model of support. *Community Practitioner* 72:168–171.

Department of Health (1995) *Health visiting: working in the community.* HMSO, London.

Department of Health (1998) *Child protection for senior nurses, midwives, and their managers.* HMSO, London.

Dingwall R (1982) Community nursing and civil liberty. *Journal of Advanced Nursing* 7:337–346.

Dolan B and Kitson A (1997) Future imperatives: developing health visiting in response to changing demands. *Journal of Clinical Nursing* 6:11–16.

Fay B (1987) *Critical social science.* Polity Press, Cambridge.

Freire P (1972) *Pedagogy of the oppressed.* Penguin Books, London.

Glew A and Heron H (1998) Child protection: developing a personal child health record. *Community Practitioner* 71:328–329.

Goodwin S (1988) Whither health visiting? *Health Visitor* 61:328–332.

Hall M (1996) *Health for all children.* Oxford University Press, Oxford.

Hall R (1968) Professionalization and bureaucratization. *American Sociological Review* 33:92–104.

Holden R (1990) Responsibility and autonomous nursing practice. *Journal of Advanced Nursing* 16:398–403.

Jackson C (1994) Strelley: teamworking for health visiting. *Health Visitor* 67:28–29.

Johns C (1998) Opening the doors of perception. In: C Johns and D Freshwater (eds.) *Transforming nursing through reflective practice.* Blackwell Science, Oxford.

Johns C (1999) Unravelling the dilemmas within everyday nursing practice. *Nursing Ethics* 6:287–298.

Johns C (2009) *Becoming a reflective practitioner* (third edition). Wiley-Blackwell, Oxford.

Kieffer C (1984) Citizen empowerment: a developmental perspective. *Prevention in Human Services* 84:9–36.

Okri B (1997) *A way of being free.* Phoenix House, London. Text extracts used with permission of The Marsh Agency Ltd.

Orr J (1990) First principles. *Health Visitor* 63:368.

Pike A (1991) Moral outrage and moral discourse in nurse-physician collaboration. *Journal of Professional Nursing* 7:351–363.

Polkingthorne DE (1996) Transformative narratives: from victimic to agentic life plots. *American Journal of Occupational Therapy* 50(4):299–305.

Roberts S (1983) Oppressed group behaviour: implications for nursing. *Advances in Nursing Science* 5:21–30.

Scott L (1999) The nature and structure of supervision in health visiting with victims of child sexual abuse. *Journal of Advanced Nursing* 29:754–763.

Singleton E and Nail F (1984) Autonomy in nursing. *Nursing Forum* 3:123–130.

Sure Start: A guide for trailblazers (1999) DfEE Publications, Suffolk.

Taylor S and Tilley N (1989) Health visitors and child protection: conflict contradictions and ethical dilemmas. *Health Visitor* 62:273–275.

Turner T (1998/9) The family way. *Community Practitioner* 71:398–400.

Van Manen M (1990) *Researching lived experience.* State University of New York Press, New York.

Watson J (1990) The moral failure of the patriarchy. *Nursing Outlook* 38:62–66.

Weinsheimer J (1985) *Gadamer's hermeneutics: a reading of truth & method.* Yale University Press, New York.

Welshman J (1997) Family visitors or social workers? Health visiting and public health in England and Wales 1890–1974. *International History of Nursing Journal* 2:5–22.

Chapter 8

Falling through the net and the spider's web: two metaphoric moments along my journey

Maria Fordham

> I feel as if I have been part of the narrative of liberation for UK (Homeless) health professionals over the past year; a huge sway, almost gathering arms to network and connect so that our (homeless) communities are also liberated and empowered in their individual life journeys. (Queens Nursing Institute [QNI] 2008:23)

In an area of practice where practitioners reported feeling isolated (QNI 2007) the above quote formed part of my response to a Homeless Health Initiative (HHI) questionnaire focusing on the way HHI had supported homelessness practitioners in the UK by networking at many levels, from professional development to political intervention. The stirring call has since been used as a backdrop canopy for speakers in the first Homeless Nursing Conference held in the UK (Opening Doors Homeless and Nursing Conference 12 May 2009 – London), as well as concluding the HHI impact report for 2007–2008 (QNI 2008). In this chapter I shall to continue using the crucial theme of *net* work in homeless health practice, viewed metaphorically as a professional 'army gathering arms to *network*' together *but* more significantly to illuminate the way homeless people *fall through the net* of health services and other local services, which subsequently further affects their health and well-being.

In the three-year narrative of self-inquiry and transformation towards self-realisation, *Falling through the net* is one of 30 stories that plot my narrative journey. Using Johns (2006) 'Six Dialogical Movements' framework throughout the reflexive narrative, I aim to illuminate the practice of health and homelessness in my specialist public health nurse role, as I tighten and weave the *net* to improve the health and well-being of homeless and vulnerably housed people in the locality in which I work. In this chapter I present *Spaghetti junction* which was presented to the PhD/MPhil reflective guidance group, which meets monthly under the leadership of Professor Johns.

The story begins …

Spaghetti junction

Wednesday, 6 March 2008

I muse on how housing, health and social care systems simultaneously curve around each other like rigid steel trajectories, entwined yet disconnected, and ponder on the ability of vulnerable or homeless people to negotiate them, particularly when they are alone and ill. So, what happens when there is a break-down on Spaghetti Junction?

Edward and Tristan are upper-middle class, intelligent men who speak with English public school accents. Both live alone in different parts of the country; both are in housing crisis, both are lost and desolate, yet one had become an unwilling and time-limited carer to the other. For nearly two months, Tristan has been stuck on Edward's grotty, 'Miss Havisham' floor; doubly incontinent, deeply depressed, continually scratching, and unable to adequately converse – broken down – physically and mentally, much like his beloved silver Porsche, which even now lies abandoned outside Edward's Victorian home. In that time, Edward himself has become *the* ghostly Miss Havisham figure, paler by the day with long unkempt hair, billowing like the long cobwebs hanging like grand chandeliers from the high ceiling of his damp bed-sit. He too had become *stuck; stuck* in a caring role which had been unwittingly thrust upon him.

On New Year's Day a crisis mental health team arrived at Edward's drab bed-sit to assess Tristan's mental health. Unaware of Tristan's abandoned silver Porche, they advised Edward that Tristan should return to his home town two hours drive away for ongoing care 'or else go to Accident and Emergency services if a further crisis emerged'. Tristan was unable to do either and continued instead, to access temporary registration with Edward's GP, who, it was reported, found Edward's caring role highly amusing. In frustration Edward had brought Tristan to my health access clinic at the homeless day centre. Over the next month my jacquard intervention sought to connect health and housing professionals to Tristan's crisis, to his aloneness and to his physical and mental inability to return to his home town. Edward had said:

> No-one has looked out for him ... no one wants to care for him. ... This man will be dead in six months. He is dying of a broken heart and loneliness.

Steinbeck's words on loneliness crossed my mind:

> A guy needs somebody ... to be near him. A guy goes nuts if he ain't got nobody. Don't make no difference who the guy is, long's he's with you. I tell ya, I tell ya a guy gets too lonely an' he gets sick. (Steinbeck 1937:72–73)

Heartache and loneliness connected these two men as e-mail companions. Perhaps, I mused, Edward is right – the spiralling effects of loneliness could cause one to die – or at least become very ill. In Tristan's case a brief but ill-fated relationship with a married woman had crushed him. At its height, he had been transported to a state of bliss and union, but unable to cope with a broken romance he had since lost his way in life, and lost his dream. The broken romance had triggered depression, and shortly afterwards, a bipolar disorder[1] was diagnosed during an acute unit mental health stay in his home town.

---

[1]Bipolar disorder is a brain disease, or group of diseases, associated with periods of depressed mood as well as periods of particularly elevated or irritable mood. Although generally episodic, it is nearly always recurrent and life-long. Recent

Discharged 'too early', in Edward's opinion, Tristan had subsequently squandered a significant inheritance in 'madness', mostly on fast cars. Yet, until his detour to Edward's house over Christmas he had still continued to be employed as a systems analyst.

During the dark, winter days of his debilitation, I continued to push through *walls of resistance* erected by the mental health team because Tristan did not live in this area and was not permanently registered with a local GP:

> Walls of resistance
> that rise
> Like prehistoric, serrated rocks
> On a silent, turbulent sea
> Walls that exclude
> Making the visible, invisible
> Walls that stop flow
> Towards healing
>
> Walls – who are you?
>
> I push you
> With soft, pointed words
> Easing your granite form
> To shift
> And create onward flow

Languishing in Lauer (2008), I pondered on the walls. Were they erected because of the mental health team's lack of compassion and understanding of the total situation (Lauer 2008)?[2] Did *their* resistance to engagement arise from a lack of resources (Lauer 2008)? What stopped them recognising the need for timely intervention to avoid involuntary hospitalisations? Lauer (2008) describes this as a form of criminalisation.

As I sought to move the mental health team's perception beyond the 'ordinary awareness of the world (which) serves as the basis of (our) responses and actions' (Polkinghorne 1983:10), I kept Tristan's needs visible, requesting a copy of the mental health assessment, and negotiating and persuading the team to support Tristan,[3] so that a period of stability could be reached, after which he would return to his home town for ongoing care. On the very day that the team agreed to do another mental health assessment, Tristan was brought into accident and emergency and admitted urgently to a medical ward – not to a mental health unit.

I approach Tristan on the six-bedded bay, wondering whether he has the cognitive ability to recognise me from those clinic meetings. Sky blue, hospital pyjamas cover much of his lean body. His head is neatly clothed by wavy, white hair and rests uncomfortably on the metal head rest. 'Hello Tristan, how are you? I'm Maria – do you remember me from clinic?' Eyes, previously lost in an unfocused gaze on a busy ward, light up as he

---

epidemiological data confirm that bipolar disorder is both chronic and disabling. Bipolar disorder is associated with significant mortality; lifetime risk of death from suicide approaches 20 times that of the general population (Perlis 2005).

[2]Citing Camilli *et al.* (2005), Lauer describes how patients presenting in mental health crisis at an emergency department were provided with adequate medical care to stabilise them, but their care often lacked compassion from nursing staff.

[3]Normally patients must be permanently registered with a local GP for the team to offer care. (Yet research clearly indicates that homeless people have difficulty in accessing permanent GP registration.)

sits forward. I touch his arm in greeting, wondering about his cognitive capacity to communicate with me. Each short reply is concluded with my name demonstrating a politeness and accent that marks his upbringing. Indeed, politeness emanates from him and through him, almost as if he were *a* lonely white cloud, floating high in the sky above his own life, high beyond those convoluted steel roadways of Spaghetti Junction – aware of his predicament and detached from it; showing passivity, and an inability to enter into the turmoil and lostness that would ground him. Edward had previously called it 'brain freeze'!

> 'I'm not too good, Maria.'
> 'Are you feeling any better than when I saw you in clinic, Tristan?'
> 'I'm not sure, Maria.'

In his debilitating depression I had expected him to be on an acute psychiatric ward but here he is on a medical ward, ready to be discharged. Can he really have made such a remarkable recovery in so short a period of time? The ward sister had phoned me asking for guidance on the discharge of a homeless person – but why had she pronounced him homeless?

It seems that Edward had ceremoniously dumped all of Tristan's belongings on the hospital ward, unwilling to provide him with further ongoing care or lodgings, and uncompromisingly declared Tristan '*homeless*', perhaps in an attempt to get him the professional care that he felt was needed. Edward had not been back on the ward to see him since. Supporting the *homeless* theme, Tristan believed that the tenancy for his flat was jeopardised because he has not been there or paid his rent since Christmas, and he felt the 'dodgy' landlord would not hold it open for him. Swirling loss and chilling words sweep around an emotional numbness:

> 'I had my credit cards stolen ... they threatened to break my legs. The landlord will have let it out now. I haven't got money. I haven't got any keys.'

Downward spirals into *homelessness* continue in his trajectory of demise caused by ill health.

> 'Is your car still outside Edward's house, Tristan?'
> 'I don't know Maria.'

In my mind's eye, accumulated parking tickets stick unceremoniously to the windscreen whilst clamped wheels deny the Porsche its freedom on the road. Worried that Tristan's financial destitution could deepen, I phone the police later to alert them to Tristan's redundant, silver Porsche.

> 'Do you think you will be able to look after yourself Tristan? Can you drive – cook meals and feed yourself – the doctors believe you are well enough to be discharged? I am just wondering how you feel about that and where you would like to be discharged too.'
> 'I don't know Maria ... I haven't any clothes.'

I sense Tristan's enormous hesitancy about going '*home*'. I am concerned, too, about his ability to cope alone, to negotiate traffic or transport to get '*home*' and, once '*home*', to negotiate and advocate for his own health needs – even though the medics feel he is fit enough to be discharged. Whilst my good practice[4] acclaimed Admission and Discharge Protocol of Homeless People (Shelter 2007) lays dust laden in the filing cabinet, I am mindful of government guidance on hospital discharge:

> Safe discharge is the duty of the hospital trust. (CLG/DH 2006:4)

And on homelessness, the Government states:

> It is vital all hospitals consider the housing situation of patients to ensure that people are not discharge to inappropriate places, homeless or become homeless as a result of their stay in hospital. (DH 2003:74)

As Tristan has nowhere to go home too the hospital discharge could be at odds with the government guidance, particularly if he is discharged to the night shelter. The creative tension I felt with mental health team stirs within me as systems again allow people to *fall through the net*. What will I do to improve Tristan's care? What would you do?

As Tristan moves on the hospital bed, the odour of sweat, scented pyjamas remind me about his entry into destitution – the request for a warm second hand jacket on that cold, January morning, in the day centre. The jacket didn't seem to quite fit, much like Tristan's awkwardness in the homeless world that surrounded him. His 'I'm not sure Maria', 'I don't know Maria' and embarrassed 'Sorry Maria' answers cement my reservations about Tristan's inability to function independently and provide me with the evidence to challenge his pending discharge. I probe the ward sister about practitioners' observations, putting the practicalities of discharging him into reality for them – changing perceptions, challenging their discharge culture.

> Do you think he can do a two-hour drive ... and care for himself now? Can he discuss his needs with you ... Does he speak with you in more than one or two sentences?
> Sister replies: No he doesn't say much at all. He does shower and eat .... But we remind him. There is no way he could drive all that way. He is having a psychiatric assessment tomorrow prior to his discharge ... just in case ... but otherwise the medics say he is well enough to go home.

'*Home*' – that word again. She uses it as if she has forgotten that she has asked me to guide the discharge process because of the possible absence of a *home* for Tristan to go to.

> She adds: He is being investigated for Huntington's chorea[5] ... such a horrible disease. We have tried to tell him but we don't know whether he understands.

Huntington's chorea – a horrible disease! So, that may be the answer to Tristan's continuing mental and physical demise. And if he is going to be homeless or vulnerably housed, it is a further major issue which triggers concerns.

---

[4]Shelter dedicated a paragraph to the developing protocol I have used in my area, developed from Homeless Link guidance on Admission and Discharge of Homeless People, but with my workload and the multi-agency co-ordination it needs I can only work on it periodically.

[5]Huntington's disease, chorea or disorder is an incurable neurodegenerative genetic disorder that affects muscle co-ordination and some cognitive functions, typically becoming noticeable in middle age. (Wikipedia)

I reply: How sad, Huntington's chorea is progressive and he is only just coping in a safe hospital environment – but what is it going to be like for him out there – especially if he is likely to become more debilitated. He will need coordinated support and secure housing. That takes time to arrange.

She nods in agreement, although timidly, and an outbreak of norovirus[6] seem to preoccupy her. 'Staff nurse,' she cries 'bed 3 is vomiting.' Acknowledging the stresses the ward staff are under, I confront and encourage their voice to be heard in this discharge process.

You must convey the nurse's concern to the medics and psych's about his discharge. He won't cope if he is homeless. I'll phone the housing departments for advice in case he can't go back to his own property.

Phone calls with housing: it takes an hour of sophisticated haggling for either the local housing advice centre or the one in Tristan's home town to own an investigatory responsibility into his housing or homelessness needs. In the event of him being homeless, neither of the housing departments will accept a homeless referral over the phone even with their homeless discharge policy in place. If our local housing agency accepts Tristan for a homeless assessment, he will be placed in temporary accommodation pending further investigation, to establish whether there is a *duty of care*. A reconnections policy will then link him back to his home town rather than rehousing in this area.[7] But the local housing advice officer wriggles saying, 'You know what it's like Maria … so many drug dealers around temporary accommodation flats … he will be very vulnerable. He should go back to his home town.'

The housing manager in Tristan's home town informs me that his landlord could have re-let the property if his rent was not paid. 'But what about his belongings?' I ask, 'Can't someone go and check?' 'No, that's not our role,' she rigidly replies. It is only later that I reconsider Tristan's legal rights[8] regarding the tenancy having trusted the housing manager to be the housing expert. If he does decide to return to his home town, Tristan will have to make the two-hour journey, not knowing whether he will have accommodation that night; present as homeless on the day of discharge. Only then will he be assessed regarding a duty to house him as a vulnerable person, 'And that,' the manager declares, 'is difficult to do without proof. Anyway he has a lot of money. Last year we investigated whether we had a duty to house him – and we didn't.'

'But,' I protest, 'his deteriorating health has apparently caused him to blow that money and his health may decline further. He needs support and accommodation and that is what I am trying to arrange with you. He is very vulnerable.'

I sense a power game, a reluctance to accept someone from hospital for a homeless assessment from either authority! Is it because it takes too long to do? Is it too complex? I argue the point with our local housing officer, knowing I have worked well with her predecessor in joint ward visits previously.

Housing is not yielding but playing a rigid power game – a reminder of Spaghetti Junction running alongside but disconnected. So where will Tristan be discharged to?

---

[6] Norovirus, an RNA virus of the Caliciviridae taxonomic family, causes approximately 90% of non-bacterial epidemic outbreaks of gastroenteritis.

[7] *Getting connected*, the CLG (2006b) guidance document on a reconnections policy states: '3.2. Outcomes for a local policy should include: ensuring that clients referred to other areas have accommodation (with support and access to services if appropriate) available when they arrive to prevent rough sleeping in those areas'. The summary of this document, however, states: 'reconnection will not be appropriate for some rough sleepers, for instance, those who are too vulnerable to return anywhere and those who do not have a connection to any particular area.' (2006:5)

[8] An eviction in these circumstances would be unlawful.

I return to his bedside. He points to a grey, hospital carrier bag where he says all his known possessions sit – all possessions, I muse, except the beloved silver Porche. At 5.45, after telling Tristan and the nurses the housing options and pathways available, I leave the ward feeling anxious and concerned with housing *and* health for not only am I concerned about where he will be discharged too but I am concerned that he is actually being discharged without his mental health needs being addressed. But if I thought today's break down on spaghetti junction was bad, then tomorrow is worse – in fact it becomes a convoluted pile up!

Thursday 7 March

The next day the psychiatric assessment confirms Tristan *is* fit for discharge. In disbelief I confront the ward sister on whether she has voiced her concerns about his discharge, but in her silence (Belenky *et al.* 1986) I am quickly passed onto the matron. Matron is insistent that the bed is freed in time for the weekend, but I am equally insistent on a case conference citing Safeguarding of Vulnerable Adults (SOVA), positioning Tristan's care needs against superficial fiscal acumen. I agree to phone all agencies for attendance at the case conference the following day – my day off[9] – especially SOVA but where are the hospital social workers and the hospital discharge planning team who should see this as part of their role? I encourage matron to invite them to the conference. That evening, at home I receive a phone call from the county SOVA lead. She listens to Tristan's discharge issue and promises to send someone to the conference the next day.

Friday 8 March

Just before 1.30, I arrive on the ward. Tristan is pacing up and down. He looks agitated. I had expected the ward office be filled with case conference attendees and I am surprised to see that that matron is alone. Her voice is now calmer; either more submissive or more compassionate than when she was looking for empty bed spaces yesterday. She has since engaged with Tristan to make her own assessment ...

'Hello Maria – he knows something is happening. He is very anxious.'
'Hello Carol! – Yes, he is very agitated. He can't even speak to me today. How can he possibly be ready for discharge?'

'Don't worry – he's not going. The psychs did the assessment but haven't written the notes up – and I want another one done. He is clearly not able to go.'

A 'u' turn – and a third psychiatric assessment! Did my liaison with SOVA reveal an unsafe hospital discharge or had Matron's personal engagement with Tristan allowed his humanity and suffering to be revealed?

I am so relieved but where is everyone? I reply, 'We still need pathways for his eventual discharge care.'

---

[9]There is no cover for the clinical aspect of my role when I am not there and I work part-time. I have requested a team of homelessness nurses (Black Monday January 2008) as a recommendation from the Health Needs Assessment and earlier approached cover from the wider health visiting team but no help was forthcoming.

Even though agencies are unaware that Tristan is not being discharged today, no one except myself, the matron and the SOVA representative (a physical disability social worker) are here for the now aborted case conference. Empty chairs lay waiting for:

- Local Authority Housing Options Service;
- The Community Mental Health Team (CMHT);
- The psychiatrist;
- The hospital social worker;
- The hospital discharge coordinator;
- The ward sister.

Assertively, I phone Housing and the Mental Health team but no one is available. I leave a message asking them to respond as soon as possible. Used to child protection case conferences where there is a statutory responsibility to attend, it causes me to reflect on the statutory obligations in regard to vulnerable adults. Yet, this vulnerable adult keeps falling through the net between gaps in assessments and between gaps in services that do not engage with him. Even the SOVA representative states that his physical disability team will not be involved because Tristan does not have a physically disability. 'It will fall to mental health teams.' But mental health teams will not offer support without a mental health diagnosis – and the psychiatrists have said he is well enough to go home.

Like Tristan we are stuck. Spaghetti junction's rigid steel trajectories clamp down on us. We invite Tristan in. He is lost and desolate. Even when he tries to speak, he is speechless. It frustrates him. 'Sorry … sorry, follows a long pause after each attempt to answer our questions. Matron tells him not to worry, 'You are not going to be discharged today.'

Sadness wells up inside me as I leave the ward. Having already said farewell to Tristan I sense him following me. I speak softly with him again and direct him back to his bed. In the car park I check that he has not followed me again but there he is, standing in his sky-blue pyjamas watching me like an abandoned child left on the pavement.

The following day, after the third mental health assessment, Tristan is finally admitted to the acute mental health unit. It is just over eight weeks since he first arrived at my health access clinic. Three months later, Tristan was transferred to a mental health acute unit in his home town.

Nine months later – Christmas 2008

Edward sends me a Christmas CD of music demonstrating his improving keyboard skills. In an accompanying letter he says, 'Tristan has now recovered but is back buying fast cars and "blowing" money.'

I surmise that a diagnosis of Huntingdon's chorea was never made.

Reflective guidance

April 2008

The need to honour chaos stories is both moral and ethical. Until the chaos narrative is honoured, the world in all its possibilities is being denied. (Frank 1995:109)

Mindful of Frank (1995), I read the story to the guided reflection group in the knowledge that this is a rolling story of chaos involving community and hospital health teams as well as housing services. The story has opened a space for the group to dwell on homelessness and the way it is perceived. CJ reminds me that Okri (1997) views storytellers as transgressors, liberators, witnesses, explorer of hidden depths, resister, sufferer, poet and writers to gain insight (pp. 1– 41). He rhetorically asks what would have happened if I had not been there. I am directed to Belenky *et al.*'s (1986) stages of voice to gauge reflexivity within the story and my narrative journey. I note my own empowerment in the process as my voice is used as a passionate knower integrated into constructive knowledge stage (Belenky *et al.* 1986) about homelessness and health as I face mental health and housing experts who are surprisingly not connected to health and homelessness but have their own agendas. Ultimately this was a successful story because Tristan was prevented from being discharged inappropriately.

Within a deepening hermeneutic circle (Heidegger 1962), other insights become clear, and together the co-creation of knowledge (Gadamer 1989) unfolds:

- Nurses working in homelessness face repeated scenarios of patient exclusion, which affects their work load, the skill level needed in negotiation and the need for personal resilience;
- The outcome *Improving access to health services for homeless people* (DH/Office of the Deputy Prime Minister 2004) will not be effective unless there is a fundamental shift in awareness that beyond *access* itself, health services are *hard to reach* – not just patients who are *hard to reach*;
- Health care professionals seem unaware that poor health is a pathway leading into homelessness. Foucault's (1973) 'narrow gaze' in mental health assessments as used in Tristan's story disconnects vulnerable people from getting health support even when it is requested;
- The line between being vulnerably housed and homeless is very fine;
- Despite having an admission and discharge homelessness policy, antagonistic and unco-operative attitudes surreptitiously arise between housing and health, preventing the streamlining of the discharge process. In the theme of *Spaghetti junction* it is like a collision of two powerful juggernauts.

AP sees the story as challenging her social perceptions that homeless or vulnerably housed people are not from the professional classes and this causes me to reflect on the value of the nursing voice as social action. Subsequently I use *Spaghetti junction* as performance ethnography (Bochner and Ellis 2002) to AP's performing arts students who develop it further into a homelessness performance. Called *No home*, the performance is seen by mental health and housing teams as well as district nurses and other third sector organisations working in homelessness – a further paper yet to be written in my narrative journey.

I conclude with Okri (1997:1) as a completion of the theme of net and an introduction to the next story called *The spider's web*.

Spiders' forge their webs in silence … where others don't care to look.

Commentary

The narrative plot *Falling through the net* is picked up again six weeks after the last practice experience in *Spaghetti junction*. In this next reflexive story, named *The spider's web*, I position myself forging links in the development of mental health service for homeless people. Transcending 'one to one' clinical encounters, the multi-faceted nature of my role is revealed where oblique rhythms of practice must be strategically travelled by the specialist public health nurse – or others in commissioning and/or providing health services – to similarly tighten the strategic net in preventing homeless people *falling though the net* of health care and other services.

Mattingly (1998) describes narrative time as 'change or an attempt to change ... an effort at transformation' (p. 94). In chronological time both *Spaghetti junction* and *The Spider's web* stories are reflexively positioned early in the third year of my narrative journey. But it is in *The spider's web* that narrative time can be seen as an 'intrinsic webbing of multiple figures' (Mattingly 1998:84) where systematic self-inquiry (Johns 2006) has led me towards self-realisation in my role with multi-agency partnerships and multi-disciplinary health services in my attempt to change and transform health care. This story can be viewed as a significant experience towards my vision of practice for homeless people as outlined in my MPhil/PhD narrative journey,[10] or as a smaller part that comprises a complex dance (Mattingly 1998); for it is in *The spider's web* that I make visible the way I seek to shift forces that constrain my realisation of desirable practice (Johns 2006) to improving access and engagement in mental health services for homeless people. Reflexivity in my journey of transformation is considered through my use of voice (Belenky *et al.* 1986) and although not overtly used in the text, Johns' (2006:33). Framing perspectives offer a coherent way for the reader to loosely gauge the complex dance (Mattingly 1998) where the experiences of *Spaghetti junction* are woven into *The spider's web*.

Imagining the dance taking place, I begin this story with thoughts of performing *The spider's web* as performance ethnography (Bochner and Ellis 2002) whilst Tillman-Healey (2002) eloquently spins the layers to metaphorically position my transformation in practice.

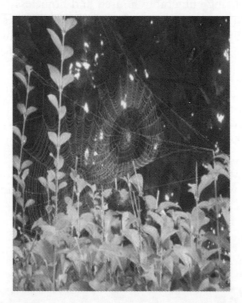

---

[10] My narrative thesis is a journey of self-inquiry and transformation towards self-realisation in being and becoming a specialist public health nurse in homelessness.

> **Dramatic backdrop**
>
> **We dizzily spun webs of significance, moving from silence, to utterance, to transcendence -- and performance. (Tillmann-Healy 2002)**
>
> **Dancers** in spider suits, perform around a circle creating a silver web, weaving in and out of the circle ... colourful streamers link people in the circle whilst stories/ideas are voiced. The structure of the newly formed web catches a homeless person, (previously seen at the side) and then another ... preventing a fall between the gaps (of service) into a void – perhaps the very void leading to cardboard city below Tristan's *Spaghetti junction*!
>
> **Web circle:**
> Senior members of mental health trusts: lead specialist mental health manager, Supporting People commissioner, housing manager, executive member of Supported Housing forum and nightshelter, specialist public health nurse - homelessness. **Vacant chair – mental health service commissioner.**

The spider's web – 18 April 2008. (Photograph by Maria Fordham.)

Intricate, delicate, systematic – I feel like a sapient, Socratic spider drawing stray strands together, spun from experience. Spider silk, twice as strong as steel thread (Gore 2005); silk experiences as precious as gold dust, gathered from day-to-day nursing practice, drawing together a sagely web that unites some of the separate, steel trajectories on *Spaghetti junction*.[11]

Seven people sit on the diameter of the web's circle, pulling it taut like guy ropes on a tent. It is an important circle;[12] one where strategic *net*works will be established to create care pathways which secure homeless people's ease of access to mental health services, as recommended by the Department of Health (DH 2007). But just at the pinnacle of the web there is a hole in the connection, marked by the absence of a mental health commissioner.[13] I ponder on whether if it is a political move – is this meeting too politically hot, exposing mental health commissioning to the scrutiny of multi-agency partners? Is she waiting for the senior provider mental health service managers to spin their own web of connection across the gap by using mainstream services removing the extra funding implications? Or is she simply so busy that this meeting holds a lower priority amongst competing tensions?

The mental health commissioner had attended the inaugural meeting of this group and disputed facts that I had presented about the experience of some local homeless people being excluded from mental health services – even when they wished to use them. I used Rudi's story from practice.[14] Rudi had a personality disorder and both extensively and seriously self-harmed, yet when I tried to refer him into mental health services, I was

---

[11]*Spaghetti junction* story, 7 March 2008.

[12]The professional gathering has arisen following the dissemination of the Health Needs Assessment (HNA) at the Health Improvement Group (HILG) meetings, which showed mental health as the area where homeless people could not fully access services.

[13]The commissioners are pivotally positioned in funding the development of additional mental health services for homeless people when services are not met by mainstream provision.

[14]Rudi's story is one of the 30 stories presented in my narrative. I was told that Rudi's care plan stated for crisis intervention only.

informed by the team that his Care Programme Approach (CPA) stated *for crisis intervention only.* Leaving hostel staff in a precarious position to care for him, the lack of mental health support led to his eventual eviction and return to rough sleeping. When the mental health commissioner attempted to undermine this experience I had calmly presented another story – that of Tristan from *Spaghetti junction.* It had silenced her. As I weaved Tristan's story from practice, I was mindful of Okri's (1997) sentiment that storytelling powerfully 'reconnects us to the great sea of human destiny, human suffering and human transcendence' (p. 47). Practice experience, coupled with government guidance (DH 2007) and critical social science empowerment theory whereby dialogue with each other about their worldview and ours (Freire 1972) had led me into Belenky *et al.*'s (1986) constructive knowledge stage of voice weaving theory and practice to connect the mental health managers and commissioners to the struggle of local homeless people. As slowly, Socratically I had begun at that inaugural meeting to spin the web of truth and justice in mental health care for homeless people locally.

Away from the Town Hall civic atmosphere of the last meeting, I underline our task today as I circulate the government guidance document about homeless people accessing mental health services (DH 2007). I am keen to bring benchmarking initiatives to this meeting early, encouraging service managers to think beyond known horizons of local practices which currently disadvantage homeless people with mental illness, creating further inequalities in their health and well-being (Bines 1994; Pleace and Quilgars 1996; Crane and Warnes 2001). Although I am not in the 'chair'[15] I am a key player, bridging health services and housing professionals, the latter of whom I work more closely with.[16] The homeless health specialism of my role has, for me, gained clarity in recent months[17] – aware now that senior health professionals need to be guided in the application of health principles in a homeless world that remains largely invisible to mainstream health services (Wilson 2002).[18]

The government document guiding the development of mental health services in homelessness is welcomed by all, pre-empting a relief-filled sigh from a new mental health executive, as if reprieved from a knowledge gap that in several instances causes him to apologise. In pointing out the models of good practice, I am priming all agencies towards a social inclusion multi-disciplinary health team which includes a dedicated community psychiatric nurse (CPN) – my optimum hope for service improvement in homeless mental health care. It is a confrontational move in a forum with multi-agency partners because it holds a heavy resource implication[19] and draws homeless people outside of mainstream service provision (DH 2007), generally viewed by commissioners in this primary care trust as colluding towards a dependency culture rather than stoking a philosophy of independence and empowerment for homeless. However, practice experience with people

---

[15] Local authority (housing) is chairing the meeting.

[16] Supported Housing Forum, Multi-Agency Panel, discharge from hospital, referring clients to their services.

[17] 'Black Monday' – the practice story written following my presentation of the Homeless Health Needs Assessment (HNA) to provider service managers which provided insights about the way homelessness is perceived by health managers.

[18] A Crisis (2002) survey found that the homeless people they interviewed were almost 40 times more likely not to be registered with a GP than the average person – they are therefore more likely to be excluded from other health services, as GP registration is a gateway to other services.

[19] I aim to explore the costing of mental health services eventually, so that the consequences of not providing dedicated homeless teams that include a CPN can be calculated against poorer health outcomes in inequalities in health, to inform my argument for future service plans.

such as Rudi and Tristan[20] has led me to believe that many homeless people are unable to engage with mainstream health services without having a facilitator who acts almost as an interpreter initially, rather than an advocate, in a two-way process of understanding that promotes engagement on both sides. In this meeting I hope to secure the netting in the 'spider's web' ensuring senior mental health managers are primed to promote a specialist model of service delivery[21] so that they, too, can also influence the partnership commissioning forums at county level (joint needs assessment feeding into the local area agreement [LAA]), although *any* improved model of service provision would currently be beneficial to me[22] and to local homeless people as well as third sector agencies.

As the meeting gains ground, a ripple of awareness echoes inwardly, that I am in *the* group position I feel most relaxed in, most powerful in; one where another person holds the structure in place by chairing, and I provide the relationship links and guidance, as well as expert knowledge drawn from practice experience – offered as affirmation *and* as challenge! I feel the *net* being created and caste beyond between myself and the other health professional managers here, who often look to me for confirmation when the local authority 'chair' is speaking. Much like the amity I feel with other non-NHS agencies that I work closely with in other homeless strategic groups,[23] I become the bridge, casting the net more securely between NHS and non-NHS partners. In this homely atmosphere it feels like campfire stories unfurling. But I am also fired up and focused, aware that individual stories set the scene so that a larger story of empowerment in the local homeless underworld is underway (Freire 1972; Kieffer 1984), including my own reflexive journey of 'being and becoming', marked largely by use of voice (Belenky *et al.* 1986) developed from homeless experience, theory and reflective practice.

It is Freire (1972:74) who offers me further insight into the current level of provision of mental health services for homeless people:

A naively conceived humanism often overlooks the concrete, existential, present situation of real people.

Today I continue to challenge perceptions by presenting real people in real health situations, highlighting to the group the daily challenges that appear.

Just today, I tell them, 'a providential experience occurred ...', which incensed me, although I do not use that phrase: 'An e-mail arrived informing me that the half day per month CPN support to the homeless community has been discontinued following a management reshuffle.[24]

Shocked stares confirm their concern. Having positively raised the profile as a valuable resource at the inaugural meeting only a month ago, this group connects more strongly to its sudden withdrawal. The CPN arrangement was not commissioned and probably viewed only as a goodwill gesture in homelessness *despite* the fact that the service began following extremely concerning mental health crisis in the local bail hostel which led to joint clinics with myself and the ex-mental health team manager. I continue.

---

[20] Stories from practice captured in my PhD thesis.

[21] A multi-disciplinary social in/exclusion homeless team is one recommendation in the HNA.

[22] Lowering stress/workloads/better patient outcomes.

[23] Supported Housing Forum/Multi-Agency Panel etc.

[24] The service was introduced following a very concerning episode where a hostel resident was eventually placed in a secure mental health unit.

The (new) manager has not entered into discussions with me and the CPN cited 'increased demands on time from homeless hostels' as a reason for discontinuing the service. The root issue has not been addressed. CPN clinics were arranged by the previous manager following a number of joint clinics we did together when increased mental health crisis needs were identified in probation approved premises and another (long-term) homelessness project. How can they simply just cease?

Inwardly I pondered on where the new manager had placed me ... where she had disempowered me in my role, leaving it to the CPN to send me the e-mail. Our organisations sit side by side and we share a health responsibility to homeless people where mental illness is greatly increased (Bines 1994).The precarious nature of homelessness and health services in our area is revealed, exposing the tension of my role – as I draw one part of the net together in health care, it loosens again. Rather humorously I am holding an audience with the most senior managers in the mental health trust, to whom I make my challenge.

Words of regret and surprise instantly arise from multi-agency partners, confronting the three mental health managers. Two of them respond affirmatively to our disappointment. They are uncomfortable. The third mental health manager is silent, holding a finger to her lip ... as if letting go of the web with one hand. ... She wants to say something and although our eyes meet she remains in sulky silence. I acknowledge her with a smile – a political smile, for I can sense too, that she does not know where to place me – who is this homeless public health specialist – as I continue to reveal the political power that my role, and voice, brings from both practice experience and partner relationships in homelessness, in which mental health managers must inevitably be accountable for mental health services.

'Increased demands in hostels ... and the removal of the CPN service has occurred at a time when these discussions seek to improve access to mental health services, not reduce it.'

My voice is strong as I focus on their accountability.

Accountability – shifting the burden – sharing the burden.

There is so much going on in this meeting with eyes: looks of tenderness versus resource limitations, need, even shame.

Homeless mental health service provision needs to be formally audited. I am not a CPN, but mental health issues continue to absorb most of my time when in fact I need to also create care pathways in primary care for families and single people. I can't do it all. Another way you could proceed if you can't continue to provide a CPN to improve mental health services would be to link CMHTs to hostels in their locality – which seems to be the way primary care is looking at providing future services.

I can not do it all ... words touch the raw, dawning reality within me that I will drop out of local homelessness health care unless more funding for health care development is offered for the homeless community. Okri (1997:67) writes:

There is great suffering that is an intrinsic part of love, the love of one's work, the love of the world, and of humanity.

Suffering which, here now, the spider's web is tentatively trying to overcome, connecting the ripped netting, setting the scene to allow me to *let go* whilst the web stays in place and my vision of practice is achieved ... *but not just yet ... first tying knots more securely in the mental health service web. ... Letting go later,* to guide other developments needed in local homelessness health care.

Supporting People and other partners heartily agree with the suggestion of linked generic mental health teams to hostels.

What will this mental health contingent put in place?

In the considered quietness, space is left for me to bring two spontaneous examples from this week's practice which would *not* fit into mainstream services[25] – illustrating the need to consider other ways of service redesign. As stories fill their gaps in knowledge of homelessness and health, my focused guidance is met with absolutely no resistance and I feel a fusion of horizons taking place (Gadamer 1989). My nursing stories have transgressed the taken for granted order of things (Johns 2006) to reveal the mental health service gaps in homelessness in which others have listened. Greeted with nods of agreement and encouragement I express solutions to problems within the stories – joint training on homelessness and mental health (HHI 2008) promoting connections between agencies, allowing mental health practitioners to integrate more easily with the third sector agencies as well as the housing authority. It seems so simple!

Yet even within this multi-agency forum, other key issues are alarmingly revealed. Housing (in the chair) pronounces that they are 'waiting to hear' from the hospital whether Tristan has been discharged. Half-alarmed; half relieved, it confirms my frustration about delays in some hospital discharges of homeless people. Housing blame late notifications from hospital. The housing manager's face reddens as I immediately but softly confront her.

'Housing has known for several weeks about Tristan and the need for a homeless interview to be made on the ward. I have made sure they are aware. I am watching Tristan's discharge closely to inform our multi-agency hospital discharge policy in the light of this experience. It has to be co-ordinated with housing services in Oxbridge.'

Faux pas revealed, she embarrassingly retracts – *the spider's web silken trap* reveals a local contention in discharge co-ordination![26] 'I haven't had anything to do with it ... I'll check it out with the senior officer when I get back.' Even in my assertive but gentle approach, seeking adult-to-adult interaction (Stewart and Joines 1987), I feel like the arch overseer with a multi-agency whip by my side; practice knowledge giving power to my role. Mental health professionals are gauging my relationship with the local authority and I am aware of it. As the housing manager discusses the planned complex needs unit with referrals via the Multi-Agency Panel (MAP) for rough sleepers *another silver strand is linked*. ... A core member of MAP recently expressed concerns about multi-agency

---

[25] A former hostel resident, a teenager, has experienced severe paranoid disturbances but is not accessing treatment. He was evicted and is now rough sleeping whilst an 18-year-old former LAC girl displays persistent behavioural problems with suicidal tendencies, climbing onto the roof of the hostel, saying she will jump off – but when police are called she says she was sunbathing.

[26] I am writing the recommended admission and discharge protocol (DH/Homeless Link 2005; Shelter 2007), chairing multi-agency meetings with housing, alcohol/drug agencies and discharge planning nurses prior to a full steering group and ratification by hospital managers.

information sharing in police presence and in front of another third sector agency fearing that information sharing could be detrimental.[27] The housing manager and I work well together in partnership working. I inform her ...

> 'Issues of mistrust are arising between some agencies in MAP. I've provided guidance and recommended documents on partnership working. If we hope to bring agencies closer in the homeless health world we need to nip it in the bud.'

> 'Oh, Maria. ... Can we talk? I had a delegation from an agency meet with me yesterday.'

We ... We ... We ... The housing manager and I. She smiles – sadly; she is very compassionate and works extremely hard on the homeless agenda of housing. She needs support, and another significant connection is made to strengthen homelessness partnership links. After the meeting we devise and collaborate on a strategy to improve trust within MAP.

And still silver links continue to be forged ... as the chief executive of a night shelter tells a concerning story about a middle-aged character resembling 'Spider', the hero in the Cronenberg and McGrath (2002) film played by Ralph Fiennes, whom she brought to accident and emergency (A&E) in a psychotic state with no string to form a web to assuage his mental distress. With extreme difficulty she contained him in A&E for six hours whilst waiting for a mental health assessment to be performed. Capturing him in A&E was an achievement requiring a quick response from the mental health team. Were they aware of the government target to reduce rough sleeping (Communities and Local Government [CLG] 2006a, 2008) and their potential contribution towards achieving that target by assessing and treating Spider's mental health illness? Or were they simply disconnected from the guidance on homelessness, busy with other life-threatening issues to see a homeless person in mental health crisis as a priority? Is the homeless world easily dismissed by A&E staff, and mental health illness not recognised as life-threatening, despite higher morbidity and mortality in rough sleepers than a housed population (Bines 1994) with a life-expectancy of 42 years of age for rough sleepers who have been on the streets from the age of 16 (Crisis 1996)?

Did the mental health team recognise that if the night shelter resident left without the assessment being done, 'Spider' would have been excluded from their accommodation that night because of the immense difficulties he presented to the staff and residents? Failure to make a connection between homelessness and mental health illness and between rough sleeping and government recommendations to reduce rough sleeping (CLG 2007) leaves another hollow space for homeless people to *fall through the net.*

The meeting considers that the same mental health team is being cited in several cases and I offer my insight:

> You see they are experts in their own field, but they are unable to make the connection with homelessness agencies. We in health work in silos and the effects of that are enormous – issues of a much reduced life-expectancy and increased mental health morbidity[28] – everything needs linking up. The staff need training to make them feel more comfortable with discharges and partnership care in the community.'

---

[27] See *Seven golden steps to information sharing* (DH 2008). Training on information sharing in the MAP arranged December 2008 to allay agencies' concerns about what and what not to safely share.
[28] Crisis (2003) *Homeless fact file.* Crisis, London.

Nods and approvals from everyone – with stories in place it feels so easy now. They murmur noisily between themselves, energy at a different level now, planning what can be done for their staff to respond differently.

We arrange another meeting to look at care pathways that have become evident from our stories for future service development:

- Care pathway for those who want to access mental health services but are unable to do so;
- Care pathway for those who do not engage with mainstream mental health services but are a concern to hostel or other homeless service staff;
- Care pathway for those who are assessed by mental health services and discharged from care.

Success!! *The silver web of silver strands has been tentatively positioned* so that mental health need in the local homeless community is linked with mental health managers who can shape service design. *Once again I feel I can begin to let go.* I have done what I can to feed into a systems change for some of the most vulnerable people in our town. This is my empowerment story. It lies in practice experience, honouring the stories of those I meet. The transformation within my role is marked too, by a growing confidence that my knowledge and experience is recognised by others, as a 'specialist public health nurse in homelessness' – *as the spider crawls steadily along collecting stories in a web of homeless health care:*

... near the gutters where the underside of dreams fester ... to be multiple witnesses around the central masquerade of reality ... (Okri 1997:1–2)

Endnote

CJ describes *The spider's web* story as a pivotal experience in my narrative journey where self-inquiry has led to self-realisation, following the process of successful reflection. Discussing Belenky *et al.* (1986), we consider how others have listened to my constructive voice as I confronted multiple systems of care in this practice story which can be positioned through the 'Framework for assertive action' (Johns 2006). I celebrate with an inner sigh knowing that a massive corner in local homelessness health care has at last been traversed with senior mental health managers. But most importantly I celebrate homelessness nursing, in the knowledge that caring and compassion inevitably leads to social action where transformation occurs. Finally, I invite you to bring your own hermeneutic (Gadamer 1975/1989) reflections about your practice to these stories and consider how your service accommodates the needs of some of the most vulnerable people in our affluent society – the homeless.

References

Belenky M, Clinchy B, Goldberger N and Tarule J (1986) *Women's ways of knowing: the development of self, voice and mind.* Basic Books, Harper Collins, New York.

Bines W (1994) *The health of single homeless people.* Centre of Homeless Policy, University of York, England.

Bochner A and Ellis C (2002) *Ethnographically speaking.* Altamira Press, New York.

Camilli V and Martin J (2005) Emergency department nurses' attitudes toward suspected intoxicated and psychiatric patients. *Topics in Emergency Medicine* 27:313–316.

Communities and Local Government (2006a) *UK homeless code of guidance for local authorities.* CLG, London.

Communities and Local Government (2006b) *Getting connected.* CLG, London.

Communities and Local Government (2007) *Rough sleeping 10 years on: from the streets to independent living and opportunity.* Discussion paper, CLG, London.

Communities and Local Government (2008) *No-one left out communities ending rough sleeping.* CLG, London.

Communities and Local Government/Department of Health (2006) *Hospital admission and discharge: people who are homeless or living in temporary or insecure accommodation.* CLG Publications, West Yorkshire.

Crane M and Warnes A (2001) The responsibility to care for single homeless people. *Health and Social Care in the Community* 9:436–444.

Crisis (1996) *Still dying for a home.* Crisis, London.

Crisis (2002) *Critical condition: vulnerable single homeless people and access to GPs.* Crisis, London.

Crisis (2003) *Fact file.* Crisis, London.

Cronenberg D and McGrath D (2002) *Spider.* Capital Films, UK.

Department of Health (2003) *Discharge from hospital, pathway process and practice.* DH, London.

Department of Health (2007) *A good practice guide – getting through – access to mental health services for people who are homeless or living in insecure accommodation.* HMSO, London.

Department of Health (2008) *Seven golden steps to information sharing.* HMSO, London.

Department of Health/Homeless Link (2005) Available at: www.olderhomelessness.org.uk/documents/older_people_strategies_final.pdf.

Department of Health/Office of the Deputy Prime Minister (2004) *Achieving positive shared outcomes in health and homelessness.* Office of the Deputy Prime Minister, London.

Foucault M (1973) *The birth of the clinic: an archaeology of medical perception.* Tavistock Publications, London.

Frank A (1995) *The wounded storyteller: body, illness, and ethics.* University of Chicago Press, Chicago.

Freire P (1972) *Pedagogy of the oppressed.* Penguin Books, London.

Gadamer GH (1975/1989) *Truth and method* (second edition) (transl. Weinsheimer J and Marshall DG). Sheed & Ward Sage, London.

Gore B (2005) *Spider silk is stronger than steel* (Wow Science). Franklin Watts Ltd, New York.

Heidegger M (1962) *Being and time* (transl. Macquarrie J and Robinson E 2008). Blackwell Publishing, Oxford.

Homeless Health Initiative (2008) *Homelessness briefing spring 2008.* Queens Nursing Institute, London.

Johns C (2006) *Becoming a reflective practitioner.* Blackwell Publishing, Oxford.

Kieffer C (1984) Citizen empowerment, a developmental perspective. *Prevention in Human Services* 84:9–36.

Lauer M (2008) Replacing the revolving door a collaborative approach to treating individuals in crisis. *Journal of Psychosocial Nursing* 46:25–32.

Mattingly C (1998) *Healing dramas and clinical plots. The narrative structure of experience.* Cambridge University Press, Cambridge.

Okri B (1997) *A way of being free*. Phoenix, London. Text extracts used with permission of The Marshall Agency.

Perlis R (2005) Misdiagnosis of bipolar disorder. *The American Journal of Managed Care* 11:S271–S274.

Pleace N and Quilgars S (1996) *Health and homelessness in London*. King's Fund, London.

Polkinghorne D (1983) *Methodology for the human sciences*. State Univesity of New York Press, Albany.

Queens Nursing Institute (2007) *Homeless health survey*. QNI, London.

Queens Nursing Institute (2008) *Homeless health initiative impact report 2007–2008*. QNI, London.

Shelter (2007) *Good practice guide: homelessness early identification and prevention*. Shelter, London.

Steinbeck J (1937) *Of mice and men*. Bantam Books, New York. (Used with permission.)

Stewart I and Joines V (1987) *TA today a new introduction to transactional analysis*. Life Space Publishing, Nottingham, England.

Tillman-Healey L (2002) Men kissing. In: A Bochner and C Ellis (eds.) *Ethnographically speaking*. Altamira Press, New York.

Wikipedia. Huntington's disease. Available at: http://en.wikipedia.org/wiki/Huntington%27s_disease (accessed 18 February 2010).

Wilson C (2002) Hidden homelessness and health care. Cooper and Wilson cited in Crisis 2002.

Chapter 9
Climbing walls

Christopher Johns

Preamble

I constructed *Climbing walls* as a performance narrative from my reflective journal notes of journeying with Ann through her breast cancer treatment. Over a 17-month period, I gave Ann 35 reflexology sessions. *Climbing walls* reflects the first six months of our journey. It is important to emphasise that this narrative is my story, not Ann's, even as I capture her experience through my eyes and hands. Ann's own journal resonated strongly with mine, reflecting my empathic ability to capture her experience beyond our actual conversations.

Amanda Price, April Nunes Tucker and Antje Diedrich are dance and theatre teachers at the University of Bedfordshire who co-supervise doctoral students within the school of guided reflection and narrative inquiry. Amanda and April became co-performers whilst Antje directed the performance.

The performance is followed by a dialogue with the audience with a view to social action towards confronting the ways medical services too often add to suffering rather than easing it.

I have also performed *Climbing walls* as a solo performance, sitting in a solitary chair with an adjacent empty chair to represent Ann's presence. I designed a series of 15 ink abstract paintings, inspired by my work with Ann, as background to the solo performance, two of which were used in the group performance suggesting a scar (see text).

Sketch 1

Thursday July 5th. Lou says goodbye outside my study. Ann hovers in the corridor. I say hovers because she seems reticent, uncertain. I am surprised to see her. I say, 'You've come for your dissertation result?'

She holds a book in her right hand. I add, 'The exam board is not till next week …?'

She says, 'I've come to return the book you lent me.'

Sensing her disturbance I ask, 'What is it?'

Her eyes drop. 'I have some news to tell you.'

She enters the study and sits on the chair I pull out for her. Her tears are close to the surface. She says softly, 'I have breast cancer … they intend to operate on July 19th … I've had the lump for 18 months … I put off going to the GP … I thought I could finish my studies first ... then the nipple became puckered ..... then I went to the GP ... I've also felt a hard lump under the axilla ... I saw a surgeon ... I need a mastectomy ... in a matter of fact way he said I would also need an axillary clearance ... he wasn't pleasant ... it wasn't easy to make a relationship with him ... his manner ... he kept me at a distance ...'

Ann's eyes meet mine. She pleads, 'Surely they can differentiate which nodes are affected and which are not and be more selective in their removal?'

Her words spin before me. She is defiant about not wanting this clearance.

I feel my along the edge of her suffering. Uncertainty lies thick between us. Ann is a lymphoedema therapist who works at a hospice. She knows what it means to have an axillary clearance. Now the shoe is on the other foot? How the tide turns. I ask, 'Why do you tell me this?'

Moving beyond our teacher–student roles, we move into another space. She knows I work as a holistic therapist with women with breast cancer. No words. She glances through the study window into the dull day. I ask, 'Do you want me to give you therapy?'

She looks up again as if not wanting to ask ... 'Yes ... if you would.'

A strong tide surges to flood my senses, her ache inside my own.

How do I respond?

I move to hold her but keep my distance, 'I will support you as much as it takes ....'

Come meet me on the dance floor.

Come ... meet me on the dance floor.

Sketch 2

Wednesday 18th July. I have just come from Gill, a woman with breast cancer I journeyed alongside for the past five years giving reflexology, from her trauma of the mastectomy when her reconstructive surgery failed, from her howl of grief at losing her breast five years after the original surgery, from the pallor of her face, from the anguished twist of mouth, from the endotracheal scar spanning from the bottom left corner of her mouth a reminder, from her raw wound sliced open.

Now I must refocus – can I clear this image to see Ann? Adjust my feet for this new dance?

Picking up a dangling thread, 'How was the surgeon when you saw him again?'

Ann twirls the thread, 'Umm, he showed no interest in me, flipping through his diary looking for a date ... avoiding my eyes ... but my eyes were probably downcast anyway.'

'I can imagine. It can't be easy facing your nemesis.'

Nemesis – the Greek god of retribution, a rival or opponent who cannot be beaten.

Is that the cancer or the surgeon? Perhaps both?

Ann demands he see her as a person rather than a breast he must hack off. Images of hacked breasts heaped high in the theatre corner – words I have used before.

What does he think as he flips through his diary to set the surgical date. Does he sense the immensity of this date for the woman? Dare he see her in her humanness? Perhaps he glances from the corner of his vulnerable eye to deflect the demand.

Another dangling thread – 'What news on the axillary lump?'

Ann replies hopefully, 'The radiologist is optimistic from the x-rays ... that maybe only one node is affected and maybe not even that. They will inject blue dye during the operation and make a judgement about what needs to be cut out.'

Her relief is tangible, crumbs of hope grasped. I wonder – does the surgeon paint a worse case scenario of clearance? Is it better to paint a worse or best scenario?

I ask, 'Are you ready for reflexology?'

Ann positions herself on the brown leather settee, lifts her feet onto the footstall, and we sink into therapy.

Before I leave I meet Ira, her husband, he appears as if from behind the screen. Small chat, his signs of fear obscured behind the banter. The way men cope? My work done for the moment, they have much to do. Ann asks, 'Will you give me reflexology after the surgery?'

'Of course,' I say with a smile of deep compassion.

I take her hand and we begin to dance. The tune is familiar. I hold her in this moment to guide her steps, our first steps faltering as we seek the rhythm, faltering as we let go of what we know in order to flow into the gathering chaos, into the mystery of the dance.

Sketch 3

1st August. Blue skies, a warm day. Ann had no blue dye injected as she had imagined to map the suspect lymph nodes. Instead she had a second stage clearance. She rages about this, for she knows and fears the consequences. Anger spilled over at herself, misplaced towards herself, she is unable to point the finger in the face of the distant surgeon.

She had asked about the sentinel node procedure. The reply – her tumour was too big, 21 cm, the size of a walnut. Evidently sentinel node procedure is considered for tumours less than 7 cm.

She had felt her fear rise in the anaesthetic room. First the theatre room glimpsed beyond where the surgeon with his knife waited. Is he patient or impatient? Do his fingers drum with the demand to get through the list?

Clock ticking ... tick tock, tick tock ...

Ann was delayed because the anaesthetist said she could have some water and paracetamol for her headache. Then they came to get her. Risk of aspiration and so it was delayed. Then the anaesthetist came prancing in some semi-god-like way, a student with him. He invited the student to insert the cannula – the big grey one. He couldn't get the vein, stabbing away until her hand was so bruised, abused ...

The injection flows through her, she felt the waves of nausea, the room spinning ....

She says, 'It was such a dreadful feeling ... I woke in recovery ... the pain in my chest told the story.'

I touch her suffering.

I venture, 'How is the mastectomy scar?'

Her reply 'I haven't given it much thought ... I've always had small breasts.' As if she's hardly noticed the missing breast, at least not yet. She feels she can live with the mastectomy. As she puts it, 'My bras have always been padded!' But she wonders what will the biopsy reveal ... fear on the edge.

I guide her to visualise a healing light flow through her lymph system – destroying, healing, reconnecting.

Afterwards she says that thought held her through the therapy ...
During the therapy I played her music by Wah![1]
[music]
She loves the music. It is sacred. She knows what I mean about the healing vibration.
We listen to *Closing* as she rests ...
lokaha samastaha sukhino bhavantu
[may all beings in the world be peaceful]

I step again into the warm day. Blue skies remain. I hope so for Ann.
We tune into the rhythm of the dance, patiently shaping each step, letting go of expectations, sensing the flow, touching chaos.

Sketch 4

21st August. The three dogs swarm about us demanding attention from the stranger. Ann says 'She likes you' as Brecon sits pressed against me.

She continues, 'I have been to a very dark place following the first chemotherapy session last Thursday ... hallucinating ... climbing walls ... vomiting ... four days unremitting ... only yesterday I managed to get up and eat a few baked beans ... umm they were lovely ... [laughs]. I can't drink green tea ... just water ... I've never been ill before like this. I thought of cancelling you but my mother, who was here, said I mustn't ... and now, today, I feel fine.'

I move my neck and feel a gentler, warmer breeze blowing.

Ann continues, 'The biopsy revealed a few grade 3 cells ... grade 3 is ominous.. just a few – what does that mean? ... 10 lymph nodes removed ... three invaded with the cancer.'

I sense its tentacles reaching out like Attila to vanquish without mercy. Can we find the sanctuary in time?

Ann continues, 'The chemo is FEC. I had no choice having it even if it improves the odds just 5%.'

I sense the statistician raises his eyebrows from across the room.

I say, 'You have your hair?'

She pulls at it ... tufts come away in her hand – 'It started coming out today ... it was on the pillow ....

Her words trail off in despair, her distress palpable ... 'Maybe I'll shave my head to spare the coming out mess.'

We choose her oils. She surprises me by choosing basil. We add thyme (linalool variety) and black pepper – a subtle herby aroma. She loves it. She loves rose but didn't want me to use rose because she was afraid she would turn against the aroma. The chemo is affecting her smell. Normal smells have become offensive.

Thyme: stimulates the production of white corpuscles, so strengthening the body's resistance to invading organisms. it stimulates the circulation generally, and raises low blood pressure.

---

[1] *Savasana*. Wah! (www.wahmusic.com).

it is particularly good for people who are fatigued, depressed or lethargic, making it very useful for convalescence and it stimulates the appetite which is so often poor after an illness. Thyme helps to revive and strengthen both body and mind. (Davis 1999:294)

Basil is described as 'uplifting' and, citing an early herbalist, it 'expels melancholy vapours from the heart' (Davis 1999:52). I sense Richard Dawkins barely containing his outrage at such nonsense. Notes gleaned from the CancerBackup website:

Fluorouracil (5FU) – floo-ro-you-ro-sill
Epirubicin – epi-roo-biss-sin
Cyclophosphamide – sigh-clo-fos-fa-mide

You may feel hot and slightly dizzy, your nose may itch, you may have a metallic taste in your mouth, or you may have the lot. And by the way drink plenty as it can irritate the lining of the bladder. peeling away the squamous cells. It can cause total hair loss – that can be one of the most distressing side effects, but you may cope more easily if you know in advance that you will lose your hair. You may get your periods back, others may not, especially if you are over 40, permanent infertility.

Not to mention the cracked nails, the loss of sensation in her lips, the tingling toes and fingers. The persistent nausea and always the fear of death.

Ann is not melancholic, yet her balance is precarious. She contains her suffering, her despair. She discreetly mops up the mess when it spills over. I am a container but I must also help her express her suffering so it might be eased.

She surrenders easily into the dance, even though her body has become awkward, self-conscious, no longer taken for granted. She doesn't know how to be ill. She struggles to accept help. I guide her, easing her suffering to flow more easily into the depths of the dance to the sacred space. She must learn to focus on each step at a time, looking at the whole mountain is too daunting.

I ask, 'Ann how do you see the future?'

She trembles, 'I had a strong fear of death when told the diagnosis … it prevails.'

Sketch 5

September 4th. Ann pulls out a clump of hair. Her despair at losing her hair thick in the air – her hair is thick so it doesn't come out so easily as if hanging in there in the faint hope it can survive the chemotherapy attack. Washing it today, piles were left around the basin.

Ann sighs, 'I should have had it shaved … I have ordered three wigs paid for by my father. I am embarrassed about them. I can't see quite see them as a fashion accessory … I feel that everyone will know I am wearing a wig. I thought I would have been more distressed about my 'boob' but my boob is hidden away, now a silicone artefact.'

[I respond] 'If I was in your position I imagine being more upset about my boob than my hair, knowing my hair will grow back and that my boob won't … although I suppose it could be reconstructed.'

I seek to fathom the feminine psychology.

Ann says, 'My left arm aches after gardening … I want to get into the garden, to get on with life.

'Touching nature nurtures my life force ... takes me outside myself. I have been thinking about the future, about the possibility of death ... that in a year's time I may not be here ... I have a premonition about that ... I'm fearful of that, and yet I accept that we only have a certain time on earth but I'm not ready for that yet!'

I listen intently for I have no advice or information to give, my presence is cathartic, supportive, encouraging her to spill her premonition into the dance.

During the therapy Ann had felt she was falling. She had resisted. I urge her next time to let go and fall, to trust and surrender, to dance into chaos to find ourselves ....

Gabrielle Roth (1997:118/9) says:

We try desperately to hold our lives together, to keep everything secure and predictable, but life is nothing of those things. Chaos teaches us how to hang in the unknown and dig it. Chaos is the wild mind fully embodied; if you release yourself into it, the world becomes transparent and you can read it like a book.

Sketch 6

14th September. Ann wears a headscarf that gives her a Parisian bohemian look

I quip, 'I love your scarf.'

'My Parisian bohemian look ...'

She twirls and laughs. She says, 'See my wig? I'm pleased with it ... it's highlighted just the colour of my hair. I haven't worn it out yet.'

She laughs but her life has not been a laughing matter. She reacted badly again to the FEC.

She says, 'I haven't seen myself with no hair ... I avoid the mirror although this morning I was tempted to have a peep ....'

She cautiously lifts the edge of her headscarf, fingers the bald scalp. A game of dare? Hair so important to her, her identity, her femininity.

She continues, 'I wore the wig once ... I felt I was wearing a hat ... I kept fiddling with it ... but then I fiddle with my hair anyway.'

Losing my hair has been much harder than losing my breast. No one can see underneath my clothes. But everyone can see my hair. I never thought my hair was beautiful: it was a simple, brown mop that I combed and washed. It grew out of my scalp. It was part of me. It was mine. But as I saw it cover my pillow, as I saw gobs of it come out on the comb, and masses of it clog the shower drain, I sank powerlessly into resignation.[2]

We let the thread dangle and pick up a new one. Ann says 'The red tide enters through my bruised skin now black and blue, red makes me feel sick ... I try to grin and bear it as it courses through my veins, veins that have become so very brittle, red hardened painful lines across my skin that aches and burns. I'm reluctant to accept the offered PIC line, anxious about it being close to my aorta with risk of infection and yet six more treatments to go?'

I whisper, 'Let me share my dark blue German chamomile secret with you, add healing colour to our dance.'

---

[2]Butler S and Rosenblum B (1994) *Cancer in two voices*. The Women's Press, London

Sketch 7

October 4th 2007. Still Ann avoids the mirror's gaze. The wig stares at us – the wig has a name I cannot recall. Social life on hold. She didn't realise how tense she was, the headaches are a give-away. I ask, 'Maybe someone in the family could massage your neck?' She looks doubtful but will ask. I wonder – can they cross the divide?

She is hit by fatigue, some gardening left her exhausted after just a few minutes. It really hit home just how tired she was, and yet those few minutes in the garden were renewing.

We stand at the window and gaze on the Russian vine, its rich red leaves, a poignant moment.

Sketch 8

Tuesday 16th October. Relentless rain falling from grey misty skies. Ellisse, Ann's daughter, is just leaving the house to go shopping with a friend, hair hennaed, afro mop, her broad warm smile. I like to dwell within the family.

The dogs shepherded into the kitchen, wild barks seeking attention, curious for the visitor.

Ann laughs as she always does. Her headscarf says 'Taliban' but still no mirror glance.

She remains very tired, pulled down into a deep weariness. She is in a dark place where she dwells with thoughts of dying.

She says, 'It was triggered shortly after your last visit, seeing the red leaves on the Russian vine, seeing the beauty of that and thinking is this the last time I am going to look out and see that. I was intuitive about the lump, I knew what it was and I sensed that I am going to die. I was right about the lump.'

'Did anyone talk to you about statistics?'

'No ... and I don't want to.'

'I know, the risk is we become the statistic.'

Sketch 9

Wednesday 21st November 2008. The light is fading, days shortening as winter beckons.

Dogs barking as I knock on the closed porch door. Becky, Ann's other daughter, answers.

She shouts into the interior, 'Mum ... it's Chris!'

Ann arrives, as always smiling, masking the despair I know she feels. The room feels different, maybe a chair moved from here to there?

To my enquiry she reveals her despair – she is fed up with talking about IT! I say I won't talk about IT but she laughs. Her face is puffy – maybe a side effect of docetaxel? She had reacted badly so they stopped. Yew tree poisoning. Images of branches spreading over grave yards casting deep shadows.

She says 'A week later they gave me a 5th cycle of FEC. I reacted as I did after the first cycle ... five days of hallucinations climbing the wall, at first vomiting and then persistent nausea ... no sleep ... HELL revisited ... and then I snapped out of it ... it just stopped. I then felt euphoric as I did before.

Perhaps I reacted more strongly because they gave me about a third of the docetaxel. The prescribed anti-emetics were ineffective, the oral ones thrown up with the vomit, just the rectal suppositories … and now I'm constipated! and I'm confused about my radiotherapy planning! My first oncologist said he would irradiate the axilla and now the new one says he will irradiate the breast site. Why is medical opinion so contradictory?'

She laughs at her predicament and for a moment it seems as if it is a tragic comedy. But her trust is dented as mine might be.

I use marjoram instead of black pepper alongside basil and thyme to boost Ann's energy and yet relax her tension, fortifying her heart and mind, strengthening Qi energy. I move my hands above her ankles to work on easing her calf muscles heavy with tension. After the reflexology, I gently work the German chamomile into her arms likewise heavy with tension, the left arm swollen below the elbow. I work at clearing energy and soothing the inflammation until the pain and swelling has gone. Ann opens and closes her hand without pain. She is amazed! I mix a pot to leave with her for her to apply.

To dance well she must first find herself. Only then can she let go and flow intuitively through the chaos, for there is no path to follow, only the music if we listen well enough.

Sketch 10

Monday 17th December. Ann proudly shows me the small tuft of hair on the back of her head, growing like an island in a bald flesh sea. She has looked at that small patch in the mirror but still avoided her whole 'bald' self. She laughs at herself – thinking of when she will be 80.

I say, 'You feel more positive about the future then?'

She remembers her gloom when the reality hit her for the first time that she might die linked to her misery over the FEC. Now she feels more positive as if making it through the FEC was bursting through a barrier. The sixth FEC complete 10 days ago. That's it, no more. The sensation of nausea still rises but nothing like it has been. The last of the poison working itself out. She vomited just thinking about last FEC treatment.

I write Ann a poem:

> Fecking fec
> leaves me a wreck
> climbing walls
> my guts spilled out
> upon the heavy blanket
> metallic taste
> numbed and tingling toes
> six cycles gone
> I hope its worth it.
> Now, the blanket's lifted
> I can breathe again
> disturbed by dreams of red tide
> flowing through brittle veins
> nausea caught in the throat
> seeing demons stare and gloat;
> but I wake
> my life still at stake
> but no longer tied
> I can move about again

sing and shout
fecking fec
fecking fec
fecking fec
X-mas will have some joy
before the x-ray mist
comes to destroy.

Sketch 11

Friday, 28th December. A warmer day, strong breeze, rain in the air. I read Ann fecking fec

She says, 'That's exactly it.'

The little tuft of hair has grown distinct above the surrounding hair growing back – her hair a mixture of dark and light grey tones. It used to be brown. She knows her hair may not grow back as it once was she had grey flecks before disguised by colour and highlights.

She says, 'I have to wait four months before I can highlight ...'

The fragility and comfort of re-grown hair.

She continues, 'Even this tiny fuzz that grew back on my head as a consequence of not having chemotherapy for a few weeks makes me feel less vulnerable, less exposed, my head covered in the presence of God and life.'[3]

Ann sends me a card.[4]

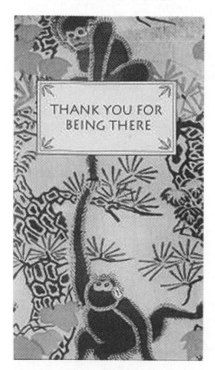

THANK YOU FOR BEING THERE

Dear Chris,
Just wanted to say
Thank you for helping me
through the last six
months your treatment
kept me calm through
some very dark days,
now that the 'fecking fec'
is done, I can see more
clearly, and feel ok.
    love + best wishes to you
        [signature]

---

[3] Butler S and Rosenblum B (1994) *Cancer in two voices*. The Women's Press, London, p. 28 read by audience member.
[4] In the performance, the card and message are shown silently on the PowerPoint.

Sketch 12

10th January 2008. A mild windy day. Intermittent rain. The three dogs leap and bark up through the glazed panels of the new sitting room door. My hand instinctively reaches towards them. My urge to leap and play with them. Moments of abandon and surrender. I sense the child within me yearn.

Ann wears a grey woolly hat, a playful grin.

She says, 'I've looked at myself in the mirror without a hat ... just a glance mind you, no more, in the mirror across the room ... nothing too close up.'

She takes her hat off.

'Can I touch your head ... run my hand across your stubble?'

'The children do that ... I like it ... it feels good ... .'

The small tuft of hair less distinguishable within the surrounding stubble. Her head is hot, sweaty.

([She says)] 'I've commenced tamoxifen! But the sweats are no worse than with the chemotherapy ... I saw Dr George again ... he is polite ... he introduces himself – "Hello I'm Dr George ..." and shakes my hand ... I'm sure he's forgotten I've met him several times before. I asked him if he wanted to examine me. He said oh he might as well ... so I stood in the room naked to the waist .... he felt the scar, around the scar, says it was ok .... he said, "I suppose you're used to it now being a patient" ... he felt my right breast ... checked it was ok ... I felt vulnerable ... it's only skin ... He doesn't make me feel at ease.'

I sense the doctor's unease ... his vulnerability nakedly exposed.

[I enquire] 'Standing naked – just one breast – are you more conscious of your loss?'

'I am but I have yet to process the loss ... about what it really means.'

'Do you remember when we looked out at the Russian vine? It had been a difficult day with the first realisation that you might die. I wrote a poem about that day. Would you like to hear it?'

From my window the Russian vine
has turned a vivid red
such beauty ...
yet a sudden sense of doom envelops me
as if bursting from the beauty
a pressure deep within
tightly contained until this moment.
I feel the red tide flow through me
a poisoning stain upon my spirit
pulling me down into this black void
past the Russian vine
that had seemed so safe
to a place I have resisted
a place where I might drown.
A place that scares me
kept at bay until now,
but now I have no energy to resist.
My panic rises like a thick morning mist
I try to turn to twist away,
grope my way along the crumbling ledge

> my small fists bleeding scraped along its edge
> grasping ...
> Can I let go of fear
> and touch again the warm fur of life?

Tears spill from Ann's eyes.
Gently I ask, 'Is this talk upsetting?'
'It is but it is ok ... my thoughts and feelings need to surface and break open ... rather than be contained.'

'I am dying' hums through my head endlessly and without relief. I hear that melody all the time. it is the beginning of me humming a lullaby to myself. What can I write about this aloneness? If you think standing by yourself waiting for someone to talk to you is lonely, if you think holidays alone are lonely, if you think not having a relationship for a long time is lonely, if you think that the long, frightening nights after a divorce are lonely – you cannot know the aloneness of one who faces death, looking it squarely in the eye.[5]

Is this why Ann averts her gaze? That she cannot look at herself naked (without hair) in the mirror because she sees her aloneness even as she is wrapped up in her loving family. Her family avert their gaze from Ann as dying. Not that she is dying but the thought is there.

We talk of the expectation to be 'normal' so as not to remind everyone else because others struggle to deal with it. It is difficult to find space to relax, meditate, listen to music. She says she will try and create space when she has time, and that is the rub-fitting it in rather than seeing it as essential work for herself. She says she is going to work on her life-style – sleep, relaxation, diet, exercise. I hear this but wonder if she will or even can. She has been the mother for these past 25 years. Patterns are set in harder stuff than sand.

I have travelled a similar road before. I find myself drawing parallels with Gill at every turn: the fatigue – Gill sitting on a wall when she couldn't walk back, her grief over her thinned hair – even a wig unworn had felt so alien, the radiotherapy journey, the silent hidden husband, girls looking after X-mas, the problem with returning to work, the disenchantment with doctors – being reduced to an object of medical gaze, the small signs of threat and that I cannot pretend to know.

Sketch 13

January 26th. Cold in the room. Ann wrapped in blankets. Her nose as always cold. The smell of the herbal oils, pungent, intoxicating.

After the therapy Ann says she was floating three times as if transcending her body. Each time she pulled herself back as if from the void.

Just a smear of the dark blue chamomile remains in the glass brown pot. Her brittle veins are much better, even her eczema has cleared up.

---

[5] Butler S and Rosenblum B (1994) *Cancer in two voices*. The Women's Press, London, p. 119 read in the performance by an audience member.

It is now six months past her surgery. Ann writes a journal.

Audre Lorde[6] commenced a journal six months after her radical mastectomy. Her first entry –

I'm not feeling very hopeful these days, about self-hood or anything else. I handle the outward motions of each day while pain fills me like a puspocket and every touch threatens to breech the taunt membrane that keeps if from flowing through and poisoning my whole existence. Sometimes despair sweeps across my consciousness like luna winds across a barren landscape. Ironshod horses rage back and forth over every nerve. Oh seboulisa ma, help me remember what I have paid so much to learn. I could die of difference, or live – myriad selves.

Seboulisa is a mythological African mother goddess who Lorde turned to comfort and guide her in her suffering. Our ancestors are moorings to hold us. The mastectomy scar is an ironshod hoof-mark.

Ann's suffering bubbles through the flimsy masks, it is not so easily contained. Yet who are her ancestors? She has no faith. What does she hold onto? Her family, her friends? Me? But is that enough? Her cry across the barren landscape is the whistling of a luna wind. Perhaps that is why her nose is always so cold?

The dance is the luna wind. Luna turns the tides. We are shapeshifters opening up the possibilities of the dance, tuning to the meanings we create deep within its rhythm.

Sketch 14

February 8th. Ann answers the door without a headscarf, her hair growing back.

'Charcoal grey,' I murmur.

'No it's not charcoal … [she laughs], it's brunette with blond highlights … those flecks of grey?'

'Cassie' – the wig is on its stand, no longer worn, played with by the girls. Even Ira wore it for a laugh.

I say, 'I love the shape of your head.'

Yet her fatigue still bites deep into her body that has suffered so much insult. Her nails a mess. The numbness around her top lip persists – it is not pleasant, sensations in her fingers and toes, the pain in right hip persists, the thousand worms wriggle relentlessly. She is anxious about it, finding it difficult to get comfortable especially in bed where she normally sleeps on that hip. Dr George is arranging a bone scan to put her fearful mind at rest. I cannot imagine a cancer has invaded there.

Ann and Ira had a weekend break in Bath. She recounts a story of being in the sauna. Another couple in there. She took of her hat to reveal her cropped hair. The other couple in the sauna went silent. They had seen Ann earlier with her wig … Ann laughs, 'She probably thought I was a lesbian.'

I ask why?

'Because lesbians have short cropped hair.'

'Did you have your doc martins on as well then?', feeding the stereotype.

---

[6] Audre Lorde (1980) *The cancer journals*. Spinsters, New York, p. 10.

'We went to bed at 5.30 with chocolate eggs and red wine.'
She gives me a knowing look. I wonder – does he run his finger along your scar line?

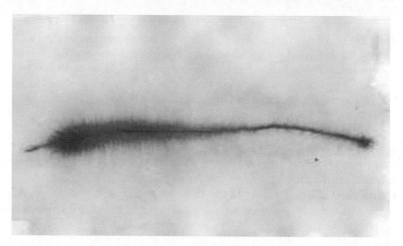

Ann has shifted. She no longer wants to return to work. Having come through the treatments she is now in a different place, no longer searching for who she was, trying to recover her old self when work was important. Maybe she will work in M&S or a bookstore for a year or more. She does not know whether she can face other woman with breast cancer, that she may over-identify, that she may not be compassionate or even be angry at them.

Shifts in life: she has been to yoga session, swimming three times a week, finding her breath. Life no longer taken for granted. Everything is more significant. She has learnt from this illness. Each step a journey into stillness and then the thoughts creep back in, emotions run high, frustration on the cusp, fears lurking. Yet stillness has been touched. It leaves a memory trace and shifts the tide slightly.

My hands move across her back as if sculpting clay, shaping beauty, easing the tension deep within the tissues. 'Those hands,' she says. And outside the Tibetan prayer flags sway gently.

I write Ann a poem:

> Do not bend for me you say
> even as you bend and sway
> to the stiffening breeze
> that takes your breath away.
>
> Do not bend for me you say
> even as the burden bends you to the ground
> where no joy is found
> amongst the fallen leaves.
>
> Do not bend for me you say
> for you have other things to do today
> than to hold me still
> even as the demons dance and shrill.

In response I bend and sway
I bend to make you whole
to lift the spirit the cancer stole
in flowing dance upon the wind.

The reed bends in the aching breeze
it gives but is not broken
nourished by a love unspoken
it dances with the swirling trees.

So like a reed I bend for you
in graceful dance and harmony
how else could I be
but toss with you on the raging sea.

Do not bend for me you say
but your eyes plead for me to stay
and bend with you as you bend
in case you break upon the wind.

Like reeds together we bend and sway
In joy-sad dance upon the wind
I bend but am not broken
Nourished by this love unspoken.

In the struggle to survive our wounds, we may adapt a strategy for living which gets us through life. Life-threatening illness may cause us to re-examine the very premise on which we have based our lives, perhaps freeing ourselves to live more fully for the first time.[7]

Thank you.

---

[7]Remen R (1994) *Kitchen table wisdom*. Riverhead Books, New York, p. 156. This quote is unspoken, read from the screen.

Chapter 10

Reflections on performance

April Nunes Tucker, Amanda Price and Antje Diedrich

What is performance and when does it occur?

I arrive at work in the morning and, having observed the rules and cultural norms governing the parking of my car and greeting of colleagues, I encounter a group of students experiencing difficulties meeting an assignment deadline. In my role as personal tutor I offer them appropriate advice and hurry to my first lecture. As I enter the room the students acknowledge that my presence heralds the beginning of a formal teaching session and alter their behaviour to reflect this awareness. I, in my turn, adopt an authoritative posture and position in order to signal the start of the class. After a few moments the students are required to begin work on a dramatic text; now they will assume the role of actors and I of the director. The relationship between us changes again; we are now less formal with each other and the spatial relationships become fluid, adaptive and unstable in place of the more fixed and formal arrangements adhering in the early stages of our encounter. Now the students take on 'characters' and play actions 'in the name' of those characters. Accordingly I sometimes address them by the name of their character and sometimes by their real name. Suddenly 'normal behaviour' becomes difficult to achieve and requires detailed reflection if it is to appear 'authentic' to an audience. The question 'How would my character sit down?' involves detailed discussion of the context in which the sitting takes place – is your character anxious, or at ease? – consideration of age, profession, gender – an old soldier would sit entirely differently from a young mother – and speculation concerning motive or intent – what does this character want to achieve from this action; ease, authority, threat, respite? All of a sudden every action involves a discussion of life itself in all its complexity and contradiction. The reproduction of 'normality' is never a simple undertaking.

In this brief example we encounter both traditional and non-traditional forms of performance. At the traditional end of the spectrum – the rehearsal – performers speak lines that have been written for them, perform actions which serve a dramatic plot, and represent people other than themselves. The non-traditional performances which precede the rehearsal are unscripted, improvisational, and are characterised by the apparent spontaneity of the performer, who performs no one but herself. A clear differentiation may be made between the two modes of performance by defining the professional performer as 'representational' and the non-professional performer (one who performs within a social context) as non-representational. The term 'performer' straddles the two modes, however, in recognition that:

> A 'performance' may be defined as all the activity of a given participant on a given occasion which serves to influence in any way any of the other participants. (Goffman 1956:15–16)

Over the past half century the term performance has become solidly located within an academic discipline and, as a consequence, has shrugged off its traditional roots invoking images of theatrical posturing and rigidly trained dancers. A newly democratised approach now recognises performance as a cultural manifestation of the knowledge we embody. In other words, the roles – both professional and private – which we perform, and – more importantly – the ways in which we perform them, make explicit our relationship to our social and cultural norms. Instrumental in this shifting paradigm has been the burgeoning discipline of Performance Studies, which acknowledges its roots in traditional forms of performances but draws on sociology, anthropology, philosophy and cultural theory in order to extend our understanding of the ways in which performance both confirms and challenges the knowledge and belief systems that underpin our everyday behaviour.

Reflective/non-reflective performance

The performance I engage in when I park my car, greet colleagues, or offer advice to students in my role as personal tutor, is non-reflective. This performance is habitual, based on learnt behaviours, which I have repeated, honed, and embodied thoroughly. Richard Schechner, a pioneering practitioner and theorist of Performance Studies describes such behaviour as 'twice-behaved behaviour':

> Everyday life … involves years of training, of learning appropriate bits of behaviour, of finding out how to adjust and perform one's life in relation to social and personal circumstances. The long infancy and childhood specific to the human species is an extended training and rehearsal period for the successful performance of adult life … In fact, the everydayness of everyday life is precisely its familiarity, its being built from known bits of behaviour rearranged and shaped in order to suit specific circumstances. (Schechner 2006:23)

These fragments of learnt behaviour, which are endlessly rearranged, are described by Schechner as 'having a life of their own' due to the fact that their origins are lost to the performer. Set adrift from the social and cultural moorings that gave life to them they continue to implicate the performer in 'causal systems' of which he or she remains entirely ignorant. In *Gender trouble: feminism and the subversion of identity*, Judith Butler examines the cultural construction of gender in Western society and suggests that repetition, rehearsal and mimicry are central to the development of gender roles:

> The subject is not *determined* by the rules through which it is generated because signification is *not a founding act but rather a regulated process of repetition* that both conceals itself and enforces its rules precisely through substantializing effects. In a sense all signification takes place within the orbit of the compulsion to repeat. (Butler 1990:145)

Butler's positioning of gender development as 'social performance' affirms Schechner's constitution of adult identity as the outcome of behaviours learnt and repeated throughout childhood and adolescence. Both Schechner and Butler concur that non-reflective behaviour developed under such circumstances will normally produce 'performances' aligned to traditionally conservative habits of thought and experience circulating within the original social context. Change within social contexts requires the facility of reflective behaviour, or behaviour which is no longer simply repeated but has been chosen for a purpose, or goal. If the behaviour which determines identity and agency in an individual is signifying non-reflective ways – ways which remain to some degree inaccessible to that individual – then the efficacy of that individual to 'act' or effect change within his or her social context must therefore be severely compromised.

Once behaviour becomes an object of reflection it immediately ceases to be considered 'natural' or spontaneous and can be recognised rather as a patchwork of copied and carefully – if unconsciously – rehearsed fragments. It then becomes possible that the 'performer' may begin be able to consider making critical or aesthetic choices about the 'material' he or she has embodied. Schechner describes the fragments of behaviour we adopt as a means of articulating our identity as 'strips of behaviour', rather like strips of celluloid film. These, he suggests, can be consciously as well as unconsciously organised.

Performers working on a dramatic script will identify Schechner's 'strips of identity' in order to develop the character they will play. Each 'strip' – which may be a gesture, a habit of speaking, or an attitude towards others – is discussed, tried out, rehearsed over and over, until it finally becomes part of the 'make-up' or identity of their role. A good performer will recognise that a believable character is made up of a broad range of attitudes, gestures and opinions, many of which sit uneasily alongside each other, or even contradict each other. A poor representation of character is one which is made up of only a few clearly indicated traits that do no more than serve the exigencies of the plot.

Performance and the nature of reflection

Richard Schechner's 'strips of behaviour' are echoed in Chris Johns' discussion of the ways in which our social and cultural context impact upon our responses to the world around us:

> You do not live in isolation from others but share a world that is largely pre-governed by cultural norms that strongly, albeit unwittingly, shape the way you think, feel and respond within situations. Reflection gives you access to understand these patterns of relationships and the ways they have influenced you within experience … reflection also helps you view or place your experience in terms of social systems that shape everyday practice. (Johns 2002:7–8)

Johns suggests that reflection upon our behaviour – our practice – in social situations allows us insight into the cultural scripts and performances we have acquired through unreflective repetition. The process of reflection, applied to this practice, raises questions concerning the originating source of the behaviour and provides the beginning of a critique of the performances these sources have engendered. Do we have set response patterns to certain types of people, or situations in our working practices, for example? Once behaviour is recognised as an habitual performance born of repetition and mimicry one may begin to enquire as to *what* or *who* is being articulated through this particular performance. This process of reflection, recognition and review is not an easy one; ingrained patterns of behaviour (like bad habits picked up by actors) can prove to be intransigent even if the will to change is strong. Changing our performances requires learning new 'strips' of behaviour that articulate more accurately our professional, social and cultural environment.

One simple example of this was suggested to me by a lecturer in Linguistics at a conference I attended. He commented, in conversation, on a common trait he had observed amongst the British to make 'heavy work' of pronouncing 'foreign' words in the course of conversation. Whilst he found that most people attributed this to their individual lack of linguistic knowledge his observation was that, as an 'island' people who had once presided over a powerful empire, the British tend to resist the penetration of foreign words into their mother tongue; they would far rather – he suggested – impose their language upon others, or anglicise foreign words which take their fancy. It was a logic which I found hard to resist and have, since then, enjoyed perfecting the odd foreign phrase which creeps into my vocabulary knowing that in doing so I am articulating a post-Empire attitude towards the new global context within which we all now live. My performed identity has changed, therefore, in response to reflection upon cultural norms, or habits.

Whilst much of our behaviour is bound up with language, there are also modes of performance we employ as a means of articulating subjective states which would appear to evade linguistic utterance:

> What has not been given sufficient consideration is that large areas and important aspects of culture, no one, not even the native, has information that can simply be called up and expressed in discursive statements. This sort of knowledge can be represented – made present – only through action, enactment, or performance. (Fabian 1990:6)

The knowledge to which Fabian refers is that described by Lockford and Pelias as a 'tacit knowledge' which 'operates from an implicit system of logic; a learned and imprinted grammar of practice ... a structure that supports each performance but typically remains hidden' (Lockford and Pelias 2004:436). What is being discussed here are the ways our bodies respond to social and cultural stimuli. How do we know that certain jokes are funny and others aren't? How do we know who we should pay attention to and who we can ignore? These are areas of knowledge that are only articulated through the body, in looks and glances, laughter, bodily posture, spatial relationships and uneasy silences. Dwight Conquergood proposes that a process of reflection on non-verbal performance (non-discursive knowledge) has the potential to unlock, or expose, contradictions or tensions in lived experience. He suggests that language may articulate one form of knowledge in the world whilst the body may be articulating something entirely at odds with this. Conquergood suggests that this potential conflict between the words we speak and the way we are is a result of objectifying systems of knowledge: 'dominant epistemologies that link knowing with seeing [and] are not attuned to meanings that are masked, camouflaged, indirect, embedded, or hidden in context' (Conquergood 2002:146). Instances of non-discursive or embodied performance tend to occur in situations where power is unevenly distributed. The powerful group will tend, in such circumstances, to dominate linguistically whilst the less powerful group will supplement its discourse with a network of signs, gestures, and glances that constitute an alternative language of resistance.

Jon McKenzie, in *Perform or else: from discipline to performance* (2001) suggests that the cultural life of a society provides an arena within which to discuss, debate and critique the relationship between discursive and non-discursive forms of knowledge; between knowledge held at the level of language and knowledge held in the body. These cultural performances can take many forms but they share the aim to 'engage with social norms, as an ensemble of activities with the potential to uphold societal arrangements or, alternatively, to change people and societies' (McKenzie 2001:30). McKenzie cites a range of cultural performance activities, which include political demonstrations, raves and rock concerts, and certainly these events have – over the past half century – changed our perceptions of ourselves as a people, and of our relationship to both our society and the broader global context within which we live. One has only to consider the impact of the

1984 miners' strike, the death of Princess Diana in 1997, the anti-war rallies in 2003, to recognise the powerful potential we have to perform our response to fault-lines in our social fabric. In each of these instances the response, at the level of performance, provided a commentary upon lived experience of the unfolding events that evaded the discursive structures operating at the level of official national debate. The urgency of these cultural performances betrayed the frustrations and anger of those participating and a desire to make visible a knowledge that evaded 'expert' commentary; they are what Lockford and Pelias would describe as an 'act of doing as a way of coming to understand' (2004:432).

Whilst cultural performances are most visible at the macro level, they also occur daily at a micro level; every meeting we attend, every professional encounter we experience exposes us to the political and cultural beliefs, or a framework of knowledge, which implicate us in the power structures operating within our social context. To return to Erving Goffman's definition, we engage in performance whenever our interaction with others exerts influence upon their behaviour or actions. Recognition of this powerful component of performance serves to remind us that we are agents as well as recipients of the structures which define social experience. The ability to change our 'strips of behaviour' in order to affect change in others is, therefore, central to an understanding of the potential political impact performance at a micro-level may have on those around us. Richard Schechner defines this type of performance mode as an 'efficacious' tendency in which efficacy overrides the more traditional attributes of performance as entertainment:

> At each period in each culture one or the other (mode) is dominant – one is ascending while the other is descending. Naturally these changes are part of changes in the overall social structure: yet performance is not a passive mirror of these social changes but a part of the complicated feedback process that brings about change. (Schechner 1977:76)

Performance as efficacy

The Brazilian practitioner, Augusto Boal, provides a model for the efficacious use of theatre, which he named 'forum theatre' (1979). The premise of this theatrical event is that it provides participants with the opportunity to place everyday behaviour in a public arena and reflect upon it in an active and dynamic way. The process is a democratic one in which 'performers' and 'spectators' combine their skills and expertise with the communal focus being upon the solving of problems through the initiation of change. In order for forum theatre to be effective a group sharing a common vocabulary – be that a profession, a living environment, or a social concern – decide upon the situation they wish to change. This may be, for example, the way meetings are conducted, or the ways in which a client group is treated by professional staff. Having articulated the 'problem' clearly, a typical scenario that illustrates the problem is chosen by the participants. This initial decision often involves detailed and complex discussion as 'problem' situations are rarely simple in their structure or content. Having decided on the scenario the 'performers' rehearse and perform it for the rest of the group. The performers may be participants, or they may be professional performers who have been invited to the event. In either case the rehearsal of the scenario is important as it needs to be detailed in its presentation of the 'problematic' behaviour, or situation, and it needs to reproduce the situation accurately – as if the scenario is actually happening in front of the group as a whole.

Once all the participants are happy with the performance, a Master of Ceremonies is elected. This person will 'chair' the event and ensure that progress is made through discussion of the 'problem' towards alternative approaches to its solution. The scenario is then played out without stopping for the rest of the participants. It is then immediately played out for a second time, but this time any participant can stop the action in order to discuss a particular aspect of the scenario, or to suggest a different way of playing out the scenario. Each suggestion will be acted on by the performers, who may also participate in the discussion as they are 'experiencing' the situation for the participants who are watching. It may be the case that a spectator may wish to take the place of one of the performers in order to clarity or provide an example of what he or she is suggesting. Boal encourages the idea that eventually the 'performers' will be replaced by the 'spectators', as he considers this an entirely positive dynamic that represents the embracing of change in action. The process continues until a solution, or alternative course of action, is agreed upon and has been enacted by the group. The Master of Ceremonies ensures that 'magical' solutions – which ignore the realities of the situation – are dismissed, and that everyone has a chance to participate verbally, if not physically.

Augusto Boal describes the process of forum theatre as a 'rehearsal for revolution'. The overtly political nomenclature reflects its beginnings in the slum dwellings of Brazil but also suggests that the democratisation of performance – he refuses to acknowledge a schism between performers and spectators, preferring to call all participants 'spect-actors' – allows for the creation of a space in which our performed behaviour can be scrutinised, critiqued and, most importantly, changed in order to effect social, cultural and political responses within the context of 'everyday' behaviour.

Performing liminal experience

The radical nature of Augusto Boal's forum theatre is based on the simple proposition that the narratives we experience on a daily basis, when performed and reviewed, can provide the potential for profound change both culturally and politically. The basis of the stories that form the material for Boal's theatre allow for the performance of cultural and social life from the perspective of the participants; the performances are, therefore, suffused with the subjective experience of those participating in them. This subjective measure of reality is often found to be in direct contestation of rules, laws or measures of behaviour extracted according to a more objective vision of reality.

Mark Johnson, in *The body in the mind: the bodily basis of meaning, imagination, and reason*, explores the ways in which we construct the meanings that define our relationship to the world around us. He suggests that *meaning* has been defined as an objective measure of reality relying upon an evidence base of 'abstract symbols and things (objects) in the world' (1987:x). This construction of reality prioritises objectively evidenced propositions over 'subjective elements':

> The world consists of objects that have properties and stand in various relationships independent of human understanding. The world is as it is, no matter what any person happens to believe about it, and there is one correct 'God's-Eye-View' about what the world really is like. (Johnson 1987:x)

Boal's forum theatre contests the 'God's-Eye-View of the world' and suggests that objectively arrived at parameters of meaning have a tendency to reduce subjective experience to a by-product of lived reality rather than a central component in our relationship to the structures that define that lived reality.

The word 'liminality' has been used by anthropologists to describe such experiences which fall between objectively arrived at categories of experience and knowledge. Anthropologist Victor Turner has famously discussed the liminal state, taking as his starting point the work of Arthur Van Gennep. Van Gennep's work on *rites of passage* in traditional pre-industrial societies identified a communally agreed process which guided individuals from one state of being to another. A common example of a *rite of passage* is the transition of the child into puberty which, Van Gennep noted, was marked by the removal of the child from the community, the initiation of the child into their new role in their community, and the reintegration of the child into the community. These three stages were defined by Van Gennep as the pre-liminal, the liminal, and the post-liminal. The pre-liminal phase is defined as a separation from community. The liminal phase is a state of non-identity in which the characteristics of the past are dropped and the future characteristics are not yet assumed, this is a state of 'betwixt and between'. The post-liminal stage sees the individual reintegrated into his or her community. Turner identified in this model the recognition of two modes of society. The society from which liminality separates individuals he defines 'as a structured, differentiated, and often hierarchical system of politico-legal-economic positions' (Turner 1969:83) and the society celebrated during the liminal process is one 'of society as an unstructured or rudimentarily structured and relatively undifferentiated … community, or even communion of equal individuals' (1969:83).

Turner notes that the process of liminality recognises that change can only occur when the human being is prioritised over the structures and frameworks which facilitate social or communal life. In order to affect change, therefore, the individual will have to be removed from the social context; removed from the systems of identification; and returned to a state of being in which the knowledge held 'in the body' overrides all social constraints and mores. Turner notes that in moments of liminality a society is able to make a symbolic return to its roots, its gut feelings and responses as human beings, as part of a process of reflection which may engender change in the society as a whole.

Anthropologist Colin Turnbull suggests that Victor Turner's definition of social, or communal experience of liminality, also exists within the individual's daily experience of the world. He highlights moments of experience when an 'intuitive', or subjective, knowledge clarifies that experience and often has the power to override the more objectively established responses to a situation or problem. Such moments are often described as 'going out on a limb' or 'having a hunch' and are characterised by individuals refusing to follow the rational, or accepted route, but rather choosing work on a more instinctive level which they 'just feel' is the right course of action. Turnbull notes that intuition often operates upon the individual at an unconscious level and is not, therefore, accorded the importance or exposure it deserves in our negotiations with lived reality.

> Liminality is a subjective experience of the external world … it is integrative of all experience; in the liminal state disorder is ordered, doubts and problems removed, the right course of action is made clear with a rightness that is both structural and moral since the inevitable discrepancies between belief and practice in the external world are among the many problems ordered and removed in the liminal state. (Turnbull 1990:80)

Turnbull proposes that this '"other" state of being' – which he calls 'the liminal' – is essential to our ability to make sense of our experience as human beings, and that its acknowledged co-existence in an objectively defined society is fundamental to the cultural, social and political health of that society.

Reflective writing dwells with subjective experience wherever and whenever it erupts in our professional lives. The writings that emerge from reflective practice acknowledge the 'liminal' being co-existing in the repetitions of our daily work as those moments in which the 'human' response must override the professional response.

Reflective performance searches for ways in which liminal experience can be shared in a communal arena of action. Once shared it becomes subject to review, discussion and critique. A performance event may be the reading of a narrative to others, the sharing of a problem using Boal's forum theatre, or the playing out of experience in order to comprehend or acknowledge that which cannot easily be translated into language.

In the second part of this chapter we will reflect upon our process of creating a performance in response to Chris Johns' reflective journal entries whilst treating a woman diagnosed with breast cancer. The text had been 'performed' by Chris Johns at conferences prior to our involvement and very few changes were made in the course of our work on it. The aim of our creative process was to enquire as to whether the inclusion of trained dancers and actors could enhance the spectators' experience of Johns' text. Amanda Price (Theatre) and April Nunes Tucker (Dance) joined Chris Johns as performers of the text, and Antje Diedrich (Theatre) worked as director on the piece.

Performing *Climbing walls*

The nature of the *Climbing walls* text written by Chris Johns[1] combines both objective and subjective knowledge. It traces the clinical process experienced by Ann and positions this as objective knowledge alongside the subjective experiences of both himself as therapist and Ann as patient.

This second section of the chapter looks explicitly at our processes of making and performing *Climbing walls* and does so through an oscillation of writing styles that include three modes: an informal account of our working processes toward the performance of *Climbing walls* (2008); a more formal discussion of theories underpinning performance practices found within our approaches to expressing Chris' text; and excerpts from reflective journals kept by Antje Diedrich, Amanda Price and April Nunes Tucker. The interweaving of these three modes of writing aims to capture a flavour of the different types of practical and theoretical processes involved in the making of our performance.

A look at process – moving into performance

Clutching our copies of Chris' text, we sat in a state of 'not knowing' over cups of coffee. Instead of going off to research breast cancer we chose to enter into a personal discussion about how the text made us feel. It was an emotional discussion not a theoretical one and we attempted to integrate the text into our own lived experience by locating ourselves in relation to it.

---

[1] *Climbing walls* text is presented in Chapter 9.

First rehearsal with April and Amanda.
Conversation over coffee.
We discuss cultural differences in our relationship with cancer and the body.
You can't say the word or you might catch it.
The unmentionable ...
The opposite in my home country.
'How are you?' – 'Oh, I've just learnt I've got cancer. Will have to have surgery and chemo.'
BANG!
Some subtle pleasure in laying bare one's suffering.
Have some doubts about these clichés and generalisations. Have been away for too long.
Things will have changed in the meantime.
Back to talking about the body and the breasts in particular.
Shared feeling that breasts are not so important to us. Don't consider them as site of sexual
pleasure. See them as something functional.
Made extensive use of them in breastfeeding.
Amanda talks about the tragic element of the text. Facing one's nemesis, facing death.
Am reminded me of my engagement with Holocaust literature and drama and of our work
on *4:48 Psychosis*.
Aspects of human life we tend to marginalise and blot out in everyday life but that inevitably
form part of our humanness, humanity.
Theatre is a good place to face these issues and to remind ourselves of what it means to be
human: suffering and death but also easing of suffering and healing.
Antje Diedrich (10 September 2008)

The pervading feeling of 'not knowing' stayed with us as we sat and shared our reflections on our responses to Chris Johns' text. This 'not knowing' could be equated with an authentic, reflective state, dwelling in an in-between that carries with it extraordinary potential. In performance, this 'not knowing' fosters a reaction to the lived moment. A situation unfolding in 'reality' makes its way into performance whereby processes of making may be exposed and mutual experiencing, based in a shared experience of 'not knowing', helps to activate an interrogation of the text that involves 'the other'.

Embodiment

To contextualise this in the situation in which we found ourselves (i.e. pouring over Chris' text, drinking cups of coffee in a state of 'not knowing'), it would be accurate to recount that this important authentic event of sharing our own lived experiences would find its way into the performance of *Climbing walls*. What we did not do was concern ourselves with was how we could apply our learned techniques in theatre and dance to the text. Rather, we as performers talked about how we could potentially embody the text. There is much debate and discussion around the term 'embodiment' in the field of dance but for the sake of clarity in the capacity of performance and reflective practice, I think it is important to highlight two facets of embodiment that were present in our working processes towards the performance of *Climbing walls*. First, that embodiment assumes that 'consciousness is not 'pure', but exists within a membrane of flesh and blood' (Bullock and Trombley 1977:264) and second, as Gail Weiss puts it, 'The experience of being embodied is never a private affair, but is always already mediated by our continual interactions with other human and nonhuman bodies' (1999:5). If our thoughts, actions and perceptions are tied up with the thoughts, actions and perceptions of others then the powerful, uncomfortable state of uncertainty, of 'not knowing' is formed and re-formed according to our mutual corporeal experiencing of each other and of ourselves. Because Chris Johns' knowledge of the *Climbing walls* text was embodied, it was important to our performance making processes that Chris' symbiotic relationship with the text remained preserved.

> I had concerns about Chris' text.
> Not quite understanding where he was coming from.
> Examining it with the critical academic mind, trained to pull things apart before they can even be whole for a moment.
> Feeling guilty and nervous about voicing these concerns.
> Chris' clear and concise answers: 'I want people to be aware of human suffering' (Not sure these were his precise words).
> Still concerned about his use of the dance metaphor. Suggesting an erotically charged relationship rather than the embracing of chaos.
> Remember that first rehearsal when we asked Chris to read the text to us and all concerns dissipated. It worked!
> The surprise and relief to find that this was totally unproblematic when he spoke the words, when he read his text to us.
> The text does not have a life of its own. It is not a piece of drama to be dissected by the critical mind.
> The text is entwined with its speaker. It is authenticated by the author's presence.
> Chris is the text and the text is Chris. The two belong together.
> He embodies intent that is not necessarily expressed in words, not necessarily written into the text. He cannot be separated from the narrative. We need to read the two together.
> The task ahead was to find out what this unity of author/text needed in addition. What could Amanda and April bring to the process?
> Antje Diedrich (23 September 2008)

There we were, the four of us in the performance space enveloped by the reality of a complete integration between text and author. Where to start? How could we best interrogate this text involving 'the other'? The other was Ann, a woman with breast cancer whom none of us had met except Chris.

Rejecting naturalism

It took us only a few hours to decide that a naturalistic approach to Chris' text was not working. We began by trying out a scene in *Climbing walls* where Chris and Ann interact. Amanda 'acted' Ann, reading Ann's words from the text as if they were her own and spatially relating to Chris in a dialogic arrangement. Something in this first stab at working with the text was unsuccessful. We tried again. In this second attempt at the same scene we asked Chris to speak Ann's words whilst I stood in the performance space as a representation of Ann. This approach also felt contrived. In fact, attempts to represent Ann and her suffering in a dramatic way felt blasphemous. The imposition of a naturalistic technique removed the immediacy of the text. This distancing effect on the text was perhaps because naturalism as a theatrical technique 'refers to an objective portrayal of daily life that appears true to the spectator or reader's actual experience' (Innes 2000:13). Nothing removed Ann further from the truth than an attempt to characterise her. Naturalism and its defining aspect of objective characterisation failed to meet the innate subjective nature of the *Climbing walls* text.

We needed to turn away from orthodox theatrical representation and offer our own authentic presence to tell Ann's story. Chris already embodied this authenticity as author, as therapist, as himself. The only way we perceived to match this truth in all its starkness on stage was to seek within each scene of Chris' narrative the essence and mood behind it. This approach meant that traditional performance techniques such as naturalism and a striving for technical virtuosity were obsolete. We therefore turned to a method of working which allowed us to express Chris' narrative through an organisation of space, body and energy.

> Not a light bulb on the stage, but a fragile, constant light – with the occasional flicker.
> Chris illumines suffering dimly – he doesn't bring it into the glare of the spotlight.
> No body on Chris – except when he's clumsy, or uneasy.
> His light illuminates his face, and energises his voice.
> The words are the carriers of energy; they are not borrowed.
> This energy has a source inside him. He has – or uses – no technique.
> Are April and I frauds beside this?
> Much of the rehearsal process was about our desire not to be frauds.
> What do we bring? Skills, presence, technique, spatial awareness, voice, focus, intention.
> But how do they become more than that?
> How can they sit beside the 'real'?
> Chris, too, is distanced from the 'real'; his aim is to ease suffering though; his vision is clear.
> What is our vision? What do we do?
> Beside Chris do we become ornamentation, aestheticisers of the dirty, rotten, stinking business of dying?
> Amanda Price (10 October 2008)

Towards authenticity

After reaching the decision to avoid the naturalistic, we faced the challenge of engaging with our work authentically. This is defined by Dwight Conquergood when he describes dynamic performance as a process of undergoing 'a shift from mimesis to kinesis' (1989:83). As the processes of making began to unfold we questioned other performance techniques present in our own specific disciplines of theatre and dance and aimed to find more authentic means of expressing the things we were discovering through our work with Chris and the *Climbing walls* narrative. We were firm in our agreement that none of us could represent Ann and therefore instead of imposing a myriad of pre-established techniques into the working processes we simply allowed the female body into the performance space. This realisation of simply allowing the female body to share the space alongside Chris' narrative was testimony to our own reflective success. The female body was in fact, what was missing from the text. As two women accompanying Chris in the telling of Ann's story, we aimed to articulate what the text as words could *not* articulate. One example of this manifested in the following scene where Chris narrates a dialogue he has with Ann about her experience of meeting the surgeon who will perform her mastectomy:

> 'How was the surgeon when you saw him again?'
> 'Umm ... he showed no interest in me ... flipping through his diary looking for a date ... avoiding my eyes but my eyes were probably downcast anyway ...'
> 'I can imagine ... it can't be easy facing your nemesis ...'
> Nemesis

The Greek god of retribution
A rival or opponent who cannot be beaten
Is that the cancer or the surgeon
Perhaps both.
I sense Ann's expectation that he sees her as a person rather than a breast he must hack off … images of hacked breasts heaped high in the theatre corner … What does he think as he flips through his diary to set the surgical date … does he sense the immensity of this date for the woman? Dare he see her in her humanness?

As Chris reads these words Amanda stands downstage and lifts up her t-shirt to reveal one naked breast. This female body exposed, standing in the space is not a neutral body nor is it Ann's body but it raises questions.

In this moment, although Amanda's body is held in stillness it is charged with vibrancy. Her presence demands that the observer reflect on the uncertainty that exists between her presence and Chris' words. In our newfound approach to the text which was to allow the female body into the actual and metaphorical space of Chris' reflective narrative we upheld the desire to stay authentic in both our approaches to making and performing.

Authenticity is a very complex issue that has fluctuated in its value across performance history. The image of the double helix is useful to illustrate this point.

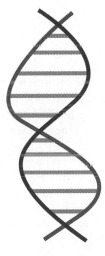

Each strand of the double helix can be taken to represent two separate but interdependent value systems within performance. The first strand of this double helix values reflection; the other, technical virtuosity and they find their definitions in relation to one another. Performance valuing technical virtuosity alone results in performance that has lost its immediacy and is remote from audiences. Yet, when the two value systems collide there emerges a state of questioning and this state of questioning is one of the defining characteristics of authenticity. Dwight Conquergood also uses a double helix to highlight the relationship between self and other.

The aim of dialogical performance is to bring self and other together so that they can question, debate and challenge one another. It is a kind of performance that resists conclusions, it is intensely committed to keeping the dialogue between performer and text open and ongoing. Dialogical understanding does not end with empathy. There is always enough appreciation for difference so that the text can interrogate, rather than dissolve into the performer. (Conquergood 1985:9)

It is in the collision of the two value systems located in the double helix, the first of which values self and the second which values virtuosity, that emerges an immediacy. Chris Johns refers to this as a 'way of being within everyday practice' (2004:1). This characteristic of immediacy which Johns describes is another defining aspect of authenticity.

Performers who 'act' inside a characterised role without reflecting upon the role they are undertaking obstruct the authentic experience. David Mamet, playwright and theatre director shares this view in challenging the performer to strip away the rigid confines that come through striving toward virtuosity via the utilisation of theatrical representation techniques:

> participate in the low, the uncertain, the unproved, the unheralded, to bring the truth of yourself to the stage. Not the groomed, sure, 'talented,' approved person you are portraying; not the researched, corseted, paint-by-numbers presentation-without-flaws, not the Great Actor, but yourself – as uncertain, as unprepared, as confused as any of us are. (1997:124)

As Mamet illustrates, in performance observers are quick to recognise an act. They are not fooled by the performer who attempts to play something other than themselves. This is the paradox that lies within performance. The performer is aware that they are not 'themselves' whilst performing and likewise, the observers are aware that they are not seeing the performer's innate personality. Despite this recognition of falsity, personas are perhaps assumed by performers as a shield against the exposure of their vulnerability in performance. As a result of this, the attention of the performer will not be fixed upon being in the moment of lived experience. Instead, they will be absorbed in a process of aesthetic judgement about their own level of success in 'playing the role' or in executing the technique measured against a virtuosic ideal. To parallel the negation of technique in the context of reflective practice, Chris Johns says:

> The idea of paying attention to self within the unfolding moment defines reflection-within-the-moment; the exquisite paying attention to the way the self is thinking, feeling and responding within the particular moment, and those factors that are influencing the way self is thinking, feeling and responding. Such self-awareness moves reflection away from techniques to apply to a way of being. (2004:2)

Mamet argues the same point in relation to theatre.

> What would the word 'technique' mean if applied to a chef? Or a lover? It would mean that their works and actions were cold and empty and that, finally, we're disappointed by them. This is precisely what it means when applied to a performance onstage. (1997:118)

Issues of the balance between technique and reflection and as a result, issues of authenticity faced us in our processes of working toward the performance of *Climbing walls*.

My own struggle with previous technical striving cultivated through years of dance training became a real hurdle to overcome in this performance process. The dance training that I experienced embraced an aesthetic ideal where technical virtuosity took priority over self. This tradition of imbalanced values, still very prevalent in dance education, manifested in me as a questioning but more than questioning. A sense of torque, a wrenching toward change began to unfold for me in this performance process. An example of this was evident in the scene that Amanda and I named 'Chaos'. 'Chaos' was a scene where the two of us propelled ourselves on stage and clambered over one another on all fours in what felt like a whirling vortex. We swept the whole space of the stage, around Chris' legs, and finally collapsed onto the floor panting with genuine exhaustion.

> Chaos doesn't work because I'm 'performing'
> The movement isn't right
> It's far too 'contemporary dance'
> And my connection to Amanda is merely spatial
> Although there is the physical connection:
> Touch, push, wait, move.
> Everything else feels arbitrary
> Maybe it's the predictable, dynamic patterning of the thing
> I feel distanced from Chris and removed from the visceral experience
> It's too organised:
> Set floor plan
> Set ending
> Set rules about how the movement unfolds.
> April Nunes Tucker (10 October 2008)

It became evident what an important role immediacy, or as Chris Johns has coined *reflection-within-the-moment*, became in the making of our work. We began to focus on the use of energy in each moment and worked substantially with a state I have called 'readiness' (Nunes Tucker 2009).

The whole process of making *Climbing walls* was involved and by no means straightforward. We went through a journey of rejecting technique and naturalism only to discover that the 'way into' Chris' narrative was to play it moment by moment, embracing subjectivity and fostering authenticity. This led us to 'readiness', a state that we felt was sensitive enough to give way to the delicate nature of Chris' text as well as being strong enough to support the subject matter and the physical demands that were required of our bodies as we met the essence of each scene.

Readiness: working with energy opposed to technique

Readiness is a description of both a physical and mental state. It is a state of alertness, likened to that of a cat preparing to pounce. There is an intensifying of mental focus and an opening of sensory awareness. Although the body may be still, it is charged with energy. This sense of engaged presence fosters immediacy by way of harnessing absolute commitment to each moment such that gaps in attention are diminished. Readiness demands cultivating a heightened attention[2] in order to feel the 'right'[3] moments for movement initiation.

---

[2] See Csikszentmihalyi (1990).
[3] See Ritsema (in Bloois *et al.* 2004) on choosing the 'right' moments to move.

Amanda stands still for a long time. It seems endless.
What's happening there?
Chris has taken position behind the table and seamlessly continues with the reading of the narrative. And Amanda just stands there.
We listen to Chris' words and we look at her. There is this living presence, a human body in all its material and non-material concreteness. It is still, but is alive.
And somehow we cannot ignore this body, we have to deal with it.
As Chris' narrative continues, we begin to make connections between his words and the person standing there.
Who is she? Ann? Chris?
A listener/spectator? A performer?
The connections are ever defined.
We cannot get past that person, that living breathing body, because we cannot define her.
And as the performance continues her presence becomes charged.
She is and is not Ann. She seems to say to us that Ann is not an abstract idea, but a person in flesh and blood that has suffered.
Chris owns the narrative. We only know about Ann through him. The person standing still in space seems to resist that ownership. She seems to say: 'I have a life of my own. And however much you try to capture me in words, you are doomed to fail. I have a life of my own.'
Antje Diedrich (17 September 2008)

The vibrancy of life that exudes from Amanda as she stands in stillness described in the excerpt above relates directly to the state of readiness. Although we brought the female body to the stage to stand alongside Chris' narrative, the body that we brought was not a passive one. In both cases of myself and Amanda, the bodies that we brought into the performance of *Climbing walls* were trained bodies; bodies that housed deeply ingrained techniques from our respective disciplines of dance and theatre. Herein lies a paradox concerning our working approach to *Climbing walls*. The cultivation of readiness and the decision to negate traditional techniques such as naturalism would not have occurred had we not both had the desire to reflect on our working practices. Yet, it was the technical training embodied within us which permitted us to access the state of readiness.

Readiness is achieved through a harnessing and directing of energy in the body and both the disciplines of dance and theatre have within them practical training mechanisms that advance a performer's work with their energy. For example, Tadashi Suzuki, founder of the Suzuki method (a psychophysical training method predominately used by actors), highlights a key concept in his training called 'animal energy'.[4]

> The audience perceives this (animal energy) as an altered mood, a precise external focus and a physical intensity…the performer is exposed and vulnerable on stage in this highly charged state. Encouraging animalistic sensitivity shifts the performance away from being an aesthetic entertainment and towards a transgressive interactive event. (Allain 2002:5)

Like Suzuki's 'animal energy', it is important to highlight that this state of readiness encompasses both technique and reflection. As a result, the state of readiness feels vulnerable, uncertain and is authentic. In the performance of *Climbing walls* we cultivated readiness between us in order to determine the 'right' moments to both move from one scene to another and to move around the performance space within scenes.

---

[4] See Allain (2002:4–5)

Stand shoulder to shoulder with someone
in complete stillness and without touching
Keep your eyes looking straight ahead
In a moment you will both move at exactly the same time
The time between stillness and movement, pregnant with potential
is what the state of readiness feels like.
April Nunes Tucker (Choreographic Journal – September 2006)

To give an example of this state of readiness in *Climbing walls*, there is a scene in the text where Ann has undergone a series of intense chemotherapy treatments and she is exhausted, absolutely drained of all energy. Chris describes his interaction with Ann on this particular day. In our devising process we found the essence of this scene to be exhaustion and how the impossibility of movement was prevalent.

In the performance space Amanda and I stand side by side facing downstage. We must feel the moment to walk together towards the little table and chair that mark our destination. We wait, both still but ready. The energetic connection grows between us, the moment arrives and simultaneously we move.

Each time we play this scene, we have to put ourselves energetically in the authentic state of exhaustion. We have to actually physically direct our energy to hang low in the body, heavy in the legs, the weight of the skull nearly unbearable upon the spine and wait for readiness to take hold, to permit that first step forward. If we force this or pretend to do it, then the vortex of meaning is lost. Even though we do not know what that meaning is, the state of readiness that rises up between us when we are true to the moment of exhaustion is what allows for this scene to unfold.

Our work together on *Climbing walls* was a journey along a search for authenticity in performance. We showed the female body without showing a particular female body and let our reflection-within-the-moment rise to the forefront of importance. Our traditional value systems underwent a shift from the technical and objective to the reflective and subjective. As a result, each performance of *Climbing walls* arises out of a genuine shared desire amongst us to tell Ann's story.

References

Allain P (2002) *The art of stillness: the theatre practice of Tadashi Suzuki*. Methuen Publishing, London.

Bloois J, Houppermans S and Korsten F (eds.) (2004) *Discern(e)ments: Deleuzian Aesthetics*. Rodopi, Amsterdam, New York.

Boal A (1979) *Theatre of the oppressed*. Pluto Press, London.

Bullock A and Trombley S (eds.) (1977) *The new Fontana dictionary of modern thought*. Harper Collins, London.

Butler J (1990) *Gender trouble: feminism and the subversion of identity*. Taylor & Francis, London.

Conquergood D (1985) Performing as a moral act: ethical dimensions of the ethnography of performance. *Literature in Performance* 5:9.

Conquergood D (1989) Poetics, play, process, and power: the performative turn in anthropology. *Text and Performance Quarterly* 1:82–95.

Conquergood D (2002) Performance studies: intervention and radical research. *TDR: The Drama Review* 46:145–156.

Csikszentmihalyi M (1990) *Flow: the psychology of optimal experience*. Harper and Row, New York.

Fabian J (1990) *Power and performance: ethnographic explorations through proverbial wisdom and theater in Shaba, Zaire.* University of Wisconsin Press, Madison, WI.

Goffman E (1956) *The presentation of self in everyday life.* Doubleday, New York.

Innes CD (2000) *Sourcebook on naturalist theatre.* Routledge, London.

Johns C (2002) *Guided reflection – advancing practice.* Wiley-Blackwell Publishers, Oxford.

Johns C (2004) *Becoming a reflective practitioner.* Wiley-Blackwell Publishers, Oxford.

Johnson M (1987) *The body in the mind: the bodily basis of meaning, imagination, and reason.* University of Chicago Press, Chicago.

Lockford L and Pelias RJ (2004) Bodily poeticizing in theatrical improvisation: a typology of performative knowledge. *Theatre Topics* 14:431–443.

Mamet D (1997) *True and false: heresy and common sense for the actor.* Pantheon Books, New York.

McKenzie J (2001) *Perform or else: from discipline to performance.* Routledge, London.

Nunes Tucker A (2009) *Revealing intersubjectivities in contemporary dance choreography.* Unpublished doctoral thesis. Middlesex University, London.

Schechner R (1977) *Performance theory.* Routledge, London.

Schechner R (2006) *Performance studies.* Routledge, London.

Turnbull C (1990) Liminality. In: R Schechner and W Appel (eds.) *By means of performance: intercultural studies of theatre and ritual.* Cambridge University Press, Cambridge, pp. 50–81.

Turner V (1969) *The ritual process: structure and anti-structure.* Penguin Books, Harmondsworth.

Weiss G (1999) *Body images: embodiment as intercorporeality.* Routledge: New York and London.

Chapter 11

More than eggs for breakfast

John-Marc Priest and Christopher Johns

Preamble

The following *performance* narrative is grounded in John-Marc's effort to become a transformational leader. It has been constructed/edited to be performed[1] from his original narrative of 22 000 words submitted as a dissertation.[2] Within the narrative are a set of 'readings' that help to emphasise what I consider significant issues of content or narrative process to engage the audience in dialogue. However, dialogue is not restricted to these readings. The readings have been changed in response to each performance, reflecting how new ideas emerge through audiencing and which become integrated into the text. The 'readings' are taken from other student narratives, my own words or from literature. The readings can be read by random audience members to engage them in performance. For the purpose of written publication (as against actual performance) I have integrated the 'readings' into the text to better illuminate their significance into the main text.

The performance is set against a PowerPoint presentation background of a set of headings (as set out in the following text) that demarcated different moments within the narrative.

The stage is set. On stage are two readers to represent John-Marc's voice. They are marked voice 1 and 2 and simply provide contrast.

More than eggs for breakfast: a narrative of becoming a leader

Reading 1

Welcome to the performance. As Alexander (2005:429) notes, 'a performance must be well crafted'. This implies craft both in poetic terms, through aesthetic language that invokes the links between felt emotion, critical thought, and understanding; as well as

---

[1] In the Toronto performance John-Marc's text was read by myself and Fran Biley as two alternating voices. The idea was to contrast different experiences through the narrative, marking distinct moments within the text, especially as the performance was an hour long.

[2] In fulfilment of the MSc in Leadership in Healthcare Practice at University of Bedfordshire.

craft in the sense that the language must be clear, effective, evocative, and more than subtly representative of the populations to which it reflects. The writing must give the audience to which it is represented access to the world of those it represents in a manner that simulates the visceral response of actual experience.

Voice 1: My narrative has been constructed to plot my realisation of leadership as a reflexive journey of self-inquiry and transformation. It has not been easy.

Reading 2

Marina wrote in her narrative – This narrative recounts the trials and tribulations encountered on that journey through the reflexive process of guided reflection. The primary aim is to explore being and becoming the leader I have come to believe I was destined to be from birth. Revelations come in many guises, sometimes apocalyptic, sometimes insidious; accompanied by pleasure, pain and paradoxes of unfolding clarity from confusion, contradiction and conflict. I learnt from the personal and the collective, from theories, histories, emotions and the discipline of guided reflection that forms the central tenant of this research.

Voice 1: Being a leader isn't accidental. Leadership is intentional. It is visionary and heart-felt. It is something lived, actualised in the moment. Leadership is not a neat set of ideas or techniques. The health care literature on leadership reveals a consensus that a *transforming* or *transformational* leadership is both desirable and necessary in the modern health care era, which is characterised by increasing complexity and change. This literature contrasts transformational leadership with a transactional-type leadership that is pervasive within health care organisations.

Reading 3

There are many images associated with leadership and most have their roots in war and conflict. It is outwitting of opponents, the convincing of people into action or the control of a crisis. I often think of special individuals like Nelson Mandela, Martin Luther King and Florence Nightingale. But what is leadership? [pause] … Bolman and Deal (1995) state that leaders are people who appeal to people's 'better nature and move them towards higher and more universal needs and purposes.' Can anyone learn to be a leader?

Voice 1: Transforming leadership was developed by Burns (1978:19) whereby one or more persons engage with others in such a way that leaders and followers raise one another to higher levels of motivation and morality.

Words like integrity, beneficence, virtue, justice, doing good, and caring come to mind. Yet, when organisational life is primarily concerned with meeting organisational objectives the moral landscape can quickly become obscured. The human factor lost in the machine. Building on the foundational work of Burns, Bass (1990) developed transformational leadership that was related more to organisational leadership than Burn's wider social agenda. He identified four inter-related essential aspects of transformational leadership – the four 'Is'.

Reading 4

(1) 'Idealised influence' – that leadership is based on genuine trust built on a moral foundation.

(2) 'Inspirational motivation' – that leadership provides meaning and challenge for engaging others in working collaboratively towards shared goals and success.

(3) 'Intellectual stimulation' – that leadership liberates the creative and responsive spirit in followers to fulfil their individual and collective aspirations towards overcoming problems in realising a shared vision.

(4) 'Individual consideration' – that leadership invests in each person towards enabling the person to fulfil their potential and needs leading to higher achievement and growth.

Voice 1: Brain food! Yet these four 'Is' are inspirational. Transformational and transactional are essentially different ways of being in the world. They are *not* different hats to wear at different times. Otherwise transformational leadership becomes instrumental and authentic. Transactional leadership is *not* a fall back position if transformational leadership falters. Or is it?

Reading 5

As Bolman and Deal (1995) write: 'to prevail in the face of uncaring and violence and the many other spiritual challenges to modern life, we need a vision of leadership rooted in the enduring sense of wisdom, spirit and heart. We need a new generation of seekers – yet … how will we develop the seekers we need? To begin with, we need a revolution in how we think about leadership and how we develop leaders. Most management and leadership development programs ignore or demean spirit. They desperately need an infusion of spiritual forms such as poetry, literature, music, art, theatre, history, philosophy, and dance.'

Beginning of the end – charge nurse – April 2006

Voice 1: Let's start with the ending. His outstretched arm held the phone receiver for me. The doctor was confused about the caller's request. I held the receiver to my ear and placed a finger in my other ear to drown the din of the emergency department. The pleading voice of a GP [general practitioner] in the home of a dying patient with cancer. The syringe driver had run dry of morphine and now the doctor was helpless towards alleviating the patient's pain. He asked for morphine for his patient. He knew and I knew it was against protocol but still he tried, just in case. After checking with the consultant of A&E [accident and emergency] I said it could not be done. Yet something triggered. I didn't want a patient to be in pain until the following day. I felt bad, angry and upset. I closed my eyes and told him that we could not give him what he needed most. The GP's anger and frustration boiled over. He had no choice then but to send the patient to A&E to receive the morphine. Would he do that? Send a dying patient in an ambulance to spend his final hours on an A&E trolley? Why did it have to be this way? Why couldn't we help? We had enough morphine here.

Why hadn't this bureaucratic NHS changed one bit since the time I was a student nurse until now, nine years later, a charge nurse in A&E. I had managed to change. I have moved away from the traditional authoritative ideology. I had grown and developed into the leader I wanted to be, or had I?

Reading 6

And so the stories begin. Yet already I hear the doubts about 'shining worlds', as if a deeply layered cynicism runs like a vein through the transactional culture defensive to outside threat ... that a culture deeply dissatisfied with its own functioning must resist or it will die ... and yet the irony is that transactional cultures, by their very nature, are withering, are dying.

Student nurse – early Autumn 1997

Voice 1: It was on my first placement as a student nurse on a medical ward that I noticed the authoritative culture of the NHS. I stood in the corridor between the two medical wards wondering why I could not obtain a bag of intravenous fluid for the patient. I was shocked, I didn't know what to think. Is this really how the NHS works? It was then that I first realised what red tape meant. One of the patients needed some fluids which the ward I was working on did not have. I asked the nurse in charge if I could go over to the next ward to see if they had any.

Voice 2: You can't, they won't give anything out of their budget.

Voice 1: To me this was essentially mindless. Why were the wards just reacting to organisational objectives instead of realising the human value of care? I felt confused. The culture allowed the nurses to feel protected by following protocols to the letter, even to the detriment of patient care. I could not see why it was so complicated, it seemed people where making it harder for themselves. However, during the course of my training, I too became institutionalised. If anyone else had the thoughts I used to have I considered them naïve and not in the 'real world'. Now, with guidance, I become more mindful.

Reading 7

Bolman and Deal (1995:174) write 'leaders learn most from their experience – especially from their failures. Too often, though, they miss the lessons. They lack the reflective capacity to learn on their own and have not been fortunate enough to find a spiritual guide who can help them sort things out through their own spiritual center.'

Staff nurse – April 1999

Voice 1: My first job when I qualified was on a medical ward where I came to understand the constraints of the nurse's role within the hierarchy of the NHS. Beds had to be made before doctors rounds, otherwise they would moan. A nurse had to follow the doctors' ward round and take notes on what was said – a daily reminder that nursing was initially organised as a submissive role, in terms of gender and professional status, in relation to doctors [Turner 2001]. Every step was to be done in a certain accordance because that was the way it had always been done. These rules were rarely written down. They were passed down by word of mouth from senior nurse to junior nurse. Thus norms, values and rules become ingrained. On occasion you were only made aware of these rules after breaking them. However, on some occasions this punitive authority caused me to fight back. On one occasion, I answered a phone call from a lady wishing to speak to the nurse in charge. I found the sister, who was drawing up some intravenous medications, and informed her that there was a phone call for her. I returned to the bay where I was working. A few minutes later the sister stood in the doorway to the patient's bay and shouted:

Voice 2: Anybody could have dealt with that call.

Voice 1: Feeling embarrassed but angry I replied, 'but you are anybody'. I enjoyed moments like that, but I also felt a little worried about my future. Not so trimmed.

Reading 8

Paramananda (2001:71) writes: 'Of course, the sad thing, the tragic thing, is that many of us do get trimmed. We all start off with real heads full of space and imagination, but slowly, somewhere along the path that we call growing up, our heads get trimmed. We become caught up in the doings of this world, the realities of adult life, and we get down to size …. without imagination the world loses its mystery and sense of depth in which we can find meaning.'

Charge nurse – Autumn 2003

Voice 1: Shortly after becoming a charge nurse in A&E I began my master's degree in 'clinical leadership'. Suddenly I was exposed to an alternative leadership ideology which appealed to my better nature. When did I get so wrapped into the transactional structure and culture of the NHS hospital, with its reliance on authoritative power of coercion and bureaucratic relationships? Of course there is another way. One in which I wouldn't have stood helpless in the corridor between the two medical wards, six years before, because the wards would all be mindful instead of mindless. When I was 'naïve' I could see so clearly. However, gradually my vision became blurred. The university lessons reopened my mind to what my real values had always been. This shift in paradigm made me aware that the move from hierarchical order to a new flatter, creative and fluid order may be difficult, as many nurses are institutionalised to the concept of order. What I have seen within the hospital is that everyone is scared of making decisions because they are unsure about accountability, frightened of treading on other people's toes and prefer to pass responsibility rather than to take initiative.

I commenced a journal to help me track my emerging leadership style. Its white pages, however, remained blank for a few weeks. I didn't want to spoil its pages with dull and uninspiring entries. I sought some scandalous event to analyse or an argument to reveal my leadership style, but little came to fruition. My mind kept returning to a sketch by Tony Hancock who excitedly bought a diary and his first entry began with *I had eggs for breakfast today.*

I made a conscious decision to write uninhibitedly, for it seemed the only way to unblock my retained self. I found it hard not to filter my thoughts because of guilt, self-righteousness and fear of fraudulent existence. In order to let the words and emotions flow onto the page I just wrote, even if it made no sense, I just wrote. Even if it made me feel stupid, I just wrote. Even if I felt vulnerable, I just wrote. I just wrote as if no one was watching. Because the truth is, when the mud settled down and the clouds cleared away, everything became a little clearer each day. I soon became involved in a, once presumed insignificant, conflict, which revealed a lot more about myself than expected. My scalpel and instrument of investigation manifested in the reflective model devised by Johns (2002). The reflective guide gave 13 questions to consider which ensured an exposed approach by including my personal emotions of the experience, the ethical considerations and reflexivity. However, like any new tool, it's only as good as the user. I found myself repeating the same answers to different questions. I also became impatient in reaching particular reflective cues, or going through the motions with others. The model was a skeleton key, opening previously locked complex events. Instead of jumping to conclusions, I found myself considering details which allowed for much richer experiences. By envisaging alternative outcomes or responses I could intertwine my desired transformational leadership ideology with personal and ethical values.

My insignificant conflict

Voice 1: I approached one of the nurses about her poor training attendance record. She responded quite sharply

Voice 2: I am not attending them in my own time.

Voice 1: I was annoyed by her attitude and I inadvertently let my feelings show. I raised my voice to her level and replied: 'it is your responsibility to attend such sessions' … she was caught by surprise because she didn't expect me to respond in such a confrontational manner that may have caused her to become defensive and seek justification for her behaviour. However, my response was out of character, for I continued to press the issue further, rather than backing down and accepting her opinions. Her shoulders shrunk and her gaze dropped as if in reverent prayer. Her silence spoke volumes of a child, caught by her dad, for not doing her homework. She may have wanted to continue her argument but feared being victimised for her opinions? The fear of sanctions may have caused her to be silent. The true issues now lay hidden inside of her. How could I now fully know the reasons why she does not attend the training provided?

This conflict made me realise I sometimes worked and behaved in a transactional manner. To be a transformational leader I need to nurture the right qualities inside of me in order to ensure their growth as depicted by a story told to children by the Cherokee Native Americans.

Reading 8

An old Cherokee is teaching his grandson about life. 'A fight is going on inside me,' he said to the boy. 'It is a terrible fight and it is between two wolves. One is evil – he is anger, envy, sorrow, regret, greed, arrogance, self-pity, guilt, resentment, inferiority, lies, false pride, superiority and ego.' He continued, 'The other is good – he is joy, peace, love, hope, serenity, humility, kindness, benevolence, empathy, generosity, truth, compassion and faith. The same fight is going on inside you – and inside every other person, too.' The grandson thought about it for a minute and then asked his grandfather, 'Which wolf will win?' The old Cherokee simply replied, 'The one you feed.' (Author unknown.)

Voice 1: Slowly, almost painfully, through reflection on experiences, usually of conflict or despair when patients suffered unnecessarily, I became increasingly mindful of myself as a leader. I am waking up. Yet feeding the right wolf is not easy.

The NHS bully – July 2004

Voice 1: Susan is a bed manager with government targets to achieve. She executes her job with vocal intensity and unprovoked aggression, regularly dismissing nurses' opinions or valid excuses. After such an occurrence of hierarchical pressure on the A&E team, she smiled, patted one of the nurses on the arm:

Voice 2: I'm such a bully

Voice 1: She laughed as she walked away. I felt irritated. I felt she was manipulating the nursing staff by sweetening her controlling personality. It did not seem sincere and her critical yet nurturing behaviour caused confusion and suspicion. Normally I would have appreciated the bed manager's honesty about her bullying tactics, even if her admission is wrapped in humour, but on this occasion I took time to think about some possible consequences. Using humour to disguise transactional authority does not remove the fact that force is a predominant force used by managers to gain control. How can nurses feel empowered to question Susan with their concerns? Sharing this experience at university, I realised that everyone has the right to express their opinions, feelings and to be treated with respect. Knowing your rights and believing in your own authority is only a step away from being able make a good argument. As an emerging transformational leader I would need to facilitate myself and the nurses to understand their rights, so that confronting Susan on important issues becomes feasible. Cliché, but knowledge is power.

Reading the following dialogue reminded me of the Cherokee story.

Reading 9

Bolman and Deal (1995:53) write

Voice 1: I want you to be the wizard. Give me the answers. You keep telling me to look inside. When I do, I hear the same voices. Be rational. Be in control. Be careful.

Voice 2: Those are messages from your head, not from your heart. It's hard to let go of old rules. It takes courage and faith.

Voice 1: Where do I find them?

Voice 2: You keep looking.

Voice 1: Where?

Voice 2: You've asked that question before. Let's try a different way …

That extra mile – October 2004

Voice 1: Apply a little stress and the person you knew becomes a stranger. Their true identity, which lies dormant, is woken to destroy their own illusion. My own perception of Anne, the ER [emergency room] lead nurse, was once built on the endearing transformational trait of charisma. I had previously perceived her to be interested in differing opinions and the investment in people. Thus I observed her in order to steal her secrets and to mimic her leadership style. Then, when I least expected it, she let me down.

The A&E department was under considerable pressure to meet the government's target of assessing, treating and discharging/admitting patients within four hours. The department was meeting 94% of the target which meant that we were underperforming by 3% to meet the set standard of 97%.

In the middle of a sisters' meeting, Anne came in looking pale and obviously with a few issues to get off her chest. She interrupted the meeting which had so far been led by the A&E matron.

Voice 2: Oh good you're all here.

Voice 1: The meeting halted and everyone turned to see her as she perched herself over the whole group. The chief executive had suggested that Anne's job was in jeopardy over the issue of the four-hour target.

Voice 2: He draws a line in the sand with me.

Voice 1: She was clearly upset that her job was at risk apparently due to our performance. It was not the fact that we had all worked very hard to try to reach the target that upset me, but that her manner had changed. She was no longer the leader who empowered her staff but a transactional leader who was turning the staff into a resource that can be used wherever needed as opposed to human beings. Before starting the course I would have accepted that Anne's management style was the correct and most appropriate way of dealing with issues. But now I can feel a distance between her behaviour and how I would want to be as an emerging leader. The way she handled this situation disappointed me. I felt uncomfortable, which I associate with a conflict between the experience and my ideals of effective leadership.

The collective – January 2005

Voice 1: I don't think many people enjoy mistakes and problems, but learning from mistakes or conflicts can help overcome future ones more efficiently. One day Anne asked me if I could implement a DVT [deep vein thrombosis] clinic. My first step was to organise a meeting with all the sisters to see how we can realise the new clinic. I wanted the nurses to own the idea so that we could create it together. From the nurses' expressions it was obvious that they were not keen on acquiring more jobs. No one seemed interested in the project. As one sister said:

Voice 2: It's just another job for the A&E to sort out.

Voice 1: It was tempting to cancel future meetings as it would have been much quicker to plan the clinic myself. Yet, on reflection, I realised that I was behaving in a totally transactional way, because I was viewing this problem as a threat to order. I felt disappointed in myself. I may fool myself by hiding behind the façade of having the organisation's interest at heart, but more accurately it was my own agenda. I had been given a job to do and I wanted to do it successfully, without unwanted interference. Unfortunately, this reaction is all too common. Previously, it seemed easy to understand the nurse's defensive routines when she was justifying her poor attendance to the teaching sessions. However, I now realise that, I too, had deep defences. I justified the reasons for my personal agenda by convincing myself that the nurses were incompetent. I need to be aware of my subconscious defensive routines and to monitor my surreptitious resistance to prevent 'inexplicable' problems. By having to let go of certain aspects of the project, it presented the opportunity to approach the rest of the department for guidance and support. Mycek [1999] reassures that by giving up the control, creativity from unexpected sources may appear. Soon enough, the meetings with the A&E nurses resulted in change and adjustment to the proposal. This opportunity would otherwise have been missed. The most surprising element was that some of the best ideas were from nurses who I wouldn't have picked for the team.

Reading 10

As Wheatley and Kellner-Rogers (1998:53) write: 'When we link up with others, we open ourselves to yet another paradox. While surrendering some of our freedom, we open ourselves to even more creative forms of expression. This stage of being has been described as communion, because we are preserved as our selves but are shorn of our separateness or aloneness. What we bring to others remains our self-expression. Yet the meaning of who we are changes through our communion with them. We are identifiable as our selves. But we have discovered new meaning and different contributions, and we are no longer the same.'

Prejudices and anger – March 2005

Voice 1: Friday nights always bring the usual suspects of alcohol-related injuries and avoidable mishaps. This night was no exception. An unconscious lady in her mid-thirties, smelling of wine, vomit and urine was brought in by ambulance. With minimal handling, the patient was tipped out of the stretcher onto a trolley. All was well, until she started to wake up. Even though the doctor had discharged her, I allowed her to stay in the department until she sobered up. She became verbally aggressive, throwing medical equipment over and intimidating other patients. I warned her that her behaviour was unacceptable. I heard her say to one of the nurses – :

Voice 2: Just look at you … you're just a black nurse … the lowest of the low.

Voice 1: I yanked the curtains back, strode in, with my finger pointing in her face. 'Out!', I shouted, 'I will not tolerate this any longer'. With my hand under her arm I marched her out of the department, straight into the waiting room, still wearing a hospital gown. The people in the waiting room all turned to see what was going on. She just giggled like a naughty school child. I went back to get her soiled clothes and placed them on the chair next to her and went back to work.

After the incident I started to think of the consequences of my actions, to myself, to the patient and to the department. This reflective question was chosen because it focuses on the human responses to the situation, by being both rational and emotional. I realised that I did not feel comfortable about what I had done. I pride myself in staying calm and dealing with situations in an adult way but instead I behaved like a strict parent who was telling off a naughty child. By being in this mode I allowed myself to punish her, by humiliating her in front of the waiting room. It would have been better to allow her to get dressed in the cubicle to maintain her dignity. My emotions swamped the rights of the patient and I swept in with 'rough justice'. I always thought I treated my patients with dignity, but since this incident I realise that loyalty to my staff may take precedence. My actions may have prevented the nurse from resolving this issue, instead I disempowered the nurse, strode in and caused a precedence by which future 'difficult' patients may be treated. Such actions may in fact cause staff dependence and create unrealistic expectations for future conflict management. I am more aware of my thinking.

Reading 11

Bohm (1996:25) notes that we could say that practically all the problems of the human race are due to the fact that thought is not proprioceptive. Thought is constantly creating problems that way and then trying to solve them. But as it tries to solve them it makes it worse because it doesn't notice that it's creating them, and the more it thinks, the more problems it creates – because it's not proprioceptive of what it's doing.

An acceptable war zone – May 2005

Voice 1: During the busy night shift we soon ran out of cubicles in the department. The staff were getting tired and stressed after working non-stop for eight hours without a break. The triage nurse, who assesses patients in the waiting room, needed a cubicle to lie a patient down. When I told her there was no room in A&E, I could see from her facial expression that she was annoyed, as I could not provide a solution for this problem. She must have considered it to be my responsibility to solve this problem. Think differently. I told her that we had to treat this area like a war zone: 'At times like these we have to do the best we can within the confines of the resources we have at hand.' In situations like these rules become redundant. You sometimes have to go with the wave or crash in its frothing roll. It seems that when we are placed in uncomfortable situations, we strive, and that is when fine moments arise. The department worked as a team, they realised this was an unusual situation, which became comical as opposed to demoralising. There were moments when we spiralled into sheer chaos. On some occasions you have to yield to the new situation.

Sometimes you cannot change the rules of the world, it cannot be ruled by interfering. Invariably new suggestions returned the team back into the complexity zone. This area between complexity and chaos is known as the 'edge of chaos', where creativity is at its most heightened. The creativity is created by providing simple rules and enabling the nurses to be autonomous in how they used the available space, by permitting them the mental freedom to organise their workload. Although the workload was just the same, they felt in control of the resources at hand, which in turn reduced their anxiety. If the traditional system had been used, patients may have sat in the waiting room, not being seen because of the lack of cubicles. It was interesting to see that even within the chaos most nurses seemed to enjoy or desired the greater responsibility of problem solving. These small changes cause a focus or 'strange attraction', which, within the world of complexity theory, initiates a movement within the system. These small changes repeat themselves, which in turn inspires self-organisation and the creation of new forms.

I realised that wanting to be a transformational leader, fostering small occurrences can cause the system to loop the information back on itself, so that the origin grows continuously stronger. The knowledge and power of teams was an essential understanding I previously appreciated when introducing the DVT clinic. Now the pulling together as a team in a unified direction allowed the ideas to flow, which just one individual could not imagine. However, not everyone was happy about working on the edge of chaos. Stories enfolded within stories. Accepting chaos as part of everyday life and to cease fighting it is mentally liberating and from this comes creativity. As Nietzsche (1986) once wrote, 'You need chaos in your soul to give birth to a dancing star'. Can I dwell in the Tao?

Reading 12

> The Tao never does anything,
> yet through it all things are done.
> If powerful men and women
> could centre themselves in it,
> the whole world would be transformed
> by itself, in its natural rhythms.
> People would be content
> with their simple, everyday lives,
> in harmony, and free from desire.
> When there is no desire
> all things are at peace.
> (Lao Tzu, Tao-Te Ching 37 translated by Stephen Mitchell)

Confidential – August 2005

Voice 1:

The 18-year-old patient did not want her family to know that she had taken an overdose of paracetamol. She looked nervous when her dad arrived.

Dad (Voice 2):	Why is she here?
My response (Voice 1):	I'm sorry, I can't disclose any information due to patient confidentiality. It may be best to speak about it to your daughter.
	[He returned a little later.]
Voice 2:	My daughter is not clear what is wrong, either.
My response *(Voice 1)*:	I can't disclose any information without her consent.
He then asked in front of the daughter *(Voice 2)*:	Is it OK for him to say what is wrong?
Voice 1:	I felt he was coercing her. There was an awkward silence. I couldn't think of a way out. I didn't have a contingency plan. Another nurse then stepped in and said that they were investigating why she had problems with her liver but as yet they were still running tests. The daughter was happy about the response and the dad accepted the information given by the nurse. This was like a band-aid to stop the dam from breaking. It might stop the pressure for a little while, but once on the medical ward the whole situation would have to be revisited. More than likely, the information would be accidentally given or suggested to the father, which may then cause greater mistrust. Having said that, when the nurse said those words it felt like a noose had been lifted from around my neck, but what remained was a feeling of guilt. I find myself cleaning the reflective mirror.

Reading 13

Pinar (1981:184) writes: 'We are not mere smudges on the mirror. Our life histories are not liabilities to be exorcised but are the very precondition for knowing. It is our individual and collective stories in which present projects are situated, and it is the awareness of these stories which is the lamp illumining the dark spots, the rough edges.'

Growling like a tiger – October 2005

Voice 1: I never really saw myself as a bully, but then again I've never really examined my behaviour to highlight the possibility. To me a bully is someone who is insensitive, instigates arguments, manipulates, loves power and is heartless. These are not characteristics which I would like to admit, even to myself. So what made me think that I may be a bully? It was, yet again, busy in the department. One of the managers was confronting a nurse who was temporarily in charge while I had been on my break. Many of the people around them were stopping their discussions to listen to what was going on. When I approached the manager she turned to face me with glaring eyes and suddenly I knew that she was not going to praise me. Pointing an accusing finger towards me, she scolded:

Voice 2: Why didn't you tell me that this person was about to breach? [With arms in the air and eyes wild with anger] This is not acceptable!

Voice 1: She looked really comical but I was not in a mood for laughing. Realising that people were watching this scene, I calmly took a step to the side to make some room between myself and the manager. Suddenly, from a calm pose, I squatted and *leapt* with demented limbs shaking in anger with growls of an angered feline protecting her cubs.
[Dance …]

Voice 1: As quickly as it began, I stopped. The manager was silent, puzzled, not a word, only ripples of laughter from the nurses and doctors. Finally the manager laughed with them. I did not exactly copy her behaviour, but the essence of what she looked like was unquestionable. Suddenly she was faced with how she appeared, somewhat ridiculous. In school, when children want to offend another person they often mimic and exaggerate the behaviour of the victim. Mimicking is a form of bullying. The next day the manager approached me to say:

Voice 2: Dr Sa'apu shouted at me today because I didn't manage to co-ordinate the discharge of two of his patients on time. You see, it's not only me who shouts.

Voice 1: I didn't respond. I looked at her and smiled, nodded, and went on with my work. Perhaps she will start to realise that her transactional way of enforcing compliance out of fear is not effective.
In response, I was being competitive. I know that to be a transformational leader I must consistently respond in a collaborative way, always seeking win-win outcomes. This means that the conflict would need to be openly discussed without using childlike mimicking. Then again, a little playfulness and silliness in the workplace allows the nerves to be relaxed. As Dahl [1973] writes, 'A little foolishness now and then is relished by even the wisest men.' Humour is a fine line.

Please do not ignore me – December 2005

One appalled little woman (*Voice 2*): You mean I have to stay here, overnight?

Voice 1: Unfortunately there are no more beds available in the hospital.

Woman (*Voice 2*): This is terrible, I mean they haven't even changed the sheets.

I think to myself [facing audience] (*Voice 1*): Do you normally change your sheets at home every three hours? [Turning courteously to woman] Would you like me to change them for you?

Woman (*Voice 2*): This trolley is too hard, do you have any others?

My response (*Voice 1*): Unfortunately these are the standard trolleys throughout the department. Would you like to sit in an easy chair to change position?[To audience] I hoped she would say 'no' because easy chairs were like gold dust. She didn't reply. She just stared ahead, contemplating, ruminating … I grappled with the blood bottles in my arms to indicate the jobs I had to do. The X-ray under my other arm started to slip out of its plastic covering and the drug chart … where did I leave the drug chart? Why couldn't she see that I needed to go? I knew that I should remain courteous and polite, I hoped that I was not coming across patronising … but yet I wished I did.

Why did I behave the way I did? Why did I try and show her that I was busy, but on the other hand, indicated that I could find her an easy chair? Maybe I was trying to disarm her. What greater way to stop her moaning but by acts of kindness. What greater revenge is there to someone exerting power, but to show gratitude – what Nietzsche (1986:44) describes as a 'wilder form of revenge'. From somewhere inside of me I found a little renewed energy. Maybe a passion for my work or just determination, I don't know, but I made my mind up that this lady needed more care. On the other hand, there could be another reason why I started to focus my care on the old lady. I am, as a nurse, accountable for my actions. By focusing on my values I found new motivation to improve this lady's care. It enabled me to find a softer spare bed that we exchanged for the A&E trolley. I brought her a sandwich and made her a cup of tea, which she found too milky. Oh well, you can't please them all. Posture is everything.

Reading 14

Shunryu Susuki (1999:28) writes: 'So try always to keep the right posture, not only when you practice zazen, but in all your activities. Take the right posture when you are driving your car, and when you are reading. If you read in a slumped position, you cannot stay awake long. You will discover how important it is to keep the right posture. This is the true teaching. The teaching which is written on paper is not the true teaching. written teaching is a kind of food for your brain. of course it is necessary to take some food for your brain, but it is more important to be yourself by practicing the right way of life.'

David and Goliath – January 2005

Voice 1: Sometimes, people at the head of a hierarchy act as though they own the individuals beneath them. If those individuals start to act on their own or question the integrity of the hierarchy, this becomes threatening. The heads of hierarchies feel they can exert their power without fear, as the individuals below them are dependent on them financially, professionally and socially. After parking the car on a dark cold morning, I listened to the handover around the nurses' station. Sleepily, I allocated the nurses with their roles for the day and the night staff soon trudged home to get some much needed sleep. I was taken aside by the ward sister who had led the night shift. Through her tiredness she explained why one of the patients was still in A&E after four hours. Shock horror!

During the night a young man was brought in by ambulance, with cuts and bruises to his head. He had been kicked and punched in the head when he was making his way home, after a night out with his friends. He had had a little too much alcohol to drink. This made it difficult to determine if his groggy behaviour was due to the drink or his bruised and battered head. Concerned, the doctor arranged a scan of his head with the consultant radiologist on call. Unfortunately, the e-mail link was down and the radiologist could not receive the scans to his home computer, therefore they remained unreported in cyberspace. Without the report we could not know the extent of the patient's injuries or plan his care. Did he need to be transferred to a specialist hospital or sent home? Annoyed, but not surprised at being in this situation, I spoke to the radiographer who did the scan. Although concerned at my plight, he could not provide any results until it had been officially reported on by the on-call radiologist. I made my way back to the nurses' station, and made a decision to phone the consultant radiologist at home, to try to resolve this situation. I was apprehensive because I believed that I would get a frosty reception. Am I normally this prejudiced about consultants' attitudes?

I phoned the switch-board who connected me to the on-call radiologist. I explained that in order to decide the patient's management we needed his report on the scans. His answer was that he does not speak to nurses but to doctors only. I replied that in this case he did need to speak to me, as it had become essential to make a decision about the patient's management. He hung up. I rang him back and asked him if he had hung up on me. He said he had. I proceeded to tell him that he needed to come into A&E and report the film, the e-mail being down was not a valid excuse and that I would make an official complaint about his behaviour. If you are going to walk on thin ice, you might as well dance!

He said 'yeah, yeah …' and hung up, again. I could feel my heart pounding in my chest. I told myself not be so stupid, after all I was in the right. Did I have the right to ring him at home, where was that protocol? My mind raced to justify my actions. What if he was to ring the A&E consultant on-call to complain about me? I quickly rang the consultant and explained what had happened. He was sympathetic and said that he would speak to the radiologist. However, when he rang back he did explain that I should not have phoned the radiologist directly, it should have been a doctor. My heart sank. I pointed out to the consultant that as part of my role of reaching A&E targets I had to ensure that doctors performed their duties and the radiologist had not, therefore I had every right to ring him at home. The A&E consultant's response reinforced the usual closing of ranks. It is a constant uphill struggle against the pyramid structure. At least he was willing to talk to me unlike the radiologist. Maybe I should count my blessings. Little did I know that the conversation I had held with the radiologist spread like wildfire throughout the department, nurses were praising me for standing up to the radiologist. Even the radiographers were saying:

Voice 2: Good for you!
Voice 1: Time had been on my side that morning. The department was not heaving with patients and therefore I could concentrate on the phone call with the radiologist. I was also fresh from just starting the shift, unlike the night sister who had become full of complacency about this situation, because she was tired. Would I have left the job for the next shift? I should like to think not, as I have developed a certain expectation of myself on how I should act. I was determined not to avoid issues and pass responsibility onto other people, even if it involved confrontation. However, when I was met by the radiologist's unapproachable

behaviour, anger rose in me. Instead of stating the issues, I started to tell him how to do his job. I became a critical parent. In turn, and to my surprise, he moved into a child-like mode by his playground attitude of 'Yeah, yeah, yeah ...' to undermine my apparent authority. Later that morning, the radiologist came in to report the film. A minor victory, I thought to myself with malicious glee. However, I did not go and speak to him. I justified myself by thinking 'Let sleeping dogs lie', but reflection highlighted that this was really a coward's explanation. The adrenaline and anger had gone from my veins and with it my drive. Now it seemed so much more difficult to approach the radiologist to discuss the situation in an adult mode. Instead I fell back on my comfort zone of avoidance. Later that evening, I tried to think why the radiologist behaved the way he did. Doesn't everyone want to be at work at 7:30 on a Sunday morning? Sure, the unsociable hour must have been a contributing factor to his behaviour, but at the possible cost of someone's life? I hope not. Perhaps a nurse calling him was so abhorrent to him that he found himself unable to continue the conversation. Most likely it was my profession, which made him feel that he had an authority over me, which he could misuse at a whim. Nursing is seen as a low status feminised profession that operates at the bottom of the hierarchical structure, with little empowerment. His way to control the *status quo* was to make sure that I know my place by stating, 'I do not speak to nurses', attempting to 'put me in my place'; a typical authoritative transactional ploy to quash autonomy. His lack of respect allowed him to hang up the phone, which gave me impetus to ring him back and confront his behaviour. On reflection, I wish I had taken a few moments to gather my thoughts to prepare a more collaborative approach, instead of threatening him with a complaint about his behaviour. Anger could be useful if channelled into constructive and collaborative forces. It can help to make you assertive. Although I responded in a transactional manner, I was able to witness and reflect upon my response. Hierarchical structures should not interfere in providing the best service that patients deserve. And at last, if I am not deluded, I sense the possibility of leadership.

Reading 15

Jaworski (1998) writes 'leadership is all about the release of human possibilities.' (Repeat four times.)

Recapturing my good will – March 2006

Voice 1: It was a struggle all day. I kept suctioning the back of his throat but it was useless. His pneumonia was so severe that he was filling up with green sputum. He was elderly with no family, had a nice neighbour, did not want any help. Old people can be like that. Unkempt, his clothes smelled and his once white shirt was yellow with a dark brown ring around his collar. His nails were silver and thick. He had a sore on his hip from lying down for three days on the floor of his old cold house which smelled of cat wee. Now he was dying in a hospital bed. His heart had stopped twice that morning and I reluctantly restarted it following protocols and procedures, which seemed unjustified.

The doctors decided that he should not be 'resuscitated' for a third time. He passed away later that afternoon with his neighbour by his side, just after the Catholic priest had given a blessing. Wrapped in white linen, the porters unceremoniously removed him from his cubicle. His bed was cleaned and re-made, the sheets all tucked neatly, fresh pillows lay where his head had rested. I turned to look at his bed and paused for a moment to consider the feelings of the other patients in the bay. In the bed to the right there was a lady with a fractured wrist, lost in a world that was for her a complete mystery, due to her dementia. To the left, a lady waiting to go home. She looked tired, after all she did not get much rest because of the old man who had had pneumonia. I noticed her looking at the empty bed so I went to sit beside her ...

[Dialogue with *Voice 2*]
Woman (*Voice 2*):   He passed away, his neighbour was with him.
My response (*Voice 1*): Yes ... isn't it sad, he had no family.
Woman (*Voice 2*):   I feel bad because he kept me awake all night and I really resented that. He was very poorly ... maybe it was for the best.

[She starts to cry. I rest my hand on her back.]
My response *(Voice 1)*: It's okay, he went peacefully with a friend by his side, who cared for him. His neighbour has known him for 21 years.
Woman (*Voice 2*)   I'm sorry about this, I didn't mean to cry, I know you are busy.
My response *(Voice 1)*: Not that busy, I'm just pretending to be busy.

I close the curtain and give her some tissues. She explains about her brothers who all died young, it seems to have brought all those memories back to her. She then shows me pictures of her grandchildren, they look like little devils but apparently they are cute. On this occasion, I took a conscious decision to allow this woman to express her feelings, which were obviously just bubbling below the surface. Even though I had other priorities regarding government targets niggling ... I made a decision to put her first. Whereas I would have previously felt disappointed at my usual institutionalised choice of attending to the government targets first, I now felt liberated at returning to my original values of treating patients with care and dignity, to fulfil Logtsrup's ethical demand.

Reading 16

Logstrup (1997:18) writes that by our very attitude to one another we help to shape one another's world, by our attitude to the other person we help to determine the scope and hue of his or her world; we make it large and small, bright or drab, rich or dull, threatening or secure. We help to shape his or her world not be theories and views but by our very attitude toward him or her. Herein lies the unarticulated and one might say anonymous demand that we take care of the life which trust has placed into our hands.

The end of the beginning – April 2006)

Voice 1: So, why couldn't I help the GP with the dying patient requiring morphine for his pain? The GP was obviously upset and was threatening to send a dying patient to A&E. Initially this made me feel angry, because the transportation of a dying man seemed inhumane. However, I focused my energy on maintaining a collaborative manner. I said, 'I understand your frustration, but I also want what is best for the patient, let me take your number and I will see what alternative solutions I can find.'

Calmed, reassured and thankful, his voice eased as he gave me his mobile number. I hung up and paused … and then turned to my colleagues around me and explained the situation to them. I required their help and I was open to as many ideas as possible for this difficult situation. One of the nurses provided me with the number of a hospice nearby. I explained the problem to the nurse in charge of the hospice, but she could not help because again it was not part of their practice to provide morphine. I thanked her and hung up. I remained calm, allowed a pause, a silence to linger among the whole group. Then another nurse said:

Voice 2: Why not try the cancer research hospital in the nearby town, they have an on-call pharmacist

Voice 1: I rang the on-call pharmacist. In the meantime the A&E department was getting rather full. I closed my eyes to remain focused on the problem at hand. I felt a tap on the shoulder. One of the nurses offered to take over being in charge. When I informed the on-call pharmacist where I was ringing from, she interrupted me to say that my hospital was out of her allocated area and that I should call someone else. She sounded annoyed and irritated that I had interrupted her Sunday afternoon. I decided that she had a right to be annoyed but I was determined not to be drawn into a win–lose confrontation. I apologised for inconveniencing her and quickly explained that I was concerned about a dying patient in pain, whom the GP had no morphine for. I remained collaborative by focusing on the patient's needs in an open but engaging manner. She softened. I portrayed myself as a nurse going out of their way to help a poor patient.

She put me on hold. A few minutes later, she returned. She had found a number of a co-ordinator who supplied morphine out of hours. I saw a glimmer of hope for the patient. All the nurses were around the nurses' station, keeping track of the development and continuing saga. I wrote the number down as a nurse held the paper steady, because I had run out of hands. I thanked the pharmacist for her help and quickly rang the GP who answered before I even keyed in the last number. His relief on receiving the co-ordinator's number was almost tangible. He thanked me for all my help and for that little moment, the A&E team felt that we had won.

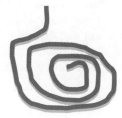

Reading 17

Margaret Wheatley (1999:89–90) writes that all life lives off-balance in a world that is open to change. And all life is self-organising. We do not have to fear disequilibrium, nor do we have to approach change so fearfully. Instead, we can realise that, like all life, we know how to grow and evolve in the midst of constant flux. There is a path through change that leads to greater independence and resiliency. We dance along this path by maintaining a coherent identity and by honouring everybody's need for self-determination. When leaders strive for equilibrium and stability by imposing control, constricting people's freedom and inhibiting local change, they only create the conditions that threaten the organisation's survival. The more I read about self-organising systems, the more I marvel at the images of freedom and possibility that they evoke. This is a world of independence and interdependence, of processes that resolve so many of the dualisms we create in thought. The seeming paradoxes of order and freedom, of being and becoming, whirl into a new image that is very ancient – the unifying spiral dance of creation. Stasis, balance, equilibrium – these are temporary states. What endures is process – dynamic, adaptive, creative.

Voice 1: Perhaps Wheatley says it all. But for me, this journey has been like standing on the shore where the ground is firm and familiar, looking out into the ocean that glimmers in the sun. But beneath the waves its true depth is hidden from view. At first you struggle against the tide, currents and waves, but upon returning to the water you have learnt a little bit more about the ocean. The more I return to the chopping waves the more graceful I move within its waters, until I swim in liquid light where I can see the shells and pearls and poisonous fish. Reflection is a skill in itself and when you finally get used to it, it usually shows that you are the root of most of your problems. With this insight I was able to nurture the good wolf. It is perhaps obvious that any person who takes himself seriously as a health practitioner must seek to realise transformational leadership as a lived reality. Such leadership is a way of being not a series of techniques. The existing transactional landscape is dehumanising and creates suffering for both patients and staff ... yet the transactional system is locked into itself. Tightly bound it cannot let go and unfold into the transformational culture it seeks rather ambivalently to be. The leaders on the course pull at the binds, first at their own binds and then at the systems ... pulling, loosening, opening a space where they can become free to continue their transgressive and transformational activity. However, it is not easy.

Reading 18

As Helen, in her leadership narrative, writes, 'I know deep down if I am honest with myself about wanting to realise transformational leadership, that this will simply not be possible if I am constantly living in this state of fear.'

Voice 1: The difference between the transactional and the transformational is a thin veil between seeing people as human and seeing them as work, aligning self to see the humanness. But there are consequences. Listening to my leadership peers in classes, I know that at times they wanted to submit and re-enter the matrix.

But after 24 months they too, like me, internalised leadership as a way of being and they breathed more easily in the transformational learning spaces that Chris opened. Education is political action.

Reading 19

Paulo Freire (1970:68) writes that 'the starting point for organising the programme content of education or political action must be the present, existential, concrete situation, reflecting the aspirations of the people. Utilising certain basic contradictions, we must pose this existential, concrete, present situation to the people as a problem which challenges them and requires a response – not just at the intellectual level, but at the level of action. We must never merely discourse on the present situation, must never provide the people with programmes which have little or nothing to do with their preoccupations, doubts, hopes and fears – programmes which at times in fact increase the fears of the oppressed consciousness. It is not our role to speak to the people about our own view, not to attempt to impose that view on them, but rather to dialogue with the people about their view and ours.'

References

Alexander B (2005) Performance ethnography; the re-enacting and inciting of culture. In: N Denzin and Y Lincoln (eds.) *The Sage handbook of qualitative research* (third edition). Sage, Thousand Oaks, pp. 41–442.

Bass B (1990) From transactional to transformational leadership: learning to share the vision. *Organizational Dynamics* 18:19–31.

Bohm D (1996) *On dialogue*. (Edited by L Nichol). Routledge, London.

Bolman LG and Deal TE (1995) *Leading with soul*. Jossey-Bass, San Francisco.

Burns JM (1978) *Leadership*. Harper & Row, New York.

Dahl R (1973) *Charlie and the chocolate factory*. Puffin Books, Harmondsworth. Used with permission of David Higham Associates.

Freire P (1970) *The pedagogy of the oppressed*. Penguin Books, Harmondsworth.

Johns C (2002) *Guided reflection advancing practice*. Blackwell Science, Oxford.

Logstrup K (1997) *The ethical demand*. University of Notre Dame Press, Notre Dame.

Mycek S (1999) Teetering on the edge of chaos. *Trustee* 52:10–13.

Nietzsche F (1986) *Human, all too human: a book for free spirits*. Cambridge Texts, Cambridge.

Paramananda (2001) *A deeper beauty: Buddhist reflections on everyday life*. Windhorse Publications, Birmingham. Used with permission.

Pinar W (1981) 'Whole, bright, deep with understanding': issues in qualitative research and autobiographical method. *Journal of Curriculum Studies* 13:173–188.

Susuki S (1999) *Zen mind, beginner's mind* (first revised edition). Weatherhill, New York.

Turner D (2001) *Liberating leadership* (fourth edition). The Industrial society, London.

Tzu L (1999) *Tao Te Ching* (transl. Mitchell S). Frances Lincoln, London.

Wheatley MJ (1999) *Leadership and the new science*. Berrett-Koehler Publishers, San Francisco.

Wheatley MJ and Kellner-Rogers M (1998) *A simpler way*. Berrett-Koehler publications, San Francisco.

Chapter 12

Shifting attitude with deliberate self-harm patients in Accident and Emergency (A&E)

Jane Groom and Christopher Johns

Background

Jane approached me to guide her undergraduate dissertation using guided reflection methodology. She was familiar with this developmental approach having studied with me previously using guided reflection.

Session 1: beginnings

Jane writes:

> In our first session, issues surrounding deliberate self-harm (DSH) patients were not on my mind or so I thought. Chris simply began by asking how I was and inquiring if there were any issues emerging from my practice in Accident and Emergency (A&E) that might be a potential focus for my study. I had not anticipated what might arise and to my surprise my anxieties about DSH patients tumbled out.
>
> Something happened a few weeks ago. I haven't really thought long and hard about it yet. I have some 'nagging' doubts about what happened, I think it's been easier to ignore it and put in to the back of my mind. On a recent shift I dealt with a man who had deliberately cut his arm. I still feel uncomfortable about the way in which I responded to him. It was a night shift at around three in the morning. I went into a cubicle to carry out a treatment. Until this point I had not met this man, all I knew about him was that he had deliberately cut his arm, he required sutures and I went into the cubicle to carry out his treatment. On reflection I am aware that I pre-judged him, stereotyped him. His deliberate act of self-harm irritated me before I met him. I went into the cubicle and communicated necessary information with him, I was professional, and I tried to hide my feelings but felt *empty*. He was excluded from any feelings of compassion that I am able to feel for other patients. Prior to treatment commencing he asked if it would hurt, I felt

this was a ridiculous question, why should he care if it hurt? I found my irritation bubbling to the surface and in answer to his question I replied, 'The local should numb the pain of the stitches, but it must have hurt when you did it!?' I wasn't asking a question that required an answer but I now realise it was a way of communicating my feelings, a reprimand for his behaviour. Although my response makes me uncomfortable I wonder if compassion would encourage him to continue with such futile acts again and again, mutilating your own body is such an alien concept. It seems such a waste of time to stitch someone that is going to repeat the injury.

Chris asked me if I had any idea why I felt this way? I hadn't really thought about it. It's frustrating when you see the same patients returning over and over again, they never seem to recover. Chris suggested that perhaps I didn't see the ones who recover because they don't come back for treatment, that perhaps my frustration lies with my inability to put things right? Perhaps these patients are manipulative. He challenged me to examine whether my role boundaries required me 'patch up the damage' or whether DSH patients require a more therapeutic approach? I had to admit that I didn't feel that I had enough knowledge to distinguish between manipulative and non-manipulative patients. I said 'They obviously have reasons for their behaviour, but I find it difficult to respond.'

Chris responded, 'What sort of reasons?'

I said I didn't know. There could be a million different reasons. The environment doesn't help. The A&E environment is very challenging, for example a nurse may find herself comforting grieving relatives one minute and the next trying to come to terms with the fact that the person in front of them has tried to take their own life, or has inflicted harm upon themselves.

Chris then challenged me, 'Are some people are more worthy of care than others?'

That put me on the spot. I know that I *should* treat everyone with the same care and compassion, but in reality I did treat these people differently. The very fact that I do this is upsetting, it doesn't meet my own philosophy of care and they are not feelings I expected to have when I embarked on my nursing career. I care that's why I entered the profession; it distresses me that I cannot be more therapeutic with this patient group.

Chris pursued the topic 'Does anything else influence your reaction to such patients?'

I had spoken about my mother in the past, she suffers with a progressive debilitating condition and I constantly witness her failing health, she doesn't deserve it, why do fit and healthy people injure themselves? CJ could see I was upset. Gently he prodded, 'Do you think this subject will be too emotive to tackle?'

I agreed it would be very emotive but that I should attempt to understand why I feel this way and change the way in which I deliver care to this patient group and hopefully deliver care in a therapeutic way.

Jane's reflection

Looking back on the session it seems amazing how talking for an hour can turn my world upside down. It was powerful! I realised that I had concerns working with DSH patients, that had laid dormant, perhaps waiting for the right time to be expressed. I suspect that if I had not been in guided reflection at this moment in time, these issues would never have been expressed. They are disturbing and difficult to face up to. Through our previous work together and somehow I had implicit trust in CJ and knew I could reveal this side of my practice. I knew he would not judge me in any way.

Sharing my experience resulted in asking various questions of myself such as – why do I have difficulty with offering the same level of care to this patient group. I realised that my negative prejudice and detachment in care giving with this group of patients affected their well-being. Watson (1999) highlights this: 'We see glimpses indicating that the nurse's presence and consciousness, attitude and behaviour can affect the patient, for better or for worse' (p. 225). Wrapped up in my self-concern I simply was not available to them. From this session I take with me the 'need' to know more about DSH. I will use my experience in a positive way and try to be more mindful of what I have learnt when faced with another DSH patient.

Chris utilised the Being available template (Johns 2000): whereby the practitioner seeks to be *fully* available to the other to help them find meaning in their health-illness experience, to guide them to best decisions about their life and assist them as necessary with skilful action to meet their life goals.[1] The extent the practitioner can be available is determine along six dimensions:

- The extent I hold the intent to realise my vision of practice moment by moment;
- The extent I know the person;
- The extent I am concerned/ have compassion for the person;
- The aesthetic response – the extent I respond to the person with appropriate and skilled responses towards enabling them to meet their health-illness needs;
- The extent I am able to manage my involvement within relationship with poise;
- The extent the practitioner can create and sustain an environment where being available is possible.

Of these dimensions, I really sensed the fundamental contradiction between my practice as it was and the holistic way I wanted it to be. To acknowledge myself as uncaring was deeply shocking and yet confessing this was a relief. I knew that my 'clinical gaze' had been on the symptoms of 'harm', averting my gaze from the person. I realised during the guided session that I do care about DSH patients, and that I wanted to develop this area of my practice. Realising that I didn't care for these patients in the way I felt I should was distressing, and even though I may find this research difficult and lay myself open to vulnerability, I care enough about my practice as a whole to eliminate this contradiction in my practice.

Concern is the motivational expression of caring. Concern creates possibility within the caring relationship (Benner and Wrubel 1989). The greater the practitioner's concern the greater the possibilities within her relationship with the patient and family. When a practitioner's concern has become numbed, then reasons for this can be explored and understood, and concern nurtured to become again a strong passion and motivational force.

The other side of 'concern' is poise. CJ expressed poise as the ability to be fully present yet without taking on board the other's suffering as my own. I could sense the possibility of emotional turmoil if I had opened myself to the DSH patient. No wonder I kept my distance and yet, I do care deeply, it is an aspect of my practice I feel I am good at with other patients. Perhaps that is why I felt bad. I know I have the potential to transform this side of me. My eyes and heart are open.

---

[1] See Appendix 1.

Reflecting on the environment I recognise that negative attitude to DSH patients is endemic. They are not popular patients. CJ points me towards unpopular patient literature, notably a paper by Hughes entitled 'Normal rubbish' – about time wasters in A&E. Do I see DSH as time wasters?

CJ also challenged me about what I knew about DSH. Not much to be honest. So, following the session, suitably motivated, I commenced a preliminary exploration of the literature.

Exploring deliberate self-harm

Deliberate self-harm is a term used interchangeably with parasuicide. Arguments surround the various terminology used. Fairburn (1995) criticises terms such as parasuicide believing they are used to suggest a person's intent to die, when arguably the range of injury a person can carry out upon themselves is wide-ranging and not always life-threatening. For the purpose of this research the preferred term will be DSH. Anderson (1999:92) also utilised this terminology in a review of self-harm and suicide, stating:

> The term deliberate self-harm encompasses behaviours where the patient can be considered suicidal, such as taking an overdose, self suffocation, self strangulation, wrist cutting, drowning, etc. However the term also used to refer to acts a young person may engage in, but where suicide may not be the intention.

Deliberate self-harm is one of the top five causes of acute medical admissions for both male and females and is a known risk factor for suicide (Hawton and Fagg 1992). With the majority presenting at general hospitals, 150 000 attendances occur per annum (Hawton and Catlin 1997). McLaughlin (1994) notes that:

> The casualty department is usually the first port of call for these patients. Such high incidence rates can cause stress on both nursing and medical staff and could influence the attitudes they hold in relation to attempted suicide.

It is estimated that in the UK one person every day contemplates suicide (McLaughlin 1991). The Government green paper *Our healthier nation* outlines targets for the reduction of suicide rates (Department of Health [DH] 1998). Research and literature surrounding the attitudes of nurses and other health professionals in both A&E and, surprisingly psychiatric units, suggest that an improvement in attitudes is needed to improve patient care and reduce suicides. I am not alone then although I take little comfort in that idea. How then is this to be achieved if the literature suggests that attitudes are incongruent with desirable practice? Alston and Robinson (1992:206) state that when responding to a suicidal patient, 'The nurse may hold attitudes which lead to fear, anxiety, absence of empathy and anger.' I can identify with that.

Whilst exploring literature I found an article by Fiona Lynn, a woman with a history of self-harm. She states:

> Needing stitches was a nightmare. I felt embarrassed and shamed about being stitched up by a nurse whose comments, or lack of comment, made me want the ground to open up to swallow me. (Lynn 1998:56)

Reading these words had a big impact on me. Lynn heard the practitioner's attitude without a word being spoken. They encourage me to view things from a different perspective, hitting home that my thoughts or anxieties about my care of DSH had lain dormant, waiting for the right time to be expressed. I have embarked on my journey and feel positive and emotional about it.

Session 2: avoidance

I met Chris again in guided reflection four weeks later. I have reconstructed our dialogue from notes Chris made during the session he gave me for verification:

Chris: What has happened since we last met?

Jane: Nothing, I have had no contact with any DSH patients.

Chris: Why is that?

Jane: I don't know really, interactions just haven't happened.

Chris: No DSH patients have been through the department when you were on duty?

Jane: Well, yes plenty of patients, there always are. I was busy with other patients. That's not really true. I suppose if I'm honest I've been avoiding them.

Chris: Why?

Jane: I haven't really thought about it, on reflection I suppose it's easier isn't it?

Chris: Perhaps you deliberately use avoidance to give you more time to unravel your belief system before you wade in again?

Jane: I admit I have been avoiding them but I haven't analysed why. I do feel that I need to grasp more understanding of the subject. I don't want to hurt anyone by saying the wrong thing.

Chris: I think this period of avoidance is a positive step towards understanding yourself. How do you feel about the two sessions we have had? Anything insights emerging for you?

Jane: I can acknowledge my negative prejudice towards DSH patients. It was a relief to admit that I feared the next interaction.

Reflection

The session began with my negative feelings about avoiding contact with DSH patients. During the session I came to realise that I had been avoiding DSH patients for a specific reason, Chris suggested that I had used avoidance as a mechanism because I needed more time, that it was a step towards unravelling my belief system. He realised this period of avoidance was a necessity and that it was significant to my journey of reflection. Carveth (1995) believes avoidance is used by nurses when the prospect of dealing with a difficult patient arises. Whilst avoidance provides a protective mechanism for the nurse from life and death issues, avoidance can be painful for the patient who may already feel isolated (Eldrid 1988).

Having explored the literature I realise that 'I am not alone'. Many practitioners have difficulty with this patient group although I mustn't fall back on that as a rationalization for my negative attitude. The work of Corley and Goren (1998) identified the way in which nurses stigmatise certain patients, including those who are suicidal. This results in nurses distancing themselves from patients and minimising the contact they have with them. Jameton (1992) described this as the 'dark side of nursing' – that practitioners can cause suffering rather than ease it.

I conclude from Corley and Goren's writing that, amongst other reasons, the overriding factor for my thoughts/feelings/actions is my upbringing, my nurse training, and my life as a whole; all have moulded my beliefs/moral opinion. I now understand that I need to view patients and respond beyond the 'label', to see these attempted suicides/self-harmers as a people/individuals needing help.

Chris has challenged me to examine my boundaries as an A&E practitioner, whether my role only required that the damage was 'patched up'? I realise now that my feelings, however well hidden, are picked up by patients and this ultimately affects their care; that they can see my negative attitude and perhaps even expect it. Corley cites Younger (1995) as suggesting that practitioners protect themselves from being overwhelmed by suffering by distancing themselves from the sufferer. I feel that I distance myself for more than one emotional reason; fear, anger, resentment and lack of empathy come quickly to mind. Distancing myself from patients has certainly been a tactic I have used in the past. I am beginning to understand that I have used this in the past as a way of protecting myself.

I felt that one significant issue was a growing sense of empowerment to act according to new beliefs and changed attitudes. As Johns (2004) understands it, reflection is concerned first with coming to an understanding of the way things are. Secondly, it is concerned with becoming empowered to change self and practice whereby I can act in tune with my beliefs and values. Thirdly, it is concerned with transformation; the realisation that self has changed and contradiction has been resolved, even as new contradictions emerge. Whilst the Being available template offers me a model to frame my transformed self, Chris suggested an 'empowerment' model might help frame my emergence. He talked several potential approaches for me to review.

I chose Kieffer's (1984) 'Attainment of participatory competence through four phases of involvement framework'[2] (Table 12.1). I am currently in what Kieffer describes as the 'era of entry'. Kieffer explains that an individual who moves through this stage is moti-

Table 12.1 Attainment of participatory competence through four phases of involvement (adapted from Kieffer 1984)

Phase	Development
Era of entry (birth of struggle against conflict)	Birth of emergence of participatory competence: realising one's integrity has been violated, provoking and mobilising a deep sense of frustration and powerlessness towards an empowering response
Era of advancement (continuing struggle)	Maturation of empowerment through extension of involvement and deepening understanding through intensive self-reflection with the help of an external enabler
Era of incorporation (continuing struggle)	Reconstructs sense of self as author and actor in environment. Learning to confront and contend with barriers to self-determination leads to a sense of mastery and competence in the individual's sense of being
Era of commitment (continuing struggle)	Adulthood of participatory competence – integrating new abilities and insight into reality in meaningful ways

---

[2] See also Latchford in Chapter 7.

vated because they have experienced an emotionally significant or symbolic episode. Particularly significant was my comment that the wound must hurt when he cut himself, so why was he worried about the pain of stitches? Kieffer states this symbolic event triggers or initiates a period of reactive engagement.

Chris is the catalyst at this stage, helping me through understanding and my new commitment, to convert my negative attitude into a positive attitude, liberating my trapped energy for the task ahead.

Session 3: Moving from avoidance towards connection

In session 3, Chris picked up on the issue of avoidance from the last session, 'when we last met you realised that you had been using "avoidance" as a coping mechanism, has anything new developed?'

I reply that I realised I was using avoidance was a step forward in itself. I acknowledge how I have been using 'avoidance time' to 'get my thoughts together'. Now I want to work out how I can learn to overcome this first hurdle and try to care for DSH patients more in tune with my holistic values. Chris presses me to be clear about my 'holistic values' – I say it is to be available to all my patients irrespective of the cause of their compromised health.

Chris asks if I have cared for any DSH patients since we last met. Yes I have. In fact I went out of my way to nurse a DSH patient. I had spoken to my colleagues on shift and asked them if I could 'take' DSH patients. It wasn't what I expected at all. I took the handover of a DSH patient and went into the cubicle explaining to him what clinical procedures were needed. I acted in a way that I wouldn't usually. I gave what I hoped was a warm smile. I pushed negative feelings to the side.

Chris interjects, 'Just remind me of those feelings you usually experience when dealing with a DSH patient?' I respond that self-harm is a cry for attention, not as 'deserving' of my attention/care as other patients. They are often time wasters; I could be helping someone who really needs it!]Chris notes that we have already discussed why I feel this way. I understand my past experiences had made me feel this way. I reiterate that I do want to do something about it, as hard as it is. I had asked Andrew, the patient, very directly why he had taken an overdose. He said his life was a mess, his mother didn't care. He was thin, a little emaciated, and I felt sorry for him.

Chris asks how I felt asking him why he had taken an overdose. I admit I had felt very clumsy. I stumbled over my words, I felt hot and uncomfortable. In fact I began to relive these feelings with Chris. He recognised and acknowledged this, simply asking why do I think you felt like that? I said I knew that if Andrew had answered my question, I wouldn't have known how to respond. I didn't do any psychiatric training; I wouldn't be able to fulfil his needs. He might ask me for something I can't give. I would have been exposed as a fraud.

Chris pushes me 'What do you usually do when you don't have an answer?'

I said 'Well I suppose I would ask someone for help.'

Chris says 'So if a DSH patient asks for something that you don't understand you could refer to a colleague who could help, couldn't you? I think your statement that "he might ask me for something I can't give" is more significant. Is this more to do with your beliefs?'

I paused before answering, pondering the depth of this question. I responded 'I suppose what I really mean is that he/she may ask me to understand them, have knowledge of whatever disorder/mental illness they have. I don't think I have it inside me to understand.

I want to change, I want to give more than clinical care, but I find these patients mentally draining. It's scary to think that someone can be so desperate.'

Chris affirmatively reflects back by words, 'Okay, so you felt clumsy but that must have been important to Andrew. Has he a past history of this type of thing?'

I responded, 'Yes, he's done it several times before.'

Chris pushes home the point: 'So what does that tell you? Do you view him less seriously? Or more seriously? You said you felt sorry for him, why?'

'Previously, before looking at the facts and figures in literature, I would have viewed him as an attention seeker, taken him less seriously than another patient. I have discovered since we last spoke that individuals may inflict harm many times, sometimes over long periods of time. Eventually a significant number will actually commit suicide, so maybe this helps me to understand a little. I felt sorry for him because, apart from his appearance he was very apologetic, he was compliant with his clinical care.'

Chris draws links with our previous discussion around the concept of the 'unpopular patient' asking, 'He was a good patient?' I had to admit reluctantly that he was.

Pursuing the point Chris said, 'It is rather interesting that you liked him and stated that he was compliant. Perhaps if he had been non-compliant in some way or abusive you may not have felt so warm towards him.' Chris reiterates the literature that explored the concept of 'good and bad' patient, notably a paper by Kelly and May (1982). Patients who comply 'do as they are told' by the nurse or doctor. He suggested I might explore this paper. As the session time was drawing to a close he asks if there is anything else I want to discuss?

I was happy with what we had covered. Anymore I think would have been too much for me to take in.

Chris recapped, 'Although you felt clumsy, you feel positive about your interaction and feel that you can learn from this experience, and move on? Perhaps you could think of a way to ask patients why they have self-harmed in a different way, perhaps you could try a cathartic approach, perhaps ask what has upset them so much today that they felt the need to hurt themselves? Or perhaps a very direct approach is appropriate for a particular patient? John Heron's work is a useful reference.'

I replied 'I think I would be happier to frame the question in a different way, but my nerves got the better of me.'

Chris sensed that Andrew didn't mind from what I had told him. He felt that the most important thing is that I wanted to ask, and I had asked, breaking through my avoidance and becoming available to Andrew.

Reflection

This was my first contact with a patient since the interaction I shared in session one. The dialogue reveals that this interaction, although not perfect, was a positive experience. The main issue is my lack of knowledge surrounding psychiatric nursing, although I do now feel empowered to change.

Picking up the issues from last session, I have read the work of Kelly and May (1982), who critiqued the idea of 'good and bad patients', who suggest that it is typically assumed that negative attitudes, held by practitioners due to educational or technical reasons, can be corrected at the training stage. However, it would appear that for many practitioners this issue is not adequately addressed. If negative attitudes had been successfully corrected surely there would not be an abundance of literature highlighting negative attitudes amongst practitioners? Sociologists such as Conrad (1979) claim patients are treated according to class/attitude or illness. Kelly and May state:

> It is unlikely that problems in nurse–patient relationships will prove amenable to simplistic prescriptions since the cause of those problems is endemic of social interaction itself. (1982:154)

The literature led me to the same answers: 'the answer is not simple', 'a wider view must be taken', 'medical models are too rigid'. I am constantly led to reflexivity, it would seem that to reflect, to know self, to be open to all the possibilities will ultimately resolve my original questions and unravel my belief system. Chris suggested that I consider why I liked Andrew and asked if this was because he was compliant and apologetic with his treatment. Trexlar (1996) described 'difficult' patients as those who are perceived to act in a deviant manner. Trexlar suggests that such patients respond by adopting expected role behaviour that results in:

> Stigma and social isolation that reinforces the original behaviour and may leads to secondary deviance and validation of the nurse's judgement of the patient. (1996:132)

If Trexlar's assumption is correct, then perhaps practitioners and society play some part in patients who repeatedly self-harm. Perhaps as nurses we perceive such behaviour as unacceptable, this is picked up on by the patients who continue with 'deviant' behaviour, or, at the very least, they do not know how to respond in any other way. Perhaps Andrew did 'tune' into me. Here was a young man with a past history of harming himself and who was familiar with the attitude and responses of medical staff. Perhaps he manipulated the situation by turning himself from what Trexlar describes as a *deviant* patient to a *compliant* patient to provoke a caring response? Nievaard (1987) cites Kiesler's (1983) classification of interpersonal behaviour, describing how attitudes of hospital patients are divided into four main groups:

- Dependant;
- Self-reducing;
- Co-operative;
- Rebellious.

Perhaps compliance is a mix of self-reducing and co-operative, whereas deviant is a mix of dependant and rebellious. Recognising my use of negative labels, all labels perverse because they are linked to a behavioural response. Whilst understanding that Andrew's *compliance* probably did affect my response to him, my response to him was empathic, and this comes with the dawning of understanding. I learn that not all individuals who attempt self-harm do so with the intent of dying. The reasons for self-harm vary and it is carried out under differing circumstances across a broad spectrum of individuals (Roberts 1996). As Hawton and Catlin (1997:1409) state:

> Someone who has attempted suicide is a hundred times more likely to commit suicide than the general population within the following year.

I may never understand DSH but I am changing my attitude and response to DSH patients as typified by Andrew. Never before have I asked a patient 'Why?' Perhaps I would have dealt with another, less compliant DSH differently? Maybe. New experiences will reveal that truth. I feel empowered to bridge the practice/theory gap, as well as being confident to examine myself. I would have said that my beliefs did not affect patient care. I now know my beliefs *do* affect my ability to care. Furthermore, I now believe that previous patients were aware of my negative feelings, something I would previously have denied.

Session 4: Confronting my resistance

In session 4 I shared my experience with a patient who made me feel really angry. Karl had taken an overdose. His notes revealed that he had taken a near fatal overdose 12 months previously. This really bought home the seriousness of Karl's feelings to me. I am attempting to view all DSH patients as *serious*, but it was easier to view Karl as *serious* because of his history. I went into his cubicle, feeling open, wanting to help, wanting to be cathartic. I asked, 'What upset you so much today? Something must have really upset you to do this to yourself.' Karl didn't want to talk to me. He ignored me, he didn't even look at me, and his face was averted to the wall. I looked at the situation and asked myself, 'How is Karl feeling, what is his main concern?' It was then I realised his mother and brother were in the cubicle, perhaps he didn't want to talk in front of them. I asked if they would mind leaving the cubicle. I asked Karl again, he ignored me. I asked could he at least look at me, I felt my anger rising, but felt that I was managing it well.

Chris asked 'Why did I feel so angry?' I didn't answer so he further asked, 'Was it because Karl wouldn't tell you why he did it?' I replied, 'Yes that's it, and he wouldn't even look at me. There I was making all the effort, a big effort. I felt like I was falling flat on my face, why was I even bothering? The fact that I wanted to help had no effect on Karl, he wasn't interested.' Chris affirmed the way I had understood and managed my anger – my development of poise within the Being available template. He asked, 'What happened next?'

I said, 'I told Karl that I could see he was upset, but if he wanted to talk later, I was there. I told him I would come back in a while and would be available to talk if he wanted to.'

Chris again affirmed my response, 'So you sent him a very positive message didn't you? You let him know that you cared, you let him know you were available to him. You told him you cared enough to go back and see him later. Are you placing too much emphasis on the fact that he wouldn't talk?'

I sensed that Chris was suggesting I had reacted to being rejected when I had made such an effort. I can see this. I replied, 'A couple of days later I reflected further on this experience in my journal. I had calmed down by then and realised that one of the reasons I wanted him to talk was because I had a need to understand. I know that Karl's reason for DSH is not the same as everyone's, but I thought he could give me some insight. The other reason for feeling angry was simply that it had taken courage on my part to offer myself, to make myself available to Karl, and yes, you are spot on, I did feel rejected. Ego stuff.'

Again Chris was affirmative: 'But you managed yourself within the unfolding moment that is a change in you, you have managed yourself with a DSH patient within the unfolding moment. You negotiated both your own resistance and Karl's resistance.'

Reflection

I now feel happier, more comfortable and appreciate my interaction with Karl through new eyes. I understand that I had rushed in with a cathartic approach with high expectations. I now realise it's all right that Karl didn't want to talk. It wasn't the right time for him, may be it was too soon, and I can reassure myself that he will have the opportunity to talk when he is ready because, in this particular case, admission to hospital was required. Again the empathy that I am beginning to feel is in itself motivating me towards achieving more. The most important issue is that Karl knew that I cared. I felt I managed my rising anger well and did not let it affect Karl's care. I reinforced the fact that I cared by telling him I was there if he needed me. My anger came from the fact that he didn't need me in the way I had anticipated I understand he just needed a caring response and nothing more. My residual negative feelings have evaporated. I can now explore my self at a deeper level and go beyond my anxiety, as if facing a great white shark in a steel cage. I utilised the Being available template (Johns 2000) as a way to view myself moving along each of the six markers that determine how available I was with Karl.

Knowing what is desirable

I have a much clearer vision of caring in my mind, and I am more aware of my vision within the moment – what Chris describes as intentionality, in particular to treat Karl in the caring way I would treat any other patient. Holding a vision is a very powerful idea. It is liberating and makes everything more meaningful. I wonder why I have not thought about this before. I sense it is because practice is driven by tasks to do around symptoms and treatments rather than by values and knowing the person.

Knowing the person

I had made a huge effort to connect with Karl. Perhaps, on reflection, it was an unpolished effort but the intent to know him as a person was there. Chris had shown me the Burford reflective cues[3]; the first two cues are:

- 'Who is this person?'
- 'What meaning does this health event have for the person?'

These cues are helpful guides. However, in A&E, when someone is admitted in a life-threatening condition, the emphasis is on saving life. In my experience with Karl, we had moved beyond that phase. Knowing the person is informed by ideas from the DSH literature, and that helps me understand why Karl may be withdrawn and turn his head away from me as he did. I shouldn't have expected him to be compliant like Andrew. All people are unique and respond differently, yet my tendency has been to categorise people – 'DSH patients'.

---

[3] The Burford reflective cues consist of nine reflective cues. They offer a dynamic reflective model for appreciating the life pattern of the patient (Johns 2004).

Concern for the person

It is interesting the way my vision fuels my concern. I was genuinely concerned for Karl. He really did matter for me and yet I could see how my own concerns were getting in the way – that I became concerned for myself as reflected through my sense of being rejected.

Poise

My experience informs me that poise is a precarious thing – why else did I feel anger and yet I could contain it within the moment. This awareness is a new thing for me. As Ramos (1992) notes, the blocks to therapeutic relationships with patients is due to issues of emotion and control. Before I had kept my distance through labelling and aversion and now I felt entangled, as if I do not know how to respond on a cathartic level. In understanding and managing my own concerns I was more able to negotiate my own resistance to Karl as well as his resistance to me. I am experiencing a great sense of motivation. As Chris suggested, I need to imagine a space between us so I can see these things unfolding, yet remain available to Karl even as he resists me.

The aesthetic response to the patient

I feel I walk a tightrope of learning new skills of being available to a DSH patient. I imagine such skills are transferable between patients but I now know otherwise because of the emotional context. I recognise that to be available to Karl, I first had to be available to myself – poised, confident and skilful, especially in catharsis.

Creating and sustaining an environment where being available is possible

I tried to provide the best environment in the given circumstances. He was in a private cubicle, I asked his relatives to leave allowing him more privacy and I let him know that I wanted to care for him. I am aware I have not yet explored attitudes to DSH patients with my colleagues, and yet that is vital to change our collective practice. I accept that responsibility at a later stage. But first I must get my own house in order.

Session 5: Nurturing my concern

I was looking forward to sharing and examining my thoughts and feelings with Chris in session 5 because I sensed I had made real progress. Chris started the session by asking what I had to share since our last meeting. First I shared my insights about the DSH literature I had explored. Then a new experience – he's a man in his forties, he had taken a large overdose. He had visited his estranged wife and when she refused to let him into the house, he sat down in her garden and took a massive overdose. She wasn't aware that he was still in her garden and some hours later a passer-by called an ambulance. To say that I interacted with him is debatable. I carried out his clinical care, but he was unconscious, quite ill in fact, so I didn't actually speak to him.

Chris asked how I felt about the man. I felt really sad, sad that he had felt so desperate, sad that he could die, sad that may be he didn't mean to kill himself but just wanted his partner to come outside and talk, sad that his ex-wife would probably feel guilty and blame herself. Just incredibly sad. Then I saw the seriousness of DSH, the desperation and the waste.

Chris said, 'This is new for you isn't it, this sympathy?'

I had felt sad when DSH patients had died in the past, but not as sad as, for example, a victim of a road traffic accident, or a child. I feel different now. Reflection has made me think differently about all sorts of things, not just in the work place, it's 'bigger' than that! A combination of these sessions, keeping a journal and learning about DSH are beginning to affect my thought processes and the way in which I interact with this patient group.

Reflection

This experience was very significant. I found myself caring for this man at a time when everything I've been thinking about is falling into place. Through understanding my whole attitude is changing. My belief system and moral opinion is being replaced by new values, brought about by these profound insights.

I have moved into Kieffer's (1984) second stage, 'Era of advancement'. Kieffer identifies three quite distinct and necessary elements needed to successfully move into this stage:

(1) The focus and stability of a mentoring relationship as reflected in my relationship with my supervisor – Chris has been extremely stable and has focused on relevant and significant issues.
(2) Supportive peer relationships within a collective organisational structure. Most of my peers/colleagues have become curious and supportive of my research. I hope that my research on an individual level will induce a collective action towards change.
(3) Critical understanding of social and political relations that I have gained though critically exploring the DSH literature, giving me a deeper understanding of DSH.

I would add that this stage is marked by a non-return to previous ways of being. I am to mindful of myself with DSH patients to revert to previous ways of being. Such is the power of insight to shift me.

Session 6: Realising right attitude

Chris started session 6 by reviewing our last meeting and asking about new interactions. I felt very comfortable, relaxed and exhilarated. I had been waiting to tell Chris about another interaction with a DSH patient that had gone very well. A young man in his twenties. He arrived in the early hours of the morning having taken some paracetamol tablets. Not many, but he was very distressed. He kept saying sorry and apologising for wasting the practitioner's time. I found that instead of offering no reply to this statement or giving a half-hearted, 'You're not wasting anyone's time', I actually wanted to talk to him. I sensed that he wanted to talk; he had financial worries and girlfriend problems. It all tumbled out very quickly. I was only supposed to be carrying out triage – a two to three minute assessment in order to categorise his problem that dictates how quickly someone should be seen by a doctor. But I found myself talking to him for at least 15 minutes. The department was not busy, so instead of handing his care over to someone else, I took him into a cubicle and continued to talk. At all times during my interaction, I was aware of my concern for him. I felt tender towards him. I had a strong desire to help by simply listening. I know that he appreciated my concern for him and I know he felt my concern was genuine. He had to stay in the department for several hours awaiting results of blood tests before he was assessed by a doctor who then discharged him. His friend was going to stay with him overnight, and ensure he attended an out-patient appointment in the morning.

Chris felt this was a very positive experience. He asked, 'Why do you think you *wanted* to talk to him, what surfaced your concern, why did you feel tender?'

I suspect my reply sounded rather glib. 'I was conscious of reflecting within the moment, of reading his pattern. The more concern I felt, the better I felt. I wasn't hiding anything from myself. I viewed him as a person, not a condition.' Using the Burford model cues, I asked myself, 'Who is this person?', 'What does he need from me at this moment?', 'How can I help him?'. These cues help me to focus on him as a suffering individual human and able to transcend any lingering prejudice I have for people who deliberately self-harm.

The word *suffering* is Chris's word – he feels suffering encompasses the whole person and doesn't discriminate in that we all suffer to varying extent. The word is evocative of compassion, that the carer's human response to suffering *is* compassion.

Reflection

I am happier I am now more available to patients. My belief system is very different from when I commenced this self-inquiry. Focusing on the third element of the Being available template, 'concern for the person' I am more motivated to care, to express my empathy, and discovering how the expression of empathy opens up new possibilities in my relationships with DSH patients. While I believe my care giving remains balanced, I am discovering the more I give the more I get from shared relationships. My beliefs and values have been exposed and examined for their meaning and relevance. My response to DSH patients has changed; there is a positive shift towards more congruent practice.

Session 7: Knock back

Commencing session 7, I was feeling quite 'down' about my recent experiences but felt comfortable enough in my relationship with Chris to discuss what I considered to be fairly negative interactions.

I said, 'I feel as if I've taken two steps forward and three back! I don't quite know where to start, I've had what I consider a very "negative" experience and a positive one, and I don't understand why. I know that I shouldn't blame myself, but I do feel guilty about the negative interaction I had.'

Chris suggested I described the negative experience first.

'Well the shift was really busy; it was over the New Year period a young girl presented in the department after taking an overdose. Her friend had recently committed suicide. She was hysterical, and I could not calm her down. At the start of our interaction, I reminded myself that here was a young girl who had lost a friend in traumatic circumstances. As I've already said, the shift was busy, and there were other patients close by who were very ill. In order to be fair to this patient and other patients in the department I needed to calm her down. I had conflicting priorities, my other patients needed a quiet calm atmosphere, but I needed to take control with this patient and I was failing. The more hysterical she became the more irritation I felt, my anger was rising up inside me. I thought she was silly, a "drama queen". Obviously, I understood she was grieving for her friend, but I was under pressure, it was 2 o'clock in the morning and I think alcohol played a part in her behaviour.'

Chris laughed, 'So she wasn't a "good" patient then?'

'No! Her father wasn't any help either, he had been drinking but their relationship did not come across as particularly close. I hoped her father would calm her down, but he seemed to cause yet more hysteria. I felt she needed to be told her behaviour was unacceptable. I told her I wanted to help but couldn't if she wouldn't let me. Nothing I tried worked. As I felt that I had made no connection with her, couldn't manage my feelings or was responding in the patient's best interest, I felt it best to hand over her care to someone else for and remove myself from the situation. She was moved away from the poorly patients, the second nurse was firmer than I was, she eventually calmed down, and I don't know what happened after that.'

Chris wondered if I had adopted a parental role with her because her mother was absent and her father 'useless'? Whether I had taken on the role of a critical mother or perhaps I had wanted to tell her off?

I felt Chris's challenge – I am learning his tongue-in-cheek style of supervision, of gentle but astute confrontation. Being positive to his challenge I respond, 'No, I wasn't conscious of taking on a parental role but, being a mother myself, it is an easy role to fall into. Anyway, if I did unconsciously take on a parental role it didn't work, did it? I hadn't even got to the point of thinking about deliberate harm!'

Chris asked about the other patient I had mentioned.

'This is where my confusion lies. A few days later another young girl, about the same age came to the department. She was at school, bought in by the class teacher; she had taken a small overdose. I was completely different with this patient, I was able to talk to her and let her know my concern was genuine.'

Chris asked what factors made this interaction so different? Was it late at night? Was I tired? Was I busy?

It was a day shift, 9 or 10 in the morning, and quiet in the department. He asked if I thought the busyness of the department made a difference in the way DSH patients are treated?

'Umm, I'd like to say no, but every ward, every department works under pressure. When it's busy it's impossible to give that little bit more. As awful as it sounds, time can be an influencing factor. We all try to make time, to make the most of our time, but sometimes it isn't enough.'

Chris asked if any research supported that idea and I was able to cite a significant literature that pointed to the influence of time on practitioners' attitudes towards DSH patients. Chris picked up on this point, noting that having time affected me with the second girl. He wondered if it being a day shift I was more receptive to her needs because I wasn't tired as I can be on night duty? Certainly having time I did not feel the pressure of competing demand. I was able to ask her why she had self-harmed and we discussed other things that she could have done instead of taking the tablets. She had taken them because her mum wouldn't let her visit her boyfriend the night before. I don't think she did it to manipulate her mother. I think she did it because she felt so desperate about not seeing him. She agreed that a preferable course of action would be to talk to someone, a nurse, a teacher, her mum or a friend. I think she actually learnt from the experience, she took something positive away with her.

Chris asked if I had adopted a parental role? In this case I had, yet this was okay because she was frightened – she needed comforting. Chris agreed, noting that parent–child pattern of communication (within transactional analysis) can be therapeutic when the practitioner is mindful is mindful of adopting that pattern rather than simply reacting to the situation because it evokes a maternal response. And yes, my response was reactive but I can see his point that emotional reaction reflects the way I absorbed some of the girl's suffering as a mother does for her child and may have obscured appropriate decision making.

So – what accounts for the difference in my response to these two young girls? What emerges is poise! The first girl outside my emotional limits and the second within them. I feel bad. Chris twists this around, suggesting that my first experience was also positive because I learn from it.

I said, 'That's perhaps a better way to look at it.'

Reflection

My response to the second patient was more congruent with my newly developed values. With the first patient, within the unfolding moment I felt that I could not manage my own concerns and care for the patient. It was in the patient's best interests to receive care from another nurse. She deserved better. I feel good about that now, with hindsight. At the time I felt I had failed her and worse, failed myself.

In exploring the variables in the session with Chris, we recognised the impact of time and workload, and time of the day as significant in my response. Greenwood and Bradley (1997) state that the majority of DHS patients present to A&E departments 'out of hours' and confirm this with an audit of DSH time presentation. They suggest this may contribute towards negative attitudes due to difficulty in accessing psychiatric services 'out of hours'. Speaking from a personal perspective, I agree that most DSH patients present during the early hours of the morning or late at night. This means on a night shift it is typical to care for at least one patient who has self-harmed. During a night shift, 'enthusiasm' may not be at the same level as during the day thus leading to a more negative approach and be less available to these patients. The human response is to critique each other on meeting for the first time. McLaughlin (1994:111) states:

> Nursing can readily lend itself to the rapid formation of attitudes towards those who come into contact with it.

McLaughlin (1994) further suggests that initial contact, in addition to confidential information about the patient, can lead to negative attitudes, resulting in influencing the quality of care and jeopardizing the practitioner–patient relationship. This I know for myself as reflected vividly through my self-inquiry.

The focus of my self-inquiry has largely been on my relationships with DSH patients and yet the environment of care – issues such as time, attitudes of staff, workload, time of day, the quality of the physical environment are all significant in my being available. Without doubt, the young girl benefited from being moved from the 'resus' room to another. The 'resus' is a large room equipped with several beds used for patients requiring life-saving interventions. The resus room may have been very frightening for her, not ideal for an intimate conversation about life and death. Moving her into a separate cubicle provided privacy not just for her and family but also for the other patients.

A few days later I met another girl, also around 15 years of age, who had overdosed and this time I was really happy with the way in which I responded and cared for her. I was able to do this because guided reflection had produced a new insight into the previous interaction, in addition to all of the other interactions. Mezirow (1981:223) states:

> Our meaning structures are transformed through reflection, defined here as attending to the grounds (justification) for one's beliefs. We reflect on the unexamined assumptions of our beliefs when the beliefs are not working well for us, or where old ways of thinking are no longer functional. We are confronted with a disorientating dilemma, which serves as a trigger for reflection. Refection involves a critique of assumptions to determine whether the belief, often acquired through cultural assimilation in childhood, remains functional for us as adults. We do this by critically examining its origins, nature, and consequences.

My belief system was not working for me, this triggered reflection has changed the meaning in the way I deal with patients. The meaning is revised and is still changing with each experience and new knowledge. This is made valid by the very fact that the next interaction provoked a caring response. Obviously variables were different. It was during the day, quite early in the shift, the workload was light and I could concentrate on her care. Throughout our interaction I remembered the other teenager. Again I dealt with a teenager verging on hysteria, quiet difficult to deal with, our interaction could easily have spiralled into a negative experience for both of us. However whilst managing my own concerns I successfully met her needs. I no longer fear involvement with such patients. As Benner and Wrubel (1989) believe, connecting with my caring is one of the most effective coping resources.

Deeper reflection

From the outset of this self-inquiry I was concerned that any changes I made to my practice in relation to my care of DSH patients would leave me vulnerable. Benner and Wrubel (1989) believe that emotions can no longer be viewed as interruptions. By this they believe emotions have significance and content in their own right and that respect for knowledge and wisdom is gained if the individual allows their emotions to direct their thoughts and attention. They state:

> Attending to emotion offers the possibility of bringing a past interpretation of the situation into the present, where past history can be reinterpreted and reconstituted. (Benner and Wrubel 1989:96)

How true. As a result of my inquiry into my beliefs, a host of factors including cultural and religious beliefs have emerged that influence my practice with DSH patients. I sense how being raised in a predominately Christian society with strong cultural beliefs about self-harm and suicide has impacted on me. As recently as 1961 suicide and attempted suicide fell into the same category as murder and there were a number of prosecutions. Decriminalisation in 1966 did not lead to any great change to the prevailing Christian ethic even as the world became more secular. As McLaughlin (1994:1112) states: 'In the Judeo-Christian cultures there has always been a belief that suicide is reprehensible and ethically wrong.' Other factors contributing to my previous belief system included my experiences with DSH patients. Now I can see these relationships were always tinged with anger. Accepting my mother's failing health and the seriousness of her condition dissolved some of my anger. I recognised that because I worked in an acute area, I had fallen into a trap of measuring, quantifying or prioritising patients and their conditions. Fear that lack of knowledge would make 'a bad situation worse' played a part in my incongruent practice.

Creating an environment

Later, I convened a debate with my A&E colleagues in response to their interest in my study. They were divided on their own feelings about DSH patients. Some felt they firmly understood and treated the patient group in exactly the same way they would any other. I wonder if they distort their reality. It is not easy to face up to being uncaring. Some found themselves, perhaps like myself, somewhere in the middle, lacking real knowledge of self-harm and experiencing difficulty with caring for such patients. Some felt that DSH patients were time wasters who manipulated both nurses and the medical system. One co-worker stated that she was 'resigned' to nursing DSH patients. I asked her to explain and she said that the only DSH patients we ever met were those in crisis. She further explained that we never saw patients who 'got better', 'recovered'. The comments made are similar to those documented by Anderson *et al.* (1999) into the attitude of medical staff towards the suicidal. These authors state: 'nurses and doctors do not support the notion that suicidal behaviour reflects mental illness' (p. 8). One staff nurse who took part in the research stated:

> Sometimes I think they are time wasters – occasionally, and quite selfish – if you have a good reason to self harm then that's that ... but if not then I think it's quite selfish. (p. 6)

These words reflect some of my own thoughts prior to my self-inquiry. The debate with my colleagues enabled thoughts and feelings to rise to the surface and whilst I was not able to change their opinion, perhaps a seed was sown, a seed that may surface later, at a time that is right for the individual to address their own contradictions. When others choose to address their own contradictions, perhaps a paradigm shift from the normal approach to a different approach will occur. The debate helped to prepare a more fertile ground for growth.

Anderson *et al.* suggest that attitudes towards DSH are complex, multidimensional and the interaction between nurse and patient will depend on their belief system of each other. Repper (1999) discusses the importance of the role of A&E staff, given that they work at the interface of all other components. Repper highlights that:

> Poor information and communication systems, lack of knowledge about suicide; negative attitudes towards people who self-harm does not help the rising number of patients presenting with DSH and advises that A&E staff become more involved with education/training and negative attitudes are challenged. (1999:11)

My insights into my practice with self-harm patients have significantly shifted my practice. I am more mindful as I interact with these patients, and more genuinely available to them. I hope that my research will challenge others towards enabling others to find a more therapeutic way of responding to DSH within A&E.

Without reflection I could go no further than to superficially question the contradiction I had ignored and which yet bubbled uncomfortably beneath my calm, confident surface. Chris challenged me early in the research to identify the practitioner's role in A&E. Is it holistic or merely physical trauma work? I take the view it is holistic, that my response to the DSH patient makes a difference; that compassion and non-judgemental acceptance works better than indifference or worse, rejection and thinly veiled contempt.

Moss (1988:616) states that, 'If nursing is to attain the status of an independent profession it must identify and rectify the factors that influence nursing attitudes'.

Only when practitioners, like myself, resolve contradiction, can they realise their visions of practice as a lived reality and lead more satisfactory lives. In acknowledging and confronting my prejudice I discovered myself as a person and have found that this, in itself, naturally leads to not just tuning into others and their needs, but also my own. It feels astonishing to realise such self-neglect and yet I sense that nurse education gives little emphasis to developing and sustaining effective therapeutic relationships, especially with what might be construed as 'difficult patients'.

All experience is positive if we can learn from it. My learning and understanding have travelled full cycle, described by Gadamer (1979) as an oscillating cycle that continuously evolves.

My empowerment to act came from within because I could no longer live with the contradiction, once the protective veneer had been torn off within guided reflection with Chris. I had a choice: to retreat or push forward. But in reality I had no choice because where could I have retreated too? My cover was blown! So I chose to push forward, to face up to my vulnerability with the challenge and support of Chris. As Kieffer (1984) clearly acknowledged in his model of participatory competence, the role of an external enabler is vital. As Johns (2004) notes it is not easy to see beyond the normal self. Emancipation, or the realisation of my changed self was affirmed quite recently. My arms around a woman in great distress, crying a steady stream of tears, suddenly I realised I genuinely cared. I had not needed to prompt myself for the best verbal response. We were talking as I carried out clinical observations, but I was so in tune with this woman I instinctively knew what she wanted from me. I sat next to her and her tears began. She physically moved towards me, I believe she sensed my empathy and the genuineness of my caring response. As I encircled her in my arms I felt emotional, I felt sadness for her, but realised the truth of Ramos's (1992:504) words 'Nurses described an emotional identification which was real, not devastating to the nurse, but a motivator'.

I feel very positive, I feel as if a burden has lifted from my shoulders. Ramos describes such a relationship as a reciprocal relationship and the very cornerstone of nursing care. I wanted to hold this woman because she needed me to hold her and I felt very comfortable doing so. With this interaction came the realisation that I had moved through the 'era of incorporation' and entered Kieffer's (1984) final stage – the 'era of commitment'. Kieffer believes individuals may struggle at this stage as they try to integrate personal knowledge and skill into everyday situations. The reader will already be aware of my struggle to integrate newly acquired knowledge through shared dialogue and patient interaction. Maybe I am optimistic about reaching this level of participatory competence. It has, after all, been a relatively short journey. My 'new self' is still to be tested for its robustness in face of more difficult interactions.

Footnote

Jane's narrative has been extensively edited from the first edition. In doing so, we gave greater voice to Chris, her guide, to emphasise more the nature of the guiding relationship. As such, it becomes a narrative of guided reflection as much as a narrative of shifting attitude to self-harm patients.[4]

The narrative itself raises fundamental and disturbing aspects of clinical practice working with a stigmatised group – notably the idea of the practitioner's role in A&E with such patients is it to patch up or care – especially considering the four-hour treatment window in line with government targets.[5] In dialogue with A&E nurses, they recognised their own attitudes within the performance and their role conflict.

Jane is able to demonstrate a transformation in her attitude towards self-harm patients whilst acknowledging that such shift is vulnerable on conditions. Using her own practice as an exemplar she begins to *agitate* with her own colleagues to set up a more collective concern, using her narrative to trigger social action.

References

Alston M and Robinson B (1992) Nurses attitudes towards suicide. *Omega* 25:205–215.

Anderson M (1999) Waiting for harm: deliberate self-harm and suicide in young people – a review of the literature. *Journal of Psychiatric and Mental Health Nursing* 6:91–100.

Anderson M, Standen P, Nazir S and Noon J (1999) Nurses and doctors attitudes towards suicidal behaviour in young people. *International Journal of Nursing Studies* 37:1–10.

Benner P and Wrubel J (1989) *The primary of caring.* Addison-Wesley, Menlo Park.

Carveth J (1995) Perceived patient deviance and avoidance by nurses. *Nursing Research* 44:173–178.

Conrad P (1979) Types of medical social control. *Sociology of Health and Illness* 1:1–10.

Corley M and Goren S (1998) The dark side of nursing: impact of stigmatising responses on patients. *Scholarly Inquiry for Nursing Practice* 12:99–121.

Department of Health (1998) *Our healthier nation: a contract for health.* DH, London.

Eldrid J (1988) *Caring for the suicidal.* Constable, London.

Fairburn G (1995) *Contemplating suicide: the language and ethics of self-harm.* Routledge, London.

Gadamer HG (1979) *Truth and method* (second edition). Sheed & Ward, London.

Greenwood S and Bradley P (1997) Managing deliberate self-harm: The A&E perspective. *Accident and Emergency Nursing* 5:134–136.

Hawton K and Catlin J (1997) *Attempted suicide: a practical guide to it's nature and management.* Oxford University Press, London.

Hawton K and Fagg J (1992) Trends in deliberate self poisoning and self injury in Oxford 1976–1990. *British Medical Journal* 304:1409–1411.

Jameton A (1992) *Nursing ethics and the moral situation of the nurse.* American Hospital Publishing, Chicago.

Johns C (2000) *Becoming a reflective practitioner.* Blackwell Science, Oxford.

Johns C (2004) *Becoming a reflective practitioner* (second edition). Blackwell Publishing, Oxford.

Kelly P and May D (1982) Good and bad patients: a review of the literature and a theoretical critique. *Journal of Advanced Nursing* 7:147–156.

---

[4] At the 15th International Reflective Practice conference in Limerick, June 2009, I performed the narrative (performance version – see Chapter 13) to open a dialogical space with audience to explore the nature of guided reflection.
[5] This was also an issue raised in John-Marc's leadership narrative (Chapter 11).

Kieffer C (1984) Citizen empowerment: a developmental perspective. *Prevention in Human Sciences* 84:9–36.

Kiesler DJ (1983) The 1982 interpersonal circle: a taxonomy for complementarity in human transactions. *Psychological Review* 90:185–214.

Lynn F (1998) The pain of rejection. *Nursing Times* 94:27.

McLaughlin C (1991) Parasuicide counselling in casualty departments. *Nursing Standard* 6:15.

McLaughlin C (1994) Casualty nurses attitudes to attempted suicide. *Journal of Advanced Nursing* 20:1111–1118.

Mezirow J (1981) A critical theory of adult learning and education. *Adult Education* 32:3–24.

Moss A (1988) Determinants of nursing care: nursing process or nursing attitudes. *Journal of Advanced Nursing* 13:615–620.

Nievaard A (1987) Communication climate and patient care: causes and effects of nurses attitudes to patients. *Social Science and Medicine* 24:777–784.

Ramos M (1992) The nurse–patient relationship: theme and variations. *Journal of Advanced Nursing* 17:496–506.

Repper J (1999) A review of literature on the prevention of suicide through interventions in accident and emergency departments. *Journal of Clinical Nursing* 8:3–12.

Roberts D (1996) Suicide prevention by general nurses. *Nursing Standard* 17:30–33.

Trexlar T (1996) Reformulation of deviance and labelling theory for nursing image. *Journal of Nursing Scholarship* 28:131–136.

Watson J (1999) *Post modern nursing and beyond*. Churchill Livingstone, Edinburgh.

Younger J (1995) The alienation of the sufferer. *Advances in Nursing Science* 17:53–72.

Chapter 13

Jane's rap: guided reflection as a pathway to self as sacred space

Christopher Johns and Colleen Marlin

I constructed *Jane's rap* as performance from the narrative 'Shifting attitude with deliberate self-harm patients in Accident and Emergency (A&E)' (Chapter 12). In preparation for the second edition (see Chapter 12), I rewrote the narrative to include my voice as guide so as to use the performance as a narrative of guiding reflection. References are included in Chapter 12.

The performance is set against a background PowerPoint presentation as follows:

(1) Slides that set out narrative approach prior to the performance (as if setting the scene) and credit slides at the end of the performance, which are read silently by the audience (not included here).
(2) Slides as photographs taken on Franz-Joseph glacier, South island, New Zealand. I chose these slides because the ice represented the coldness, isolation and fragmented life of self-harm patients. Fissures in the ice resembled cutting. These are not shown here.
(3) *Ensos* that contained six-word narratives which capture the key insight within the self-harm person's story. *Ensos* are Zen circles of enlightenment pained with one brush stroke and one breath (see Chapter 4). I painted them in different colours to represent something of the feelings I sensed. These are included in the text.
(4) Slides that set out self-harm theory representing Jane's dialogue with a wider body of knowledge to inform the development of her insights – these are included in the text and begin 'I read'.

The text also contains eight empathic poems written by Colleen Marlin (CM) to represent the voices of the self-harm patients that Jane reflects on. Giving voice to these people counters Jane's own voice, revealing the empathic plight – what does a self-harm think and feel?

The stage is set with eight chairs symbolically arranged in a reflective spiral. Each chair represents one of the eight self-harm patients reflected on within the performance. In some performances I use one poet who moves from chair 1 to chair 8, in which she reads the empathic poems. In other performances I recruit eight people to represent each self-harm patient – this creates a more powerful image for the audience. I can use students and audience to play these roles besides real actors. I find involving audience within the performance adds drama, as if the whole audience becomes a part by proxy, adding to the reflective moment. I move between the chairs positioning myself to touch the left shoulder of the poet as she reads each poem.

On completion, the performance opens into a dialogue with the audience – this may include the content of the performance or the process of constructing narrative. As with *Climbing walls*, the intention is to move the audience to social action.

Audience read:

Jane's rap is a performance narrative based on her practice with self-harm patients in ER – an aspect of her practice that concerned her.

Through seven guided reflection sessions Jane reflects on her negative attitude towards people who harmed themselves through overdose or cutting.

Guided reflection opens a space for healing dialogue where Jane reveals and confronts her negative attitude that added to the suffering of self-harm people rather than eased it, finding a better, more therapeutic way to be with these people.

The performance may show others how to bring new and sacred meanings to a previously marginalised and stigmatised public site as social action towards creating a better world for self and others and truly realising sacred space.

Session 1

I tell Chris a story, a reflection on my practice. Night shift, around 3 in the morning. He's deliberately cut his arm. Deliberate self-harm. Needing sutures. I recoil. Try to hide my feelings but feel empty. No compassion. He asks if it would hurt. My irritation bubbling to the surface.
'Must have hurt when you did it,' I spit.
Such a waste of time stitching him up. Can't waste compassion. Would only encourage him to do it again and again …
Would I act differently? I ask 'cause I feel discomfort. Prejudged him. Stereotyped him.
Chris challenges, 'Are some patients more worthy of care than others?'
Puts me on the spot. I know I should treat all with compassion. But that I don't upsets me.
Chris comforts, 'Is this too upsetting?'
Maybe … but its gotta be done … can't live my life like this.
Chris challenges, 'What is my role, what are my values? Do you merely patch up or care?'
I squirm. Mumble something like 'the environment doesn't help'.
Chris informs, 'Let me tell you about poise, the other side of compassion'
This becomes a love story.

Chair 1

CM poem 1

I find myself here, bleeding and scared,
Wondering if I've gone too far.

'Will it hurt' I ask,
unable to bear more pain.
Too much already
An interminably long night of it
Until the blade offered respite
Sweet, however briefly

She gives 'the look'
I can't alienate her
Fear I already have
She thinks I must like pain
To do this,
But she sleeps at night
Soft, empty,
In a peace I rarely touch
Voices in my head won't let me
Images I can't shake
Somersault of flailing limbs
Kick my feet out from under
Until I look to the blade
To find where I am
In the heart of the mess

She probably takes an aspirin for her rare headache
Aspirin doesn't begin to touch the roar in my skull
No volume button on the noise
Too loud too much too hard

That determined black dog,
I'm at its mouth, in its bite, vulnerable …
The blade
The only tool to cut myself loose from
Being chewed to death

She probably thinks I want to die
When all I want is peace
A minute without
The press of what comes at me …

She thinks I like pain
In truth, I can't stand any more
And to silence it,
I cut, I tear, decidedly, determinedly,
To feel something
As normal and comfortable
As the touch of metal to skin
Cold sharp
Beautiful, for a second to feel that …

With the blade in skin, the roar softens, bearable ....
And now, I want to disappear myself
Or her, looking at me as she is
As if I am scum
And have no right to drip my blood
On her polished, pristine floor

Between sessions

Looking back – it's amazing that – talking for an hour can turn my world upside down.

Dormant concerns spring to life. I realise my negative prejudice to DSH (deliberate self-harm) patients affects their well-being. Wrapped up in my self-concern I was not available to them. I need to know more about self-harm. Chris challenges, 'How much do I know?'
Not a lot I say.
I read:

Anderson notes: 'The term deliberate self-harm encompasses behaviours where the patient can be considered suicidal, such as taking an overdose, self suffocation, self strangulation, wrist cutting, drowning, etc. However the term also used to refer to acts a young person may engage in, but where suicide may not be the intention.

I read:

McLaughlin notes: 'The casualty department is usually the first port of call for these patients. Such high incidence rates can cause stress on both nursing and medical staff and could influence the attitudes they hold in relation to attempted suicide.'

I read:

Fiona Lynn a woman with a history of self-harm writes: 'Needing stitches was a nightmare. I felt embarrassed and shamed about being stitched up by a nurse whose comments, or lack of comment, made me want the ground to open up to swallow me.'

Fiona Lynn's words speak to me. She heard the nurse's attitude without a word being spoken. Helps me view things from a different perspective, hitting home the point.

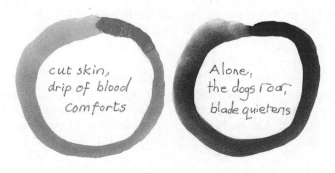

cut skin,
drip of blood
comforts

Alone,
the dogs roar,
blade quietens

Cut skin, drip of blood comforts
I have embarked on a path. I feel positive, emotional about it.
Chris calls it a pathway to sacred space.

Session 2

Chris: 'What's happened since we last met?'
'Nothing, I have had no contact with any DSH patients.'
Chris: 'Why is that?'
'I don't know really, interactions just haven't happened.
Chris: 'No DSH patients have been through the department when you on duty?'
'Well, yes plenty of patients, there always are, but I was busy with other patients. No, that's not really true. I suppose if I'm honest I've been avoiding them.'
Chris: 'Why?'
'I haven't really thought about it, on reflection I suppose it's easier isn't it? I haven't analysed why. I need more understanding of the subject. I don't want to hurt anyone by saying the wrong thing. Cock it up.'
Chris: 'Avoidance is a positive step towards understanding yourself. What insights emerging for you?'
'Acknowledging my negative prejudice towards self-harm patients. It is a relief to admit that I feared the next interaction.'

I read:

Carveth notes: 'avoidance is used by nurses when the prospect of dealing with a difficult patient arises'.

I read:

Eldrid notes: 'Whilst avoidance provides a protective mechanism for the nurse from life and death issues, avoidance can be painful for the patient who may already feel isolated'.

Voices ring in my ear. The dark side of nursing. Chris shines a light. Lends me the torch.
I am motivated to change, to live my holistic values without contradiction.
Reflection is first understanding, second empowering, third transforming. I step along the path.
Chris holds my hand, the catalyst liberating my energy for the journey ahead.

Session 3

I had gone out of my way to nurse this self-harm patient – Andrew. Not what I expected at all. I took the handover and went into the cubicle explaining to him what clinical procedures were needed. I acted in a way that I wouldn't usually ... viving a warm smile, pushing negative feelings to the side.
Chris interjects, 'Just remind me of those negative feelings?'
'That self-harm is a cry for attention, not as "deserving" of my care as other patients. They are often time wasters; I could be helping someone who really needs it! I asked Andrew very directly why he had taken the overdose. He said his life was a mess, his mother didn't care. He was thin, a little emaciated, I felt sorry for him.'

Chris challenges, 'How did you feel asking him why he had taken an overdose?'
'Very, very clumsy. Stumbling over my words, feeling hot and uncomfortable.'
Now – reliving these feelings with Chris.
Chris pushes, 'Why clumsy?'
'If Andrew had answered my question, I wouldn't have known how to respond. I didn't do any psychiatric training; I wouldn't be able to fulfil his needs. He might ask me for something I can't give. I would have been exposed as a fraud.'
Chris challenges, 'What do you usually do when you don't have an answer?'
'I would ask someone for help.'
Chris challenges, 'That he might ask for something you can't give is significant?'
I pause before answering, pondering the depth of this question ...
'I mean he may ask me to understand him, have knowledge of whatever disorder or mental illness they have. I don't think I have it in me to understand. I want to change, I want to give holistic care, but these patients drain me. It's scary to think that someone can be so desperate. He's done it several times before.'
Chris challenges, 'So what does that tell you? Do you view him less seriously?'
'Previously, before dwelling in the literature, yes an attention seeker, that individuals may inflict harm many times, sometimes over long periods of time. A significant number will commit suicide. I felt sorry for him because, apart from his appearance, he was apologetic, he was compliant with his clinical care.'
Chris challenges, 'Perhaps if he had been non-compliant you may not have felt so sympathetic towards him?'
How true. I squirm. I need to develop cathartic and catalytic skills. And poise. Chris points me towards John Heron's work – the six category intervention analysis.

Between sessions

I read:

> Kelly and May write: 'it is unlikely that problems in nurse–patient relationships will prove amenable to simplistic prescriptions since the cause of those problems is endemic of social interaction itself'. (1982:154)

I read:

> Trexlar notes that 'difficult' patients as those who are perceived to act in a deviant manner. She suggests that 'such patients respond by adopting expected role behaviour that results in stigma and social isolation that reinforces the original behaviour and may leads to secondary deviance and validation of the nurses judgment of the patient'. (1996:132)

Andrew had been compliant, perhaps through experience of his many A&E visits. Perhaps I was manipulated? I may never understand self-harm but my attitude and response to self-harm patients is changing. Never before had I asked a patient 'Why?'. Perhaps I would have dealt with another, less compliant DSH differently? Maybe. New experiences will reveal that truth. I now know that my beliefs and attitude *do* effect my care. So many patients must have suffered because of my ignorance.

Chris says that's a powerful insight. Facing the truth is not easy. This work is hard.

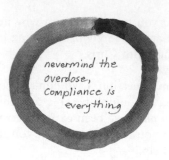

nevermind the
overdose,
compliance is
everything

Chair 2

CM poem 2

The great pass-off, 'I don't want him you can have him,
he's too dark for me'
The new nursey face lunging in at me
A mask of warm smile
She's been practicing in the mirror
And her words, awkward, scripted
'why did you take an overdose?'

Why do you think?
'Cuz I'm so g-d happy,
'cuz I'm living such a brilliant f'n life ...

I can't answer, you wouldn't want me to
This dark of mine, risky, infectious

Tighten your mask, nursey,
Keep your distance from the germ of my substantial discontent

She asks as if she wants to know
But she doesn't ...
The truth would crack her mask

She's vaguely afraid of me
I can sniff it
And my life, like my fridge,
Smelly, empty, save for the sodden take-away containers

In the eyes behind the mask
I see her judgment,
She thinks I want attention ...

I must be good now
Give her something of what she wants.
So maybe she can do something
For me
If I'm very good

I'll be good.

Session 4

Karl has taken an overdose. I'm upset. He nearly died a year ago. The seriousness of self-harm hitting home. I move into his cubicle, being open, wanting to help, using catharsis, 'What upset you so much today? Something must have really upset you to do this to yourself.'

I ooze compassion …

He rejects me. His face averted to the wall. His mother and brother watch me. I ask them to leave. I ask Karl again and still he ignores me. I feel my anger rising … I am falling flat on my face …

Chris picks me up. He enquires, 'What then?'

I said, 'I am available if you need me.'

Conveying my concern for him. Finding poise. My experience says poise is a precarious thing.

On reflection some days later I feel happier. I recognise I cannot dictate the pace or expect his compliance. I move to a deeper level beyond my anxiety. Moving through the emotional and power impasses that impede genuine therapeutic relationship.

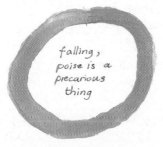

Chair 3

CM poem 3

Walls tighten
The press of your diagnostic gaze
My head in a vice

You, in nurse fashion, ask
'What upset you so much today?'
Today …
Not only today … every day.

You want me to talk,
I can't, can't breathe
Can't risk wasting precious air on stupid words
They won't be enough for you anyway

You send my family away
Thinking now I'll talk

To you?
In your peach polyester uniform?
So you can do, what,
Feel better about your own sweet life
Tell my woes at your dinner table and tsk tsk
At the hardship that doesn't touch you
All safe, smug, employed ... loved.

You press again
I turn away, conflicted
Don't want to answer and
Satisfy your curiosity
As you crane your neck
At me, poor victim of an awful accident

And yet
To answer ... to dislodge this stone blocking my airway
Inch it in your direction,
What it would unleash,
A geyser of bile would land on your hospital frock
And never wash out
With all the chemical laundering
It's just not safe ...

I turn to the wall
So you can't see
I want to cry

'I'm here if ...' you say, before leaving
As if ...

Session 5

A man in his forties. Taken a large overdose. He had visited his estranged wife and when she refused to let him into the house, he sat down in her garden and took a massive overdose. She wasn't aware that he was still in her garden. Some hours later a passer-by called an ambulance.

To say that I interacted with him is debatable. I carried out his clinical care, but he was unconscious, so I didn't actually speak to him.

Chris challenges, 'How did you feel about the man?'

I felt really sad, sad that he had felt so desperate, sad that he could die, sad that maybe he didn't mean to kill himself but just wanted his partner to come outside and talk, sad that his ex-wife would probably feel guilty and blame herself. Just incredibly sad. *And then* I saw the seriousness of self-harm, the desperation, the waste.

Chris enquires, 'This is new for you isn't it, this sympathy?'

I had felt sad when self-harm patients had died before, but not as sad as say a victim of a road traffic accident, or a child. Now I feel different. Reflection has made me think differently about all sorts of things, not just in the work place, it's 'bigger' than that! Things falling into place. Through understanding my whole attitude is changing. My prejudice slain, brought about by these profound insights.

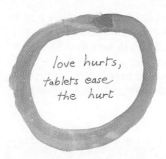

love hurts,
tablets ease
the hurt

Chair 4

CM poem 4

I can breathe underwater
Weight of cool liquid on me under me in me
Can't open my eyes
Yet I see
I was walking through her garden
To her door
There to tell her of my love
My continuing astonishingly intense love
Unprepared for her face, cold at her door,
Her finger
Pointing me away ...

I thought we could work it out try again

And I think I sat down in her garden
On a chair we'd picked together ...
Weary
Smell, sickly sweet
Can something smell purple?
My insides bruised purple
By the bash of heart on ribs
So uncomfortable
That look
Eyes, steeled blue

I waited
For her to remember she loves me
And now, under water, my lungs full
Storm warning ...
I near drown in tears ...
Taste salt or something

Some sounds far off
Roar of motorboat ...no,
Wheels rolling ... away

Why is everything going away?
And off there
As far away as the sounds, a shimmer ...

Someone has come to fetch me
Wish someone here
Could reach out
Hold me, save me
My wait over

Between sessions

I plot my empowerment using Kieffer's model for participatory competence. I move into the second stage 'Era of advancement' characterised by three quite distinct and necessary elements needed to successfully move into this stage:

- The focus and stability of a mentoring relationship as reflected in my relationship with my supervisor – Chris has been extremely stable and has focused on relevant and significant issues.
- Supportive peer relationships within a collective organisational structure – most of my peers/colleagues have become curious and supportive of my research. I hope that my research on an individual level will induce a collective action towards change.
- Critical understanding of social and political relations – I have gained this understanding by critically exploring the self-harm literature.

Stream entry. No turning back now simply because I have changed.

Session 6

A young man in his twenties. He arrived in the early hours of the morning having taken paracetamol.
Not many, very distressed. He kept saying sorry, apologising for wasting the nurse's time.
I sense he wants to talk. He had financial worries and girlfriend problems. It all tumbled out very quickly. I was only supposed to be carrying out triage but talked to him for 15 minutes.
The department was not busy, so instead of handing his care over to someone else, I took him into a cubicle and continued to talk.
I feel tender towards him. I have a strong desire to help by simply listening. I know he felt my concern was genuine. Being mindful, reading his pattern. Focusing on him as a suffering individual human transcending any lingering prejudice I have for people labelled as self-harm.
Suffering is Chris's word – he feels suffering encompasses the whole person and doesn't discriminate in that we all suffer to varying extents. The word is evocative of compassion, that the carer's human response to suffering *is* compassion.
I wasn't hiding anything from myself. I am vulnerable, powerful, more available. Finding my way.

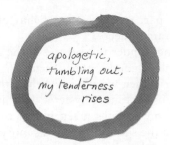

apologetic,
tumbling out,
my tenderness
rises

Chair 5

CM poem 5

I took a few pills
More than I intended
But sleep wouldn't come …

I'm sorry I'm taking your time
Sorry you're looking at me
All solicitous and concerned

I took a few tablets too many
Sorry … I have financial troubles
Sorry … my girlfriend would rather be
With him or anybody but me

I have such a sorry life
And you see how sorry it is
And feel sorry for me

I've swallowed bitter poison
Now my blood is sharp with it
And I messed up your day
Sorry I caused you to miss coffee break.

Sorry, most, perhaps,
That I am still alive
And aware of all this …

Session 7

And just as I was feeling confident … knock-back. Two steps forward and three back!
Where to start?
Two experiences – one negative, one positive one.
Chris attentively, 'Tell me about the negative one.'
Busy shift over the New Year period. A young girl overdosed. Her friend had recently committed suicide. She was hysterical. I could not calm her down. Pressure from within to calm her down. Reminding myself that here was a young girl who had lost a friend in traumatic circumstances.
Conflicting priorities, other patients needed a quiet calm atmosphere. I needed to take control with this patient and I was failing. The more hysterical she became the more

irritation I felt. Alcohol a part to play in her behaviour. Anger rising up within me. I thought she was silly, a 'drama queen'.

Losing sight of her 'grieving', under pressure, 2 in the morning, I'm tired ...

Chris laughs, 'So she wasn't a 'good' patient then?'

Tension broken! 'No! Her father wasn't any help either! I hoped he would calm her down, but he seemed to cause yet more hysteria. Nothing I tried worked, no connection with her, couldn't manage my feelings. I felt it best to hand over her care to someone else, to remove myself from the situation. She was moved away from the poorly patients. The second nurse was firmer than I was, the girl eventually calmed down, I don't know what happened after that.'

Chris challenges, 'Had you adopted a parental role with her because her mother was absent and her father "useless"?'

Being positive to his challenge, 'No, I wasn't conscious of taking on a parental role but, being a mother myself, it is an easy role to fall into. Anyway, if I did unconsciously take on a parental role it didn't work, did it?'

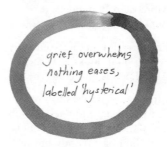

grief overwhelms
nothing eases,
labelled 'hysterical'

Chair 6

CM poem 6

The nurse tries to quiet me,
With a 'there, there, pat pat' of words and hand

I might have died
It happens
My friend did,
An error in judgment
Consumed enough to take her out
I almost went too
Unwittingly, unwillingly,
Oh God oh God oh God ...
I need to cry, get it?
Like the newborn, shocked, relieved
To be here after all ...
Slapped up side the head.
Oh, the nurse is truly annoyed now.
She feels powerless against
My waves of hundred proof emotion,
Drop a match and see what happens.
Her anger nothing compared to the fire of my fear

I could have died
And she wants me to calm down ...
Then frustrated, hands me over to
A tough cookie, too like my own mother
One whose look demands, insists
There's no more consoling ...
Instead, an unspoken
'shut up, or else ...'
I understand.
I slam my mouth shut.
Hysteria, locked in, blows air bubbles in my
Churned-up cells.

Chris shifts, 'Tell me about the positive experience?'

'A few days later another young girl, about the same age. She was at school, bought in by the class teacher; she had taken a small overdose. I was completely different with her. I was able to talk with her, let her know my concern was genuine.'

Chris leans forward, 'So what made it different?'

'It was a day shift 9 or 10 in the morning and quiet in the department. I had time, no competing demand. I wasn't tired.'

Chris notes, 'The impact of the environment seems significant on your attitude.'

'She had taken the OD because her mum wouldn't let her visit her boyfriend the night before desperate about not seeing him. Apologetic but in the spur of the moment I *was* the parent ... this was okay because she was frightened – she needed comforting.'

Chris informs, 'The parent–child pattern of communication within transactional analysis can be therapeutic when the practitioner is mindful of adopting that pattern rather than simply reacting to the situation because it evokes a maternal response.'

And yes, my response *was* reactive – I see his point that emotional reaction reflects the way I had absorbed the girl's suffering as a mother does for her child. Does this distort my decisions and actions? No, not if I am mindful enough. So – what accounts for the difference in my response to these two young girls? The first girl was outside my emotional limits, the second girl within them. Poise in the balance. I confess my guilt. Chris twists this around, suggesting that my first experience was also positive because I learn from it.

Now that's a better way to look at it!

Nurturing my poise, feeding my concern, being present. A love story.

   I read:

Poise, compassion, intention and aesthetics, are the primary qualities for enabling the practitioner to be fully present to the other within the unfolding moment.

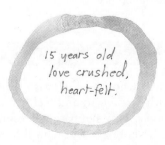

Chair 7

CM poem 7

My mother asked where I was going,
I told her, was told, 'No.'
'But'
'No'
'But'
'No'
Captive in the cell of my bedroom
Unable to go to my boyfriend
But I needed to talk to him

My thoughts, loud, crowded, hurt,
In my drawer I had something
To help with the pain
More will be better to numb
I swallow
My words
Feel poison in me
Go weak, world tweaked gray
My sluggish feet carry me
To school
Teacher sees what isn't in my eyes
Sends me to the big house
Where people in coats look into me

No scurrying
Not like on TV
All in slow mo
Except for my brain,
Up on two wheels
Careening around corners
And the nurse listens to me
Perhaps she remember what it's like
When life gets too hard
Ball and chain around my ankles
Tripping me up

I am frightened
Have never felt this before
Wish I could puke
Empty my gut of all that has choked out
My innocence

A few days later

Another deeply distressed girl who had OD, also around 15 years of age. Verging on hysteria, difficult to deal with. I listen to and feel her suffering – my empathic appreciation. I listen to my own response – my sympathetic resonance. I respond with care without judgement, more mindful ... more poised. The difference is palpable. Variables were different. It was during the day, quiet early in the shift, the workload was light and I could concentrate on her care. Dwelling with her I remember the other teenager, remembering the lessons.

I hear Chris whisper – 'you are dwelling in sacred space?'

What does that mean?

I read:

> Repper writes: 'Poor information and communication systems, lack of knowledge about suicide; negative attitudes towards people who self-harm does not help the rising number of patients presenting with DSH … A&E staff must become more involved with education/training where negative attitudes are challenged'. (p. 11)

Three weeks later

I convene a debate with my A&E colleagues – they are interested in my study. They are divided on their own feelings about self-harm patients. Some feel they firmly understood and treated the patient group in exactly the same way they would any other. Listening – I wonder if they distort their reality?

It is not easy to face up to being uncaring.

Some found themselves, perhaps like myself, somewhere in the middle, lacking real knowledge of self-harm and experiencing difficulty with caring for such patients.

Some feel that self-harm patients are time wasters who manipulate both nurses and the medical system. One stated that she is 'resigned' to nursing self-harm patients. I ask her to explain … she says that the only self-harm patients we meet are those in crisis, that we never see patients who recover.

I wonder – What does recover mean?

I had read:

> Anderson *et al.* investigated the attitude of medical staff towards the suicidal. They state 'nurses and doctors do not support the notion that suicidal behaviour reflects mental illness'. One staff nurse who took part in the research stated 'Sometimes I think they are time wasters – occasionally, and quite selfish – if you have a good reason to self harm then that's that … but if not then I think it's quite selfish'. (Anderson *et al.* 1999:6–8)

Words that reflect my own thoughts prior to my self-inquiry.

The point – the debate with my colleagues enabled their thoughts and feelings to surface and, whilst I was not able to change their opinion there and then, perhaps a seed was sown, a seed that may surface later, at a time that is right for the individual to address their own contradictions. Perhaps then a paradigm shift.

Chris is an agitator. I will also become one.

About reflection I read:

> Mezirow states: 'Our meaning structures are transformed through reflection, defined here as attending to the grounds (justification) for one's beliefs. We reflect on the unexamined assumptions of our beliefs when the beliefs are not working well for us, or where old ways of thinking are no longer functional. We are confronted with a disorientating dilemma, which serves as a trigger for reflection. Reflection involves a critique of assumptions to determine whether the belief, often acquired through cultural assimilation in childhood, remains functional for us as adults. We do this by critically examining its origins, nature, and consequences'. (1981:223)

Umm. Chris says that more simply!

The meaning of my practice shifts with each new experience and insight. Most significantly I no longer fear involvement with self-harm patients. Breaking through the fear barrier.

From the outset of this self-inquiry I was concerned that any changes I made to my practice in relation to my care of self-harm patients would leave me vulnerable.

Benner and Wrubel (1989) inform me that emotions can no longer be viewed as interruptions. By this I mean that emotions have significance and content in their own right and that respect for knowledge and wisdom is gained if the individual allows their emotions to direct their thoughts and attention.

Yes!

As a result of my inquiry into my beliefs, a host of factors including cultural and religious beliefs have emerged that influence my practice with self-harm patients.

I sense how being raised in a predominately Christian society with strong cultural beliefs about self-harm and suicide has impacted on me. As recently as 1961 suicide and attempted suicide fell into the same category as murder and there were a number of prosecutions. Decriminalisation in 1966 did not lead to any great change to the prevailing Christian ethic even as the world became more secular.

I read:

> McLaughlin states: 'In the Judeo-Christian cultures there has always been a belief that suicide is reprehensible and ethically wrong.' (1994:1112)

Reading the newspaper recently I sense that attitudes have not changed:[1]

homedigest

Spokesman David Laws said: 'The government has missed its target to get more pupils to take school meals by well over 1million children.'

Church softens its approach to suicide

SUICIDE should be greeted with compassion rather than blame, according to the Catholic Church in England and Wales. Teaching on suicide has not changed but the Church's understanding of mental health has altered, said the auxiliary bishop of Westminster, the Rt Rev Bernard Longley. 'God does not condemn anyone not fully aware of what they are doing,' he added. His remarks came as the church prepared to deliver 350,000 leaflets on suicide to parishes for its Day For Life on July 26. It is part of a campaign to soften its stance over what it regards as a grave sin.

---

[1] *Metro*, Friday, 10 July 2009, p. 6.

I can see the way my past relationships with self-harm patients have always been tinged with hostility.

Is that Christian? My contradiction, ignored yet bubbled uncomfortably beneath my apparent calm and confident surface. Chris had challenged me early in the research to identify the nurse's role in A&E. Is it holistic or merely patch work?

I know better now that my response to the self-harm patient makes a difference; that compassion and non-judgemental acceptance works better than indifference or worse, rejection and thinly veiled contempt. Only when practitioners, like myself, resolve contradiction, can they realise their visions of practice as a lived reality and lead more satisfactory lives. In acknowledging and confronting my prejudice I discover myself as a person and have found that this, in itself, naturally leads to, not just tuning into others and their needs, but also myself.

It feels astonishing to realise such self-neglect and yet I sense that nurse education gives little emphasis to developing and sustaining effective therapeutic relationships, especially with patients experiencing self-harm.

All experience is positive if we can learn from it. My learning and understanding have travelled full cycle, described by Gadamer (1979) as an oscillating cycle that continuously evolves. My empowerment to act came from within because I could no longer live with the contradiction, once my protective veneer had been torn off within guided reflection with Chris.

I had a choice: to retreat or push forward. But in reality I had no choice because where could I have retreated too? My cover was blown! So I chose to push forward, to face up to my vulnerability with the challenge and support of Chris. Without doubt, the role of an external enabler is vital. As Johns (2004) notes, it is not easy to see beyond the normal self. Emancipation, or the realisation of my changed self was affirmed quite recently.

My arms around a woman in great distress, crying a steady stream of tears. Suddenly I realised I genuinely care. I did not need to prompt myself for the best verbal response. We talked as I carried out clinical observations, but I was so in tune with this woman I instinctively knew what she wanted from me. I sat next to her and her tears began. She physically moved towards me, I believe she sensed my empathy and the genuineness of my caring response. As I encircled her in my arms I felt emotional, I felt sadness for her, but realised the truth of Ramos's words, 'Nurses described an emotional identification which was real, not devastating to the nurse, but a motivator'.

Ramos describes such a relationship as a reciprocal relationship and the very cornerstone of nursing care.

I wanted to hold this woman because she needed me to hold her and I felt very comfortable doing so. A burden had lifted from my shoulders. I get a sense of what poise might mean. I sense sacred space.

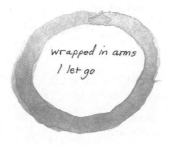

wrapped in arms
I let go

Chair 8

CM poem 8

I mean to be strong
With this nurse though,
No need.
I see in her eyes
Some understanding of the pain
I must have endured
To go so far this far
I feel she cares wants to help
And the knowledge of that
That I am not invisible
That maybe just maybe
I matter
Have worth
Undoes me
And the tears come
The years of tears
The pain that's been growing festering
Rising to boil
And now
Valve on pressure cooker adjusted
So I can safely spend
Some of this gunk inside of me

And I cry and I cry and I cry
And the nurse's arms are around me
And I can feel she wants to cry too
And sharing it
It's not so heavy
Sharing it
The tears fly out faster
And I can feel the beginnings of places, spaces inside me
Where maybe the light can come in

For so long
Hopeless
So long
I thought that's all there was
I have always been depressed
I am depressed
I always will be depressed
So I thought so I knew
And then her arms
Nudging the pain out of me
And in the space
Maybe
Maybe I can feel something other than
The grip of inevitable death

I sense her heart beating
In time with my own

It has been a relatively short journey. The terrain has been tough. My 'new self' is still to be tested for its robustness in face of more difficult interactions. I hope that my research will challenge others towards enabling others to find a more therapeutic way of being with self-harm patients in A&E; of creating sacred space *as* everyday practice.

I read:

By our very attitude to one another we help to shape one another's world. By our very attitude to the other person we help to determine the scope and hue of his or her world; we make it large or small, bright or drab, rich or dull, threatening or secure. We help to shape his or her world not by theories and views but by our very attitude toward him or her. Herein lies the unarticulated and one might say anonymous demand that we care for the life which trust has placed in our hands. (Knud Ejler Logstrup 1997:18)

[Credits]

Chapter 14

Audiencing

Christopher Johns

I take the expression 'audiencing' from a paper by Linda Park-Fuller titled 'Audiencing the audience: playback theatre, performative writing, and social action'. Park-Fuller comments on the paucity of studies on the efficacy of performance on audience especially with a view to ensuing social action.

Reading Park-Fuller reminds me to consider the purpose of narrative and performance. I have already made the point that a performance attitude or consciousness has shifted the way I write narrative; I have become more mindful of the impact of words, more empathic of my audience, as I write. Narrative is no longer the domain of the individual looking in and making sense for self, it is also a looking out at the world as an invitation to dialogue and social action.

Audiencing links with the sixth dialogical movement (see Fig. 2.1). In dialogue with the audience after performing *Climbing walls* (Chapter 9), in a public theatre to a mixed professional and non-professional audience, the question of *medical language* within the performance was noted. Being used to performing to professional audiences I had not considered the issue of language for different audiences. I realised I had taken the use of medical language for granted even as I endeavoured to write in an accessible and engaging way.

After the dialogue, I was approached by a non-medical man who praised the performance for being engaging and provoking. He felt his non-understanding of some of the language added an authenticity to it, simply because lay people experiencing medical care are confronted with a language that they do not understand. I hadn't seen that possibility within the narrative and yet the point had been inadvertently well made within the performance. A moment of insight.

The performance of narrative opens up a more profound way of communicating the author's meaning through use of the body and voice, simply because people listen more with their heart than with their minds. Yet, the author also invites the reader or listener to interpret the text and find their own meaning. This is the point of narrative and its performance.

Published narrative always seeks to move readers to social action through identification with the situation described and the insights within the narrative, and yet I recognise the limitations for published narrative to do that in ways that reading or performing narrative can realise. The idea of narrative as performance ethnography/social action (Denzin 2003) to open a potential dialogical space towards *disturbing* the audience has influenced me significantly. Saying this, I wonder to the extent performance is geared to a specific audience and yet, as *Climbing walls* showed, the invisibility of living with cancer treatment is a societal issue. It touched real nerves.

Perhaps it is Ben Okri's essay 'A way of being free' that has most influenced me, or enchanted me; the idea of enchanting the audience with poetry, and yet at the same being transgressive, revealing the horror and injustice of normal patterns of organised life and living, of time planting seeds to explode at a later time within the reader's mind. Okri writes (1997:65):

> The joy of transgressing beautifully, of taking readers to places they wouldn't willingly go, this joy of seducing or dragging readers in spite of themselves to places deep in them where wonder lurk besides terrors, this delicate art of planting delayed repeated explosions and revelations in the reader's mind, and doing this while enchanting them – this is one of the most mysterious joys of all.

Stories must always be challenging, unsettling. As you feel the struggle of the story-tellers, you begin to absorb the tensions as you begin to relate the story to your own experiences. Then the story begins to live within you and, in being lived, it changes you.

I am told repeatedly by audience (both readers and listeners) that my stories enable them to be present within the story, that they can imagine being there, living it, more so with performance than with reading narrative.

I sometimes wonder if my narratives are unnecessarily long to those readers used to being presented with the facts. Yet stories have no facts, nothing can be presented with any certainty. The facts are those perceived by the reader open to his or her experience in the juxtaposition of self and others' own experiences, a fusion of horizons.

I find myself informing readers of the rules for dialogue – to listen with an open heart and mind, not to take offence, to suspend their assumptions in order to be open to what the text might have to say and indeed, the way the text says it, to loosen their attachment to their preconceptions. Weinsheimer's (1985:166–167) interpretation of Gadamer notes:

> Understanding is projection and what it projects are expectations that precede the text. They 'jump the gun' as it were because they anticipate meaning before arriving at it. What the interpreter projects in advance is what he understands already – that is, before beginning. He tries out meaning already familiar to him and proposes it as a possibility. This projected meaning is his own possibility in that he has projected it; it is part of the world he already knows his way around, and it is something he can and does understand ... yet since we are prepared for the text to say something new, we read we stand ready to revise them – and not because we are prepared to believe anything, nor because we merely want to know what the author has to say on the topic, but instead because we want to know and learn about it ... we hold our own opinions open to disconfirmation and place them at risk not because we are neutral but, quite the opposite, because we too are interested ... Because we are concerned and interested, our receptivity implies that we are willing to integrate the meaning of the text with our previous preconceptions by making them conscious, bringing them into view, and assimilating them to what the text reveals.

Weinsheimer invites the posture of the hermeneutic reader and yet to hold this posture requires the text or performance must engage the reader. It must be crafted to enable this. Hence Richardson's (2005) injunction that narrative must be aesthetically credible to be narrative (see Chapter 15).

Matthew (1995:15), in citing St John of the Cross, captures this essence eloquently:

And I think that this is better. When words are born of love, it is better to leave them open, so that each person can benefit from them in their own way and at their own spiritual level – this, rather than tying the verses down to a meaning that not everyone could relish.

Ruth Morgan (2004) writes:

The construction of my autobiographical narrative has taken many twists and turns demonstrating the complex and changing nature of my daily practice. The penetrative process of unravelling my own thinking and committing reflections to paper has in itself altered my perceptions and created change. I have discovered that challenge is not to be feared, life need not be static and mountains can occasionally move. I invite my readers to ride in tandem with me viewing the moving scenery through the filter of their own experience and applying it to their own lives. I depend on you, the reader, to move the narrative beyond an articulation of personal experience into the realm of wider interpretation and social relevance (Pinar 1981). It is from you that the text gains its validity and movement. Stories can infect perceptions, invade complacency, amplify conscience and change lives. As Okri (1997:44) writes – 'stories are living things; and their real life begins when they start to live in you'.

Again, Okri writes:

Storytelling is always, quietly, subversive ... when you think it is harmless, that is when it springs its hidden truths, its uncomfortable truths, on you. It startles your complacency. And when you no longer listen, it lies silently in your brain, waiting. Stories are very patient things. They drift quietly in your soul. They infect your dreams and perceptions, occupying your spirit. Stories are living things; and their real life begins when they start to live in you. Then they never stop living, or growing, or mutating, or feeding the groundswell of imagination, sensibility, and character. Stories are subversive because they always remind us of our fallibility. The subversion in storytelling is an important part of the transformation of human beings into higher possibilities. (1997:43–45)

The power of the stories is the truth they speak to the reader. The stories are a both a window for the reader to view the lives of those within the stories and as a window or mirror to her or his own soul. Stories are compelling because they capture the complexity of everyday practice without fragmenting it. Indeed the stories are a testament of uncertainty: within the apparent fragmentation of everyday life is found the wholeness of experience.

To open a conversation with the text requires the reader to understand the question to which the text is an answer. Yet the question has to be an open question, and being an open question the text is not definitive. And even if the text offers an answer that answer is still open to discussion, the text is never authoritative but itself opens more possibilities. Similarly, the text asks questions of the reader, a reciprocity of questioning is realised when the interpreter puts a question to the text by which he or she in turn is put in question. Thus the question raised by the text merges with the reader's own questioning in dialectical play, which Gadamer (1975:210) calls the 'fusion of horizons' as explored in Chapter 4 between practitioner and guide. The hermeneutic spiral continues to deepen and expand. As Weinsheimer writes (1985:211):

The finality of dogmatic assertion is always premature for meaning remains in process, open to interpretation ... it is always to be realized.

Gadamer (1975) emphasises that the reader knows that the text does not have the last word but then neither does the reader. Weinsheimer (1985) continues:

> Moreover the reader needs the text to put his own prejudices at risk and to point out the dubiousness of what he himself has taken for granted, thus disclosing new possibilities for questioning and extending his own horizon by fusing it with that of the text.

> Knowing that he do not know, being cognizant of his finitude, and realizing that he do not have the first word or the last, the reader [interpreter] holds himself open to history, that is, to the continuing event of truth.

Narrative is art and art makes demands on us. One demand is to get it right. It is characteristic of artwork to invite the reader or listener to interpret it appropriately because what it has to say is too important not to do so. That interpretation is possible must be explained before addressing the problem of the multiplicity of interpretations (Gadamer 1975).

In her fictional novel about ethnography Caroline Ellis (2004:194) constructs a dialogue between herself and a class student:

> Laura says 'Stories are theoretical in the sense that they help me understand aspects of my own life. We expect that of theory. On the other hand – and I guess I'm sill caught up in my social science training, you can't generalize from a story as you can from theory.'

Ellis responds:

> 'if you think of theory in terms of empiricism, where the purpose is to represent, generalize, control and predict, then, Laura might be right ... stories and theories have different purposes. Even so, I would argue that a story's generalizability is always being tested, not in a traditional ways through random samples of respondents, but by readers as they determine if a story speaks to them about their experience or about the lives of others they know. Readers provide theoretical validation by comparing their own lives to ours, by thinking about how our lives are similar and different and reasons why.

In the ensuing conversation, Ellis writes:

> If we think of theory as social, as Art says (Bochner 1997), then the concerns become less of representation and more those of communication, Do our stories evoke readers' responses? Do they open up the possibility of dialogue, collaboration, and relationship? Do they help us get along with each other? Do they help us change institutions? Promote social justice and equality? Lead us to think through consequences, values and moral dilemmas?

Frank (1995) makes the distinction between thinking with a story and thinking about a story. In thinking with a story, considers the impact of the story on her own experience, whereas in thinking about a story, the reader tends to reduce and analyse the story into themes or patterns.

Ellis (2004) makes a similar distinction between narrative analysis and analysis of narratives. Each position reflects a reader's orientation to story and theory. In a theoretical dominated approach to health care, the natural tendency is to critique story for its validity rather than take it on face value and ask how can this story inform my practice. Because story is contextual and subjective, it is easier for readers to make comparison with their own practice in contrast with theory that tends to be abstract with its claims to impartiality and generalisability.

Pinar (1981) notes, narrative is written for self. It is not autobiography or autoethnography even as these ideas influence the shaping of narrative. It is a reflexive account of being and becoming who the narrator seeks to be, of a journey moving towards realising a vision of self and practice. For myself, this vision is framed as easing suffering. My narratives reveal the complexity of suffering yet without defining it as more than a disruption of the spirit that reflects something unsatisfactory about the person's life. Hence my narratives seek to reveal the nature of suffering as the basis for responding to it. Yet suffering is deeply embodied, shaped through tradition and life patterns. It is unique to the person even as I recognise its underlying currents. In revealing the person's suffering I open a space for the audience to reflect on their own suffering. In dialogue, I continue to investigate the nature of suffering and the conditions under which it might be eased. Whilst the application of theoretical models such as the 'Being available' template are helpful to explore easing suffering,[1] it risks imposing a particular perspective on the reader. One troubling distinction with using such frameworks is that they do impose an authority on the work that governs the way the text is viewed. The reflective or hermeneutic reader will naturally be sensitive and wary of such imposition. Even so, the narrative writer naturally problematises his use of any frameworks, inviting the reader to be creative to see other ways to frame the reflexive journey.

Performance turn

The awakening of the performance turn, shifts the focus of narrative from representation of the narrator's own journey to its presentation. Increasingly I perform narratives at conferences rather than talk theoretically about guided reflection and narrative research. Initially I simply read the narrative as I had written it, usually with accompanying images and music that held meaning in themselves and heightened a sense of drama. Such accompaniment is an art form in itself in blending media presentation to find synchronicity. It is a sort of 'trial and error' artistry for there are no theories on how best this can be achieved, and even if there were, it would remain an experiment to find the particular media blend to realise synchronicity.

I know through experience that the stories trigger the reader's or listener's own stories and facilitates the sharing of stories and the development of communities of learning, what I have described as 'camp-fire' teaching (Johns 2004a:256). I know from performing many of the stories in the narrative at conferences and from reader response to *Being mindful, easing suffering* (Johns 2004b), that my narrative resonates deeply with the audience. When I shared my narrative on 'being with Carol and her family' at a recent critical care conference, I was approached by a practitioner who said she had never thought of asking relatives to bring in photographs of the dying person. It seemed a revelation to her that photographs could open a way for her to dwell with the relatives around the dying person and to humanise the dying patient in the stark surrounds of the intensive care unit. So simple, and yet so profound.

As such, the stories change lives as they have changed my own life. They are a mandate for social action towards a greater humanity.

---

[1] The Being available template offers the practitioner to know and mark self as holistic (see Appendix 1).

I would argue very strongly that the self that is writing the story is changed by the process of writing it. (Laurel Richardson cited by Flemons and Green 2002:91)

And here we might say that the self that is reading or listening to the story is changed by that process if readers and listeners are engaged enough with the story.

References

Bochner A (1997) Its about time: Narrative and the divided self. *Qualitative Inquiry* 3:418–438.

Denzin N (2003) *Performance ethnography*. Sage, Thousand Oaks.

Ellis C (2004) *The ethnographic I*. AltaMira Press, Walnut Park.

Flemons D and Green S (2002) Stories that conform/stories that transform. A conversation in Four Parts. Part 1: Autoethnographies: constraints, openings, ontologies, and findings. In: A Bochner and C Ellis (eds.) *Ethnographically speaking*. AltaMira Press, Walnut Park, pp. 87–94.

Frank A (1995) *The wounded storyteller: body, illness and ethics*. University of Chicago Press, Chicago.

Gadamer HG (1975) *Truth and method* (transl. G Barden and J Cumming). Seabury Press, New York.

Johns C (2004a) *Becoming a reflective practitioner* (second edition). Blackwell Publishing, Oxford.

Johns C (2004b) *Being mindful, easing suffering*. Jessica Kingsley Publishing, London.

Matthew I (1995) *The impact of God: soundings from St John of the Cross*. Hodder and Stoughton, London.

Morgan R (2004) *Realising transformational leadership*. Unpublished dissertation, MSc in Leadership in Healthcare Practice, University of Bedfordshire, Bedfordshire.

Okri B (1997) *A way of being free*. Phoenix Books, London. Text extracts used with permission of The Marshall Agency Ltd.

Park-Fuller L (2003) Audiencing the audience: playback theatre, performative writing, and social activism. *Text and Performance Quarterly* 23:288–310.

Pinar W (1981) Whole, bright, deep with understanding: issues in qualitative research and autobiographical method. *Journal of Curriculum Studies* 13:173–188.

Richardson L (with Pierre AS) (2005) Writing: a method of inquiry. In: N Denzin and Y Lincoln (eds.) *The Sage handbook of qualitative research* (third edition). Sage, Thousand Oaks, pp. 959–978.

Weinsheimer J (1985) *Gadamer's hermeneutics. A reading of truth and method*. Yale University Press, New Haven.

Chapter 15

Coherence and ethics

Christopher Johns

Narrative is a journey of self-inquiry and transformation towards self-realisation, presented as a reflexive and *coherent* narrative.

> Coherence – logical and consistent
> Cohere – form a unified whole. (*Compact Oxford English Dictionary* 2005:204)

Reason and Rowan (1981) suggest that *coherence* is a more appropriate word than 'validity' in an attempt to move away from the meanings generally associated with 'validity' in terms of an empiricist paradigm. Hence the idea of a 'new' paradigm that reflects human inquiry. Coherence sets the tone of the hermeneutic spiral of being and becoming, where insights gained through the dialogical movements are woven into the reflexive narrative. It is more than an assembled collection of criteria. There are no fixed rules of coherence to be applied. As the Dalai Lama (1998:140) astutely comments:

> The ultimate authority must always rest with the individual's own reason and critical analysis.

As Weinsheimer (1985:164), in his reading of Gadamer (1975), notes:

> There is ultimately no method of understanding, no formalizable system of individual rules which if rigorously applied could prevent misunderstanding, guarantee objectivity, or obviate the ad hoc guesses, premonitions, and projections of meaning that continue to mark the historicity of understanding.

Rules or even guidelines do not ensure coherence. Smith and Deemer (2000:889) consider that rules must always be worked out and judged in response to the particular research project as *actual inquiries*. From this perspective, criteria are constructed within the narrative process. Whilst that is indeed experiential, I feel that guidelines, held loosely, as with all reflective frameworks, are necessary to help the narrator realise coherence, notably in response to scholarly and social scrutiny.

Coherence is vital because it creates a security that the narrative can be trusted. Perhaps the most helpful approach to consider narrative coherence is *authenticity* – to pose the question – 'What would most convince a reader or listener of the narrative's authenticity?' Wilber (1998) identifies *authenticity* as the key criteria, or rule of injunction, for subjective-individual knowing that characterises reflexive self-knowing gained through reflection or self-inquiry (see Figure 1.1).

Within his four quadrant model of ways of knowing in the world, Wilber (1998) identified that each quadrant or conception of truth has its own paradigmatic injunctions or what Wilber called the *eyes of knowing*. He argued that people have available to them a spectrum of different modes of knowing, each of which discloses a different type of experience; the eye of flesh, the eye of mind, and the eye of contemplation. Wilber considered the way each type of knowing can be apprehended as valid. He suggests that all valid knowledge has the following strands:

- Instrumental injunction – this is always the form – if you want to know this, do this.
- Intuitive apprehension – this is an immediate experience of the domain disclosed by the injunction; that is, a direct experience or data-apprehension.
- Communal confirmation – this is checking of the results – the data, the evidence – with others who have adequately completed the injunctive and apprehensive strands.

Wilber identifies *authenticity* as the truth injunction for the subjective-individual quadrant. Other paradigms have their own claims for truth. Wilber urges caution, that because these quadrants are all intimately related, the subjective path has tended to be aggressively reduced into the objective path. reflected in such ideas as objectivity, validity, reliability, generalisability, and significance. None of these fit reflective knowing. Indeed reflective knowing is likely to be dismissed as largely anecdotal and not research at all. A long way down the gold standard as what counts as research. Wilber (1998:84) notes that:

> The strength of empiricism is its demand that all genuine knowledge be grounded in experiential evidence. As such, if we use experience in its proper sense as a direct apprehension, then we can firmly honour the empiricist demand that all genuine knowledge be grounded in experience, in data. Data is simply not lying around waiting for anybody to see, but rather are brought forth by valid injunctions.

Thus, to gain access to any of these valid modes of knowing, the person needs to be adequate to the injunction. By this Wilber means needs to be able to use the tools of the paradigm. It is important to use these tools otherwise the results cannot be confirmed within the communion of confirmation. Wilber emphasises this point with regard to contemplation and knowing mysticism. Hence experience can only be adequately apprehended by the person experiencing her or his own being. Understanding and learning through lived experience would fit into the subjective-individual quadrant. Experience cannot be observed. Wilber (1998:14) writes:

> The only way you and I can get at each other's interiors is by dialogue and interpretation. And yet when you report to me your inner status you might be lying. Moreover, you might be lying to yourself.

Authenticity must be the marker of coherence for self-inquiry, for what would be the point of constructing a narrative of lying or deliberate false consciousness? (Lather 1986a). Self-inquiry must always be a *genuine* self-inquiry. Perhaps another pertinent word is *worthiness* – 'What makes a narrative worthy?' Can the reader *trust* the narrative? Mishler (1990:429) writes:

I am not arguing that my methods and procedures *validate* my findings and interpretations. That would be counter to my basic thesis that validation is the social construction of a discourse through which the results of a study come to be viewed as sufficiently trustworthy for other investigators to rely on for their own work.

Mishler considers that a focus on trustworthiness rather than truth displaces validation from its traditional location in presumably objective, non-reactive and neutral reality and moves it into the social world constructed through experience. Another way of saying this is to replace truth with truthfulness. He writes:

> Reformulating validation as the social discourse which trustworthiness (truthfulness) is established elides such familiar shibboleths as reliability, falsifiability, and objectivity. These criteria are nether trivial or irrelevant, but they must be understood as particular ways of warranting validity claims rather than as universal, abstract guarantors of truth. (Mishler 1990:420)

Mishler helps position coherence in tension with validity (rather than in opposition to it). Validity is just fine for Wilber's right-hand paths. Indeed it is the only way IT can be held as truth (albeit only as a significant rather than absolute truth). I sense that trusting the text is primarily a question of the text feeling right, that it speaks to the person, an intuitive connection with the text. More cognitively, some fundamental questions might be asked of the text to judge its trustworthiness (following Mishler 1990):

- What are the warrants for the narrator's insights?
- Can I or other investigators make a reasonable judgement of the adequacy of these insights?
- Can I determine how the narrator's insights were produced?
- Can I determine if the insights are trustworthy enough to be relied upon in relation to my own work?

Coherence is both a dialogical and experimental space or clearing in which no one is the master, and perhaps never can be, for then narrative would have given up its dialogical and experiential essence.

Besides, there is never one *true* narrative of self-inquiry. All narratives reflect the way the narrator has paid attention to aspects of the whole against a background of the whole. And even in the paying attention to an aspect of self within the whole, that aspect itself is only sketchily drawn given the relative obscurity of self to self. Narrative is constantly reconstructing ways of being in the world. A snapshot that captures a moment in time. When read, the snapshot has already changed. Fay (1987:168) notes how:

> The results of human activities are forever occurring, so that any narrative about them must be inherently fragmentary and tentative.

Understanding is subjective although the rigor of reflection and guidance within the dialogical movements gives understanding an objective-subjective tension. With narrative there is no attempt to guarantee objectivity. It doesn't figure in the equation in any shape or form. There are no recipes or formulas, no checklists or expert advice that describe reality (Wheatley 1999). Wheatley writes:

> If context is as crucial as the science explains, then nothing really transfers; everything is always new and different and unique to each of us. We must engage each other, experiment

to find what works for us, and support one another as the true inventors that we are. (1999:9)

Everybody will have blind spots, that insights are selective and partial. It is impossible to pay attention to the whole of experience or reality. It would simply be overwhelming. As Fay notes:

> it ought to be obvious that a narrative cannot consist of a portrayal of all the acts people perform and all the causal outcomes of these actions. There must be a principle of selection in terms of which some acts and outcomes are included and some included. The principle most generally employed for this purpose is one which says that those events ought to be included which, when related together, form a recognizable pattern by which the nature of a person's life, or an important feature of them is depicted. Such a pattern is the plot of the narrative. (1987:171–172)

Reflecting on my own reflection, I recognise the way I pay attention to aspects of experience that *seem* the most significant at that particular time. Other aspects of the experience lay like ripe plums waiting to be picked at a later time as I patiently dwell within the hermeneutic spiral. Guides are indispensable to help the narrator recognise their partial focus (see Chapter 3). Similarly, dialogue with readers or listeners will often reveal and challenge claimed insights perspectives in context with the readers' own diverse experiences and interpretations.

As I have explored, the methodology of narrative as self-inquiry and transformation towards self-realisation is influenced by diverse philosophical ideas, all of which represent different and yet synergistic views of the world or what can be characterised as an *amalgam* of interdisciplinary analytic lenses that characterise contemporary narrative inquiry – all revolving around an interest in biographical particulars as narrated by the one who lives them (Chase 2005:671).

Chase (2005:671) asserts that 'narrative inquiry's contribution to social science has to do with concepts and analysis that demonstrate two things:

(1) The creativity, complexity, and variability of individuals' (or groups') self and reality constructions
(2) The power of historical, social, cultural, organisational, discursive, interactional, and/ or psychological circumstances in shaping the range of possibilities for self and reality construction in any particular place and time.'

What Chase doesn't identify is the reflexivity of transformation through self-inquiry because social science sets out to understand what is and the possibilities of a future. A reflexive approach is grounded in an individual's particular experiences towards realising a desirable state of affairs set against a historical background. It is primarily concerned with the individual within the specific context, not the context as something separate. Every situation or experience is an opportunity for the practitioner to look at herself through a critical lens of self-inquiry to gain insight. It is the background that gives shapes and gives meaning to her experience. Thus, the social and historical are always present within the individual's narrative and become a proper focus for study but only in terms of self-realisation, not as a focus for study in isolation, for then the ontological would give way to epistemological demand for reason and rationality. Self-inquiry is human inquiry. It is not abstract inquiry into phenomenon.

Coherence through the six dialogical movements

Narrative is patterned through six dialogical movements. Each dialogical movement has its own injunction for coherence (as summarised in Table 15.1). These movements are not separate but patterned to shape the unfolding reflexive narrative.

First dialogical movement

Self-inquiry is exploration of new terrain. It is inventive, simply because experience has never happened before. It is *being* concerned with *being* and becoming, an ontological inquiry into self in relationship with others, shining a light on the dark chamber of human spirit. Self-inquiry is not primarily concerned with social and historical movements as things in themselves.

Self-inquiry reveals knowing that is particular, subjective and contextual. As I have noted, its truth claim is *authenticity* – that the narrator genuinely intends to be authentic even as the whole truth may be obscured because of the very nature of self-inquiry. *Authenticity* requires a curiosity and commitment to the truth. It is writing self. In self-inquiry it is the practitioner/narrator who seeks emancipation so the narrative is her voice being spoken in a language that owns the text. Although she is not inquiring into others, her experiences are always in relationship – so as she expresses her own voice she expresses the voice of others in a dialogical form. She may even return her text to those she has been in relationship with not so much for their validation although the person may contest perspectives but as recognition of the collaboration. For example, as a consequence of sharing my performance text of *Climbing walls* with Anne (the woman in the performance experiencing breast cancer treatment), I felt better. She also affirmed my interpretations and added her own, including sharing her personal diary.

Table 15.1 Coherence through the six dialogical movements

Dialogical movement		Key criteria
1st	Dialogue with self as a descriptive 'spontaneous' account paying attention to detail (*story* text);	Authenticity
2nd	Dialogue with the story as an objective and disciplined reflective process to gain insight (*reflective* text)	Systematic process of reflection
3rd	Dialogue between tentative insights and other sources of knowing to inform insights and position within the wider community of knowing (*informed* text)	Construct validity
4th	Dialogue with guide(s) and peers to check out, deepen and develop insights (*co-created* text);	Co-creating meaning
5th	Dialogue with the emerging text to weave a coherent and reflexive narrative text that adequately plots the unfolding journey (*narrative* text)	Reflexivity; catalytic validity; rhizomatic validity; narrative criteria
6th	Dialogue with others (through appropriate forms of presentation) towards consensus and social action (*evolving* text)	Authenticity/ worthiness/ engagement performance criteria

Second dialogical movement

Reflection is more coherent if systematic. Hence, well-developed frameworks such as the Model for Structured Reflection and Framing perspectives strengthen coherence because they give depth and breadth to reflection and widen the scope of insights. Reflection is meaningless if the person was to deliberately distort their truth for whatever reason. Perhaps if I felt I was being judged against what I write I might be tempted to distort the facts, or avoid writing about certain experiences or omit certain detail. As Walt Whitman writes (1855/2005), 'be curious not judgemental' of self.

Reflection has been questioned in the light of a psychological theory which suggests that people do not recall accurately (Newell 1992). However, the issue is not one of accuracy of recall but on the meaning of events for people. People reflect on events in the present. If practitioners distort events, then they do so for reasons which are part of their reality, or to deliberately create a false impression. Albright (1994:32–33) notes:

> How much of our remembered self is carefully, scrupulously edited in order to conform to some vision of how we would like our self to appear? If we speak of a remembered self, we should also speak of an editorial self that consciously or unconsciously selects the memories that wrap us around with the sense of our dignity, our erotic power, our nonchalance, our good will toward mankind, all those pleasures that our self-consideration craves.

The very nature of reflection is to surface and explore contradiction and to reveal self to self, if it is significant in becoming an effective practitioner. We do not live in a perfect world with perfect answers to situations. As such, failure of correspondence between 'what I say' and 'what I do' remains a potential yet acceptable flaw. The ability to recall more accurately and penetrate self-distortion is enhanced by using models of reflection that give the more novice reflective practitioner access reflection in a systematic way. The use of such models gives confidence to the reader that reflection is not merely haphazard and dismissed as anecdotal in its most pejorative sense.

Third dialogical movement

Lather (1986b) identifies the idea of a construct validity that demands the researcher ensures her emergent tentative insights are grounded within a wider community of knowledge. This condition is met through theoretical framing, or construct validity, in which the researcher/practitioner frames emerging insights within extent theory as a dialogical process. The truth is not 'out there' as some objective reality that the personal notion of truth must be judged against to qualify as the truth. Neither is it simply subjective, because people are not isolated. They exist in communities where some common understanding of what counts as truth is adhered to; a constant interplay between knowing as revealed through reflection and extant theories towards co-creating meaning that is always unfolding and evolving within the reflexive spiral of being and becoming.

Fourth dialogical movement

Coherence is enhanced through co-creating meaning, where meaning is negotiated through 'free and open dialogue' (Elliott 1989) so that agreement as to what would count as a more truthful description of work–life can be reached (Kushner and Norris 1980–1981). From this perspective, coherence is properly concerned with processes of engagement and dialogue, and an emergent reflexive sense of what is important rather than on outcomes. The guide and practitioner must reflect on their relationship in ways 'living contradictions' (Whitehead 2000) are revealed and worked towards resolving. In other words, a particular focus of guided reflection is a mutual reflexive self-consciousness on the guided reflection relationship itself.

Fifth dialogical movement

> The understanding which we can have of ourselves is always 'in the middle of the way': there are no absolute beginnings and no absolute endings; there is no closure when we can know for certain who we are and what we have done. The process of understanding ourselves can never achieve finality, but is always unfolding and always being revised. (Fay 1987:174)

In weaving the narrative, the narrator ensures reflexivity – the 'looking back' through the narrative to see the emergence of self-realisation through a series of experiences. So, if I seek to become a transformational leader then I might utilise a valid leadership framework, for example the work of Schuster to frame this (see Appendix 1). If I seek to become a holistic practitioner I might utilise the Being available template (see Appendix 1). However, I might construct my own framework based on emerging issues, or indeed use to no framework at all, simply letting the unfolding of experiences to capture transformation guided by the plot. For example 'easing suffering' is not easily reduced into a framework, as evidenced within my own narratives (Johns 2006).

Agar and Hobbs (1982) identify *catalytic validity* as illuminating the way practitioners come to see themselves reflexively. This requires the narrative to represent adequately what took place without textual distortion. Steele (1986:262) notes that:

> All narratives leave out people, events, or ideas which if included would cast doubt on the truth of the theory being expounded or the story being told. Textual distortion by omission of relevant data is difficult to see when reading a work because there are only often obscure signs in the text that point to what is missing from it.

Steele emphasises that 'textual distortion' is difficult for the reader to perceive and perhaps can only be challenged through a reflective scepticism. Are the 'results' well founded in and consistent with the dialogue? Are the results systematically connected within a coherent sense of the whole? Where research intends to be empowering, then clearly the construction of the narrative that represents the practitioner's experiences must have been negotiated as a continuous process, not just at the end, when the account has largely been formulated.

In the first edition of the book I was influenced by Lather's earlier work (1986a,b) in terms of new criteria for 'validity' congruent with a post-modernist version of truth. These validity criteria included face validity, construct validity and catalytic validity.

In her later work, 'Fertile obsession', Lather writes:

> Extending my earlier work towards counter practices of authority that are adequate to emancipatory interests, my primary desire here is to rethink validity in light of anti-foundational discourse theory. Rather than jettison 'validity' as the term of choice, I retain the term in order to both circulate and break with the signs that code it ... of doing the police in different

voices ... positioning validity as an incitement to discourse ... What might open-ended and context sensitive validity criteria look like? ... like Woolgar (1988), my own position is that the most useful stories about science are those that interrogate representation, a reflexive exploration of our own practices of representation. (1993:674–676)

As such, coherence is itself a reflexive exploration of the narrator's practice of finding an adequate form of representation. This may be unsettling for those who seek firm guidelines to be convinced of the narrative's truth. Yet, to return to the simple idea of authenticity – authenticity is no more than finding a form of representation that reflects the complex and contradictory nature of experience itself. In her exploration Lather identified four approaches: ironic validity, paralogic validity, rhizomatic validity and voluptuous validity. Of these, I find rhizomatic validity the most compelling. Lather (1993) writes:

> As a metaphor, rhizomes work against the constraints of authority, regularity and common-sense and open thought [space] up to creative constructions – which mark the ability to transform, to break down present practices in favour of future ones.

The roots of the holly tree serve well to illustrate the complexity of self-inquiry narrative as a mass of interconnecting 'roots' that grow organically and which have an intrinsic wholeness. Imagine such a root system within the narratives. Narrative needs to capture something of the actual lived reflexive experience – contradictory, fragmented, complex, unexplained and yet have a natural wholeness – literally as if a journal as a drama unfolding, yet held together by the plot.

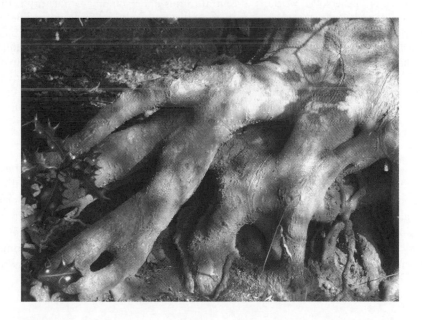

Madden (2002), writing from a feminist perspective of a woman (midwife) working with women to ease their suffering following traumatic childbirth, was guided to explore the possibility of rhizomatic validity to help frame the coherence of her reflexive narrative. She writes:

Lather (1993:680) advocates an anarchistic view of the growth of knowledge that denies the idea of a smooth, orderly progression from ignorance to knowing, she argues that 'there is no trunk, no emergence from a single root, but rather arbitrary branchings off and temporal frontiers which can only be mapped, not blueprinted'.

Any consensus of what it is that we know is, for Lather, a 'temporal contract'. Her notion of validity, rhizomatic validity, is both post-modern and feminist in that it refuses to fragment the narrative into forced codes and categories. Rhizomatic validity refers to new knowledge that 'taps underground', and in so doing creates new locally determined norms of understanding. It is based not on criteria of permanency and rationality, but on its power to open up new discourses, and subvert taken-for-granted ways of interpreting the world. Irigaray (1987) adds that women need to pay special attention to the language of science, stressing how such language forbids the first person, the subjective, as a way of masking the agents through whom it is propagated. Thus the political effects of the discourse are blurred behind a screen of neutrality. If one accepts these arguments, at least in part, then the notion of 'validity' within research (even our notions of what 'research' is, and is not) loses a certain degree of power. It can itself be viewed as an oppressive technology, as it serves to downgrade the personal, the subjective, the untidy story within each of us. The crucial distinction that marks feminist research from other forms is that it is carried out for women, that it is self-consciously partial. Admitting the impossibility of impartiality and neutrality, it seeks instead to own its political core.

The rejection of the traditional concepts of validity within research; those built around ideas of objectivity, impartiality and rationality, opens the door to a different frame of meaning – one that accords with the greater eclecticism of much feminist research (Webb 1993). For Weir (1995), those different frames of meaning are to do with self-identity, and the ways in which it is constructed. Weir looks to a concept of self-identity that sees women as active participants in the social world, and central to this understanding of identity is the capacity to sustain, and resolve, multiple and often conflicting identities. To do this we need cognitive and practical capacities for self-knowledge, self-realisation and self-direction. Combining the critical theory of Habermas (to visualise the interested nature of knowledge), and Kristeva's emphasis on the power of affective relationships (to facilitate feelings of participation in the world), Weir (1995) talks of a responsibility 'to problematize and define one's own meaning (and identity) (which) is both the burden and the privilege of modern society – as a subject who is relatively free to determine, through my own practices, who I am and who I am going to be. The flip side of this is the burden of self-definition – every action, every decision becomes self-defining – every position is open to question.' (Madden 2002: 26–29)

Madden positions rhizomatic validity within a feminist perspective. It made sense for her, liberating her from the constraints of what is generally termed a 'masculine' narrative that demands logical progression. Her approach convinced examiners of her dissertation – she gained the highest mark. You might argue she beguiled her markers but I do not think so. One reason for her success was her debate around validity, i.e. she had addressed validity in a reflexive way and justified her position. The emergence of rhizomatic validity subsumes catalytic validity, in creating a non-contradictory way to express reflexivity as experienced.

The performance turn

The performance turn reveals new possibilities of considering narrative coherence. Richardson (2000) reveals the idea of CAP ethnography (critical analytical processes), whereby the narrator moves outside conventional social scientific writing, adapting to a world of uncertainty into a tentative positioning of self to represent their journeys of reflexive of self-inquiry, patterning the narrative through various techniques and medium to adequately *tell* the story. Richardson suggests that 'there is no such thing as getting it right'. However, she does set out some evaluative criteria for reviewing the adequacy of narratives reflecting the balance of 'analytical' and 'creative', what Okri (1997) describes as 'discipline' and 'play'. Richardson's (2000) criteria for CAP are:

- Does the narrative make a substantive contribution to an understanding of social life; does the narrative seem real and true?
- Does the narrative have aesthetic merit – artistic and engaging?
- Does the narrative reflect the narrator's reflexivity in telling her story of being and becoming in *ways true to herself and her reality*?
- Does the narrative have emotional and intellectual impact moving the reader into self-reflection, new perspectives and action?

These criteria pattern coherence, incorporating many of the ideas previously explored. I added in ways *true to herself and her reality* to capture something of the essence of rhizomatic validity, given the significance of rhizomatic validity in constructing narrative.

Holman Jones (2005) uses Richardson's criteria as the basis for her own investigation. She writes 'they [the above criteria] are changing. They are generated in the doing of this writing rather than outside or prior to it' (p. 773). Put another way, in the process of interpreting and assimilating Richardson's criteria she finds her own meaning as she moves from narrative to performance reflecting a demand that performance be responsible, reciprocal, critical, dialogical, embodied and an incitement to social action. As with Denzin, she uses an evocative radical language that I feel ironically marginalises performance as being a certain type of revolt against normal practices, whereas simply exposing and transforming normal practice however mundane is equally valid. Perhaps the common root is the effort to ease suffering towards a more satisfactory life, however mundane that might seem. I suspect 'good' theatre likes drama – but that would miss the point.

Denzin (2003:123), in synthesising the work of Conquergood (1985), Madison (1998), Bochner (2000), Clough (2000), Ellis (2000), Richardson (2000) and Spry (2001) (among others), notes that narrative/performance should:

- 'Unsettle, criticize, and challenge taken-for-granted, repressed meanings;
- Invite moral and ethical dialogue while reflexively clarifying their own moral positions;
- Engender resistance and offer utopian thoughts about how things could be made different;
- Demonstrate that they care, that they are kind;
- Show instead of tell, using the rule that less is more;
- Exhibit interpretative sufficiency, representational adequacy and authentic adequacy (following Christians);
- Present political, collective and committed viewpoints.'

Of these criteria, show instead of tell – whereby the narrator crafts the narrative or performance to reveal her insights yet without imposing them or explaining them.

The criteria are similar to those of Holman Jones and Richardson. All might be considered an effort to grasp at the idea of knowing narrative and performance. As such, it is vital to take heed of Clough's (2000:278) concern, that is by setting criteria for judging what is good and what is bad in experimental writing or performance ethnography, we may only conventionalise the new writing 'and make more apparent the ways in which experimental writing has already become conventional'. As such a tension always exists between a demand to know a thing and letting a thing emerge in its own form. Criteria can only ever be guidelines. I feel the professor snap his measuring rod in frustration whilst trying to remain earnest.

Sixth dialogical movement

The ultimate test of coherence lies with the reader – the extent to which the reader relates to the text. As Okri (1997:41) writes:

> The story writer does one half of the work, but the reader does the other. The reader's mind becomes the screen, the place, the era. To a large extent readers create the world from words, they invent the reality they read. Reading, therefore, is a co-production between writer and reader.

Narrative has a social function in terms of helping people (readers and listeners) to reflect on their own experiences, leading to individual and collective social action towards creating a better world – the consensus point of dialogue (Bohm 1996). Narrative intends to show the possibilities for different interpretation rather than trying to pin the reader down into an explanation. The readers (as interpreters) will approach these narratives with their own horizons, and whilst they may not share the narrator's insights, they should be able to make sense of it. Gadamer (1975) expressed the hermeneutic belief that the reader projects, in advance, a sense of the whole as soon as an initial sense appears. This is because the reader brings to this text a viewpoint on what to expect from the text, i.e. his or her own meanings and experiences with the world. Simon and Dippo (1986:199) argue that this position assumes that:

> The audience is not composed of isolated, passive consumers of social spectacle but is in a position to use this work as a resource, critically appropriating aspects of it to help them to clarify the basis of everyday life and the possibilities for its transformation.

The reader is the final arbiter of truth and is invited to close the hermeneutic circle. The responsibility of the narrator is to write the story in such a way that the reader is able to make sense of it. Yet, the reader or listener must be open to what the text has to say. Open to its possibilities. This may be difficult because of the way readers tend to project a meaning into the text. 'We praise our capacity for reason but are unreasonably intolerant of other people's validity and reasons' (Okri 1997:34). Narrators must find the balance between communicating the meaning of the text and opening a door for others to find meaning. This may not be easy because stories are in themselves contradictory and complex, reflecting the nature of clinical practice.

Readers resonate to the narrative simply because they share common meanings and experience similar situations made accessible because they are subjective and contextualised. I know that some readers will dismiss the narrative as narcissistic, self-gratifying nonsense. It may give offence to those hardened to caring and love in the seemingly harsh world of everyday practice.

Perhaps the stories will destabilise your taken for granted perspectives and create small explosions in the mind. Arthur Frank (2002) makes the distinction between disruptive and destabilising narratives. Disruptive narratives make the reader pause before continuing in their normal way, perhaps making slight adjustments along the way. Destabilising narratives are transforming. They turn the world upside down. Reflection is always disruptive in that it cuts across the taken for granted and thus always has the potential to destabilise, which I suspect is subtly reflexive because transformation comes dripping slowly with patience.

A coherent narrative will point out the scratches, the deep etches, the flaws that flow across the polished surface of life, even as the practitioner endeavours to put on a polished face to the world. The fragility of our competence lies just below the surface waiting to be revealed. Narrators are open to themselves in authentic ways to move beyond ourselves towards self-realisation. The stories do this beautifully. This is their magic. And at the end of it all, readers will be closer to themselves, will have become more open to their own experience and will know themselves better. They will be touched by the wonder and terrors within the stories. They will feel their compassion tingle and flow more freely as the reveal themselves to themselves, lifting the masks that have clouded their vision as they reconnect to the essence of caring. They will identify the factors in their own practices that constrain realising desirable practice and understand the way these factors work and ways these factors might be swept away. In doing so they will continue the flow of their own experiences yet more consciously, more reflectively, more knowingly, and so begin to change the tradition's trajectory. The reader may even pick up a pen and begin to reflect or more formally undertake such research as advocated in the book. Reading the stories is to participate in research because it triggers powerful reflectors within each reader. That is why such stories are such powerful learning opportunities for all levels of practitioners.

I share a partial account of Ruth Morgan's exploration of coherence (from her master's in leadership dissertation) to give an impression of the way one narrative writer begins to work with criteria to shape a unified (coherent) whole. She writes:

> Traditional criteria for validation, used to justify technical, scientific studies, have found the reflective researcher to be lacking in scientific rigor (Rolfe 2002). Rolfe asserts the inappropriateness of traditional rules and procedures as measures of validity for inquiry based work. The nature of my research is inherently disorderly as it is rooted within the confusing arena of a chaotic world that limits the ability to rigidly measure its effects. The very activity of reflection serves to alter the state I am trying to reflect on (Rolfe 2002). Studies that focus on the actual practice of scientists reveal science 'as a human endeavour marked by uncertainty, controversy, and ad hoc pragmatic procedures': a far cry from the rigid logic of technical discoveries (Mishler 1990:417). Mishler (1990:416) concludes that we might do better to apply scissors to the knotty problem of validation within inquiry based, reflective studies and look for new ways of assessing their reliability: 'validation is a mess of entangled concepts and methods with an abundance of loose threads. Sophisticated, technical procedures pulling out and straightening each thread, one at a time, seem to leave the knot very much as it was.'

Lather (1986a) considers the best tactic to ensure valid new learning is to construct a research design that demands rigorous self-reflexivity. It is my view that guided reflection, as my methodology, fulfils that criteria for this research. My work demonstrates the critical levels of self-reflection achieved with the enabling support of a perceptive and experienced guide. His facilitation has helped me embrace Mezirow's (1981) state of *perspective transformation*, recognising and liberating myself from old constraining influences (Boud *et al.* 1985:23). Rolfe (2002) describes the nature of reflexive research as a type of reflection about reflection, a meta-reflection that increases knowledge and therefore develops practice. It can be said to have 'a very effective validity check built into it' (Rolfe 2002:191).

The activity of reflexivity presumes a commitment to challenge dominant norms and beliefs, to resist limiting forms of power and open up paths of new possibilities (Freshwater and Rolfe 2001). The robustness of my efforts is demonstrated in Chapter 3, outlining the methods and tools used to carry out this research. Validation should be a process through which the *trustworthiness* of interpretation is evaluated (Mishler 1990). Mishler (1990:419) gives the assessment criteria as the extent to which *concepts, methods and inferences of a study* are an acceptable basis for ongoing interpretation and empirical research of others. Integrity can be judged on the conviction imparted that what is written must be the truth (Woolf 1928). She writes: 'One holds every phrase, every scene to the light as one reads – for Nature seems, very oddly, to have provided us with an inner light by which to judge of the writer's integrity or disintegrity' (1928:84).

Since there can be no single authoritative interpretation of any text (Freshwater and Rolfe 2001), I therefore place my research into the hands of the readers for challenge, dispute and deconstruction. My use of the first person throughout the narrative is intended to facilitate this process since writing in the third person is more suggestive of a single correct interpretation (Freshwater and Rolfe 2001). If the overall assessment of trustworthiness is high enough for others to act on insights gained from the text; if their perceptions are altered and they are willing to invest time and energy on relating these to their own ways of practice then the findings are being granted validity. If the new perceptions and different ways of responding are found to work in other areas of practice then the findings take on an *aura of objective fact*. They become entrenched in changed practice.

Rolfe (2002:191) states that in practice-based disciplines 'the ultimate measure of validity has to be the extent to which the research study improves practice'. My work is a dynamic, ongoing cycle of action research with the potential to transform the researcher, researched and readers. Therefore the field is vibrant, changing and undergoing constant development for the purpose of improving practice.

Perhaps an over-focus on coherence may distract from something more significance, that is drama (Mattingly 1998). Narrative is fashioned through lived experiences connected with a sense of drama, of things unfolding with uncertainty, rather than as a neat procession to predicted outcomes.

Ethics

To be coherent, the narrative must be ethical. Responsible professionals, whatever discipline, actively ensure their own professional effectiveness. The idea of effectiveness is marked against some remit of professional role and vision, which for many professionals is a contested space between professional and organisational life concerning autonomy. For example, as a practitioner, I claim I am primarily accountable to my clients to act in their best interests or to the society to promote nursing as a caring profession, or to the organisation for being a good employee how ever that might be construed, or to the profession of nursing to act with virtue and integrity as a 'nurse'. Rationally, you might expect congruency between these aspects of accountability. Yet, there seems to be real tension between professional and organisational expectations. The patient expects a practitioner to be both competent with technical aspects of nursing and caring. Anything less is a failure. Yet organisations do not necessarily provide the resources whereby practitioners can be either competent or caring. Practitioners lack integrity when they do keep themselves fit for practice. Self-inquiry and subsequent transformation is always a moral endeavour towards self-realisation. It is concerned with realising visions of self (as a practitioner) and of practice as a lived reality. Self-inquiry is developed as an unfolding reflexive narrative that reveals the transformation – a public testimony of the practitioner's effort to become a more caring and competent practitioner. Along the journey she meets barriers to becoming, barriers that are embodied within self and embedded within organizational and professional culture. She can understand these and work towards shifting these as appropriate to enable her to realise her vision. However, in making such barriers visible she runs the risk of incurring organisational wrath that prefers her to keep the 'dirty laundry' hidden, often with a veiled threat of sanction if she makes herself visible above the parapet. The point is that practitioners have a professional responsibility over an organisational responsibility. Clearly patients have a right to confidentiality. As such, if in my self-inquiry, If I reflect on myself in relationship with you, you might expect me to ask your permission to reveal aspect of yourself in a formal ethical sense. Retrospectively, I could do that if it was possible. As a professional concerned with maintaining rights of confidentiality especially for vulnerable groups, I can ensure your identity is hidden or perhaps even construct fiction based on experiences. In my own narratives I increasingly obscure identity and place and often reshape the circumstance to become fiction. This does not make the reflection any less real, yet helps offset possible criticism of ethical violation, for without doubt an ethical tension exists regards ethics of narratives of self-inquiry linked to the positioning of self within contested discourses of the locus of responsibility. These spaces are contested based on contradictory ethical principles despite partial voices to the contrary. Partial voices react with force to ensure compliance to self-interest and dominant pattern for relationship, for example transactional organisations and the make-up and decisions of ethical committees that often bias traditional forms of empiricist research and frankly do not appreciate approaches to research such as self-inquiry. Indeed, they may dismiss such claims that self-inquiry is research at all.

Research – a careful search, systematic investigation towards increasing the sum of knowledge. (*Chambers Dictionary* 1999:1404)

In the post-modern era, the gates have been flung open leading to experimental forms of research. The idea of knowledge is also diverse and contested. So I argue that development of personal knowing (insights) through self-inquiry is increasing the sum of knowledge in the world, notably when such forms of knowing are disseminated through publication and performance. The process of self-inquiry through the six dialogical movements demonstrates its careful systematic, and inquiring nature.

So, no doubt, self-inquiry is research, within the broad parameters of what counts as research. As Schön (1983:viii) asks, 'What is the kind of knowing in which competent practitioners engage?'. Through self-inquiry I pursue this question, with the intention of developing this type of knowing or professional artistry, a knowing as Schön (1983:viii) puts it that is 'more than they can say'. Through reflection I lift some of this tacit knowing to the surface as I become more mindful of my patterns of knowing. In her narratives within the book, practitioners from diverse clinical backgrounds engage in this common idea. As practitioner/researchers this must be the focus of their attention. And, as the reader will discern, from careful reading, the narratives have a similarity in their difference.

I prefer to say systematic inquiry than systematic investigation. Perhaps that is simply a semantic thing but investigation at least in my mind is laden with a certain weight of objectivity whereas 'inquiry' is more personal, more subjective. To reiterate, narrative is a systematic process of self-inquiry and transformation towards self-realisation. It is a process of being and becoming who I want to be. The process is not determinate, for in the process ideas of what is self-realisation are always shifting within the reflexive process. As such, it is not possible to say exactly what is being researched except self.

Researching and developing self in the context of self's own practice demands no ethical approval from others. Indeed it is a mark of responsibility to take self so seriously and develop self's potential to realise desirable practice. However, self is always viewed in relationship with others as illustrated through the narratives. As such, others become visible within the narrative, and because the narrative is subjective and contextualised, the other is more easily recognised. Where the relationship is critical of others, they may recoil from the light, unable to tolerate being seen in a 'bad light'. Where others are generally perceived as more powerful, such exposure is likely not to be tolerated. Such is the abuse of patriarchal power that the 'research' is suppressed because the views expressed are 'subjective' and therefore are less easy to justify as factual.

In terms of protecting patients and families, the use of pseudonym is adequate because the intent is always to realise caring and that such stories are valuable to others to learn from.

I am not trying to write their story. I am writing my own and claim autonomy to do so. Organisations might counter claim that in revealing clinical information about patients I work with I am breaching confidentiality. Without doubt this is a concern no matter how hard I try to protect them by changing names and places and clinical information, even to the extent of fictionalising the patients. An organisation's likely objection to narrative as self-inquiry are seemingly three-fold:

- It accepts a vicarious liability for the actions of its staff;
- It holds to the idea of patient confidentiality;
- It would object to any threat of exposure that might disrupt its own smooth running.

As such, whilst it is not essential to seek permission from patients and families whom I write about in my narrative, it is preferable. However, from a holistic perspective I am in dialogue with them and, as such, it is possible to involve them in the study or to express their viewpoints sensitively. Wearing my critical social science hat, the narrative is an expression of emancipation. As such I have no hesitation in exposing conditions of practice that constrain this realisation, and would indeed hope that organisations would appreciate this feedback if they are truly patient centred. In other words, complaint that such research breaches ethical codes of research conduct is merely another constraint on practitioners to have a voice.

In *Climbing walls* I shared the performance with Anne, the woman I had been working with. In response she shared her secret journal with me. She approved both the performance and the narrative. In *Jane's rap*, Jane asked me to change one word she took offence to. Morgan (2005) writes:

My stories present living, breathing people who touch my life and influence my actions. They have an individual right to anonymity which has been observed by the use of pseudonyms throughout this research. Johns (2002) considers this to be adequate protection for patients and families within the context of a study that complies with the other guiding principles of beneficence and non-malevolence. Johns points out the greater good of exposing poor or uncaring practice rather than allowing ourselves to be silenced by the restraining voice of confidentiality.

I have made every effort to mask the identity of others and my place of work within my narrative. However due to the contextual and subjective nature of the writing I realise that some may become visible (Johns 2002). I consider this to be acceptable within the overall purpose of developing nursing practice since it is without any critical intent towards individual practitioners.

My role as a clinical leader has clear implications for high quality patient care and therefore it could be deemed unethical *not* to critically examine and develop my practice. Freshwater and Rolfe (2001) consider individual critical reflexivity to be central to the success of clinical governance. Through it the researcher-practitioner challenges the dominant paradigms and makes personal practice available for scrutiny. Johns (2002) considers it a mark of maturity to research and develop self in the context of clinical practice and one that requires no ethical approval from others. Therefore I have not felt it necessary to seek formal ethical approval for this research proposal.

The ethical principle of non-malevolence requires that I as a researcher must ensure that no harm befalls any of the research participants, including myself at the centre of the research. My commitment to guided reflection provides a means of safeguarding against this danger as it opens the door for self distortions to be exposed and motives to be scrutinised.

In her narrative study (Jarrett 2009), Lou sought ethical approval from her local committee. They insisted she sought written approval from patients who were involved in her reflections. Their position reflects a traditional orientation to medical ethics based on the patient's rights to confidentiality. The committee did not insist that approval should be sought from her colleagues who were involved. Lou's patients all gave their approval. Indeed most wanted their real names used in the narrative, raising another ethical challenge. I had written a research proposal to monitor the impact of reflexology on the well-being of people who had Parkinson's disease. In the ethics form I noted that I would use patients' real names if they requested this. The ethics committee insisted that this be changed. What rights of patient autonomy are being respected here? It was a significant realisation that malevolence is the dominating principle of medical ethics not autonomy.

I had a word with Clare, the chairperson of another local ethics committee, asking if she would mind if students undertaking self-inquiry could approach her to check out whether ethical approval was required. This was like playing a game to counter any challenge that ethical approval could simply not be assumed. We met and she gave her opinion that self-inquiry did not require ethical approval, that the focus was self-inquiry not inquiry of others, but names of patients and colleagues and places involved in the reflection should be changed to protect identity. Where contentious situations were reflected on this would be written about in judicious manner. This is a vital point. Within Wilber's four-quadrant model, the truth criteria for individual subjective knowing is authenticity. The subjective essence of reflection is mediated firstly through the hermeneutic idea of standing back and objectively asking questions of the text, and secondly through the guidance with peers and guides whereby emotional tension around difficult or contentious issues within reflection is converted to creative tension. In doing so, 'offensive talk' is converted into insights.

Writing judiciously can be re-phrased as a duty of care or virtue to do no harm. However, at a later point, one student received a response from Clare that suggested she would need to seek approval if it was possible that people within her narrative could recognise themselves or others, however remote that possibility.

My response is to draw a line, that even though that was possible, it would do no reasonable harm except for someone who was very sensitive. The writer is mindful of malevolence and ensures no intended harm through her words. I have written myself of contentious issues around differences of opinion with staff but never with patients. Conflict is part and parcel of everyday life and cannot become precious. Besides the threat of harm, Clare's response is also based on autonomy, the rights of the individual to confidentiality. I appreciate this, yet it does not outweigh the rights of the person reflecting to have a voice not censored by an inappropriate medical ethical stance.

Within a guided reflection approach to self-inquiry there is no formal contract with people mentioned in reflections. There is no intent to do research on them or with them. No formal observation, measurement or interviews take place. I sense that part of me wants to rebel against what I see as the tyranny of a partial view of medical ethics, of the way ethics committees are oriented towards a traditional objective perspective.

Indeed self-inquiry might be viewed from such a medical science perspective as not research at all, little more than dressed-up anecdote. Self-inquiry does not fit within scientific paradigms and hence its rules of injunction as to what counts as validity and ethics must be viewed differently. Presumably, if someone were to read something that they believed was about themselves and took offence they could proceed with a libel action, in much the same way I might take offence if someone were to write something about me that I felt was unjust. The role of ethics committees is not to be parental, to take away rather than enhance autonomy.

If each person involved in reflection were asked, such work would prove to be untenable. Reflection takes place either within-the-moment or following a situation. Hence permission to include the other in my reflection would always be a retrospective event. The idea that a person might say, 'No, you cannot write about me', or demand power of censureship shifts the emphasis of reflection from me to you. It misses the whole point of the reflective endeavour. Asking patients and colleagues for consent to reflect on my relationship with them might in itself distort relationships and disrupt both the therapeutic and inquiry process. What I reflect on is natural, it is integral to the flow of relationship. Reflection is itself therapeutic, changing myself and reflexively informing the next encounter. Consent changes the nature of the relationship. It may lead to a self-consciousness that alters the experience.

The result would not be a reflection of how I was thinking or feeling. It is also very clear that practitioners do hold negative feelings about patients and colleagues. This is natural. Revealing such situations through reflection opens up the learning potential to learn through such situations to resolve them and create better worlds and more effective practice. Hence reflection can claim a utilitarian function of greatest good.

Looking back through my own writing and publication I have rarely informed people I am reflecting on and writing about my relationship with them. I have never sought ethical approval and I have never been challenged that I should do so. I can remember only one situation that has caused me concern about writing, where I actually posed the question was a nurse 'a bad nurse' countering the idea that this nurse labelled a patient as 'a bad patient'.[1] I was uncomfortable about this, yet why should I be? I think it is a reflection of the transactional demand that conjecture is hidden from public view. The illusion of smoothness. I know I am contaminated by such culture. Yet I did write about it and feel cleansed in doing so, to raise it into the public domain for others to learn from. It was an act of integrity grounded in a primary demand to care for people and confront abuse where ever it exists. It was an act of commitment and transformation.

Sandelowski (1993) writes of member threat to validity. Reflection reveals the practitioner's effort to make sense of the world. It is a universal subjective experience for all practitioners. Clearly those people included within my reflection cannot be asked to verify the accuracy of my interpretations. The interpretations are mine, and mine alone, irrespective of controversy. Sometime I make lousy judgements or respond in a mistaken way but that is the nature of human encounter work. It is not predictable and practitioners do err. Reflection is the means to learn from this and so it is always a virtuous activity.

Issues of ethics in narratives of self-inquiry are inevitably complex. I suspect it comes down to a question of authority. The bureaucratic organisation demands its servants to obey, and seek ethical approval because it a way of imposing social control. What are these practitioners writing about? Does it impact badly on the organisation/will it lead to litigation? Can the practitioner resist or must she yield to such demand? The threat of sanction typical of bureaucracy may be difficult to resist. Making the choice is ultimately an issue of commitment. Do I surrender to the transactional culture or do I surrender to the transformational flow? Jaworski captures this notion:

> As Varela[2] spoke, I thought about the way both Buber[3] and Greenleaf[4] described the moment of commitment. This is the ground of being that enables the free will that is not 'controlled by things and instincts' to operate. Francisco continued 'we take a stand and make a declaration to create a new reality. This is not an arbitrary statement, for in our being we have this inner certainty we can reinvent the world to this extent. We sense the time is right; the reality is already in the system waiting to be brought forth'. (1998:179)

I say to the students you have choice. My facilitative voice says you do not need to seek ethical approval. The extent you inform others that you have talked about them in your reflections is your decision to make, just as the way you have written about them, remembering the primary intent of guided reflection is to create better, more authentic worlds (i.e. the extent the inquiry is coherent).

Ethical tension

Using ethical mapping I can plot the tension within an ethic of narratives of self-inquiry.

---

[1]See Johns C (2006) *Engaging reflection in practice*. Blackwell, Oxford.
[2]Conversation with Francisco Varela, co-author of *The tree of knowledge and the embodied mind*. Shambhala, Boston (1992)
[3]Buber M (1970) *I and thou* (transl. RG Smith). Scribner Classics, New York.
[4]Greenleaf R (2002) *Servant leadership*. Paulist Press, New Jersey.

Practitioner's perspective	Tension	Medical ethics perspective
Self-inquiry through reflection is researching self/autobiographical. Truth value of self-inquiry is authenticity with checks to ensure this Claim for autonomy to write about self (challenge to servant mentality of working within bureaucratic organisations) No formal contract to involve others in the inquiry Duty of care to mask identity of name and place to protect others mentioned in reflections (do no harm/confidentiality) Strong emphasis on beneficence-- that self-inquiry leads to positive outcomes for practitioners and others Emphasis on utilitarianism – that some risk can be tolerated in terms of the greater good	Ethical principles: Beneficence Malevolence Autonomy Utilitarianism Virtue/duty of care Ethical dilemma Should the practitioner seek formal ethical approval for self-inquiry through reflection?	A bias towards a scientific approach to research and ethics that imposes its rules of injunction on subjective approaches to research Essentially bureaucratic that seeks to minimise risk of complaint (primacy to smooth running) Parental perspective to protect the patient from harm (strong emphasis on principles of beneficence and malevolence/seeks to protect patient's rights) People involved in research must give consent

Each side has a partial view that is difficult to integrate. I advise leadership students to have a word in the ear of the ethics committee chairperson. Always the question asked: 'Does the "research" involve investigation of patients?'

The answer is 'No – it is self-inquiry – it is investigation of self.'

'Then there is no need for ethical approval' (with the provision that any reference to patients must be adequately protected).

Helen Blunn (2004) writes:

Of course although this research is primarily focused on self in the context of my own practice it cannot be ignored that it also involves intense interest in other people, my relationship with them, their views and circumstances. Within my narrative I have attempted to pay careful attention to not being overtly critical of colleagues even though anonymity is achieved within the text using pseudonyms. However, within this paying attention I have been careful not to sacrifice or compromise the honest reality of the experiences. Rather I have walked carefully along the line between what Johns (2002) describes as asserting self and marginalising self. As the course has been a very new experience for me so as a consequence has been the construction and writing of this narrative. Without doubt the whole experience has changed how I see self and others.

Susan Brooks writes:

Effective transformational leadership skills have implications for the standard of patient care delivered and it could be argued that failing to reflect upon and develop my own transformational leadership practice would be an *unethical* activity (Parahoo 1997, Cook 2001). Johns (2002) writes that researching and developing self in the context of one's own practice even when viewed in relationship to others as proposed here, needs no ethical approval. Indeed, he argues that the intent of such research is to realise caring in practice and claims that the argument that such research breaches ethical codes of research serves merely to constrain the voice of practitioners (Johns 2002). Accordingly, formal ethical approval for this research proposal has not been sought.

The fundamental ethical principles of confidentiality and non-malevolence have, however, been considered. Pseudonyms have been used for any persons featured in the research although it is noted that where narrative is necessarily subjective and contextualised as here, others may become visible and recognisable even when so masked. As Johns (2002) notes, the key to ethical management here is to ensure that negative criticism is avoided and where criticism is necessary it is worded in a non-threatening manner. The ethical principle of non-malevolence requires me as researcher to ensure that no harm should be caused to participants – in this case myself as subject (Beauchamp and Childress 1989). Rich and Parker (1995) and Hulatt (1995) note that reflection can be a painful experience, which may bring to consciousness issues, which, if unresolved, have the potential to cause psychological harm. Schön (1987) advocates that reflection should therefore always be supervised or coached in order to support the practitioner on their journey. In consideration of the ethical principle of non-malevolence to myself, I ensured that alongside my reflective guide, I developed and maintained a close and therapeutic guiding relationship with my informal clinical supervisor to support me through the process. (2004:33–34)

Ethics is a contested space within narratives of self-inquiry. The narrator is mindful of the tension and works its margins to be authentic yet in ways that do not harm others. The issue of autonomy to make the decision not to seek ethical approval is itself an issue of self-realisation.

References

Agar M and Hobbs J (1982) Interpreting discourse: coherence and the analysis of ethnographic interviews. *Discourse Processes* 5:1–32.

Albright D (1994) Literary and psychological models of the self. In: U Neisser and R Fivush (eds.) *The remembering self: construction and accuracy in the self-narrative.* Cambridge University Press, Cambridge, pp. 19–40.

Beauchamp T and Childress J (1989) *Principles of biomedical ethics* (third edition). Oxford University Press, Oxford.

Blunn H (2004) Exploring the process involved in the emergence of self as a transformational leader within a reflexive model approach. Unpublished dissertation, MSc in Leadership in Healthcare Practice. University of Bedfordshire, Bedfordshire.

Bochner A (2000) Criteria against ourselves. *Qualitative Inquiry* 6:266–272.

Bohm D (1996) *On dialogue.* (Edited by L Nichol). Routledge, London.

Boud D, Keogh R and Walker D (1985) Promoting reflection in learning: a model. In: D Boud, R Keogh and D Walker (eds.) *Reflection: turning experience into learning.* Kogan Page, London, pp. 18–40.

Brooks S (2004) Becoming a transformational leader. Unpublished dissertation, MSc in Leadership in Healthcare Practice. University of Bedfordshire, Bedfordshire.

Buber M (1970) *I and thou* (transl. RG Smith). Scribner Classics, New York.

Chambers Dictionary (1999) Chambers Harrap Publishers, Edinburgh.

Chase S (2005) Narrative inquiry: multiple lenses, approaches, voices. In: N Denzin and Y Lincoln (eds.) *The Sage handbook of qualitative research* (third edition). Sage, Thousand Oaks, pp. 651–680.

Clough P (2000) Comments on setting criteria for experimental writing. *Qualitative Inquiry* 6:278–291.

Compact Oxford English Dictionary (third edition) (2005) Oxford University Press, Oxford.

Conquergood D (1985) Performance as a moral act; ethical dimensions of the ethnography of performance. *Literature in Performance* 5:1–13.

Cook M (2001) The renaissance of clinical leadership. *International Nursing Review* 48:1, 38–42.

Dalai Lama (1998) *The Dalai Lama's book of daily meditations*. [Complied and edited by R Singh]. Rider, London.

Denzin N (2003) *Performance ethnography*. Sage, Thousand Oaks.

Elliott J (1989) Knowledge, power and teacher appraisal. In: Carr W (ed.) *Quality in teaching*. Falmer Press, London.

Ellis C (2000) Creating criteria: an ethnographic short story. *Qualitative Inquiry* 6:273–277.

Fay B (1987) *Critical social science*. Polity Press, Cambridge.

Frank A (2002) Relations of caring: demoralization and remoralization in the clinic. *International Journal of Human Caring* 6:13–19.

Freshwater D and Rolfe G 2001. Critical reflexivity: a politically and ethically engaged research method for nursing. *NT Research* 6:526–537.

Gadamer HG (1975) *Truth and method* (transl. G Barden and J Cumming). Seabury Press, New York.

Greenleaf R (2002) *Servant leadership: a journey into the nature of legitimate power and greatness*. Paulist Press, New Jersey.

Holman Jones S (2005) Autoethnography: making the personal political. In: N Denzin and Y Lincoln (eds.) *The Sage handbook of qualitative research* (third edition). Sage, Thousand Oaks, pp. 763–792.

Hulatt I (1995) A sad reflection. *Nursing Standard* 9:22–23.

Irigaray L (1987) Is the subject of science sacred? (transl. C Mastrangelo). *Hypatia* 2 No 3 (Fall 1987):66. Cited in Tong R (1989) *Feminist thought: a comprehensive introduction*. Routledge, London.

Jarrett L (2009) Being and becoming a reflective practitioner, through guided reflection, in the role o a spasticity management nurse specialist. Unpublished PhD thesis, City University, London.

Jaworski J (1998) *Synchronicity: the inner path of leadership*. Berrett-Koehler Publishers, San Francisco.

Johns C (2002) *Guided reflection: advancing practice* (first edition). Blackwell Publishing, Oxford.

Johns C (2006) *Engaging reflection in practice*. Blackwell Publishing, Oxford.

Kushner S and Norris N (1980–1981) Interpretation, negotiation, and validity in naturalistic research. *Interchange* 11:26–36.

Lather P (1986a) Research as praxis. *Harvard Educational Review* 56:257–277.

Lather P (1986b) Issues of validity in open ideological research: between a rock and a soft place. *Interchange* 17:63–84.

Lather P (1993) Fertile obsession: validity after post-structuralism. *The Sociological Quarterly* 34:673–693.

Madden I (2002) Working with women following traumatic childbirth. In: C Johns (ed.) *Guided reflection: advancing practice*. Blackwell Publishing, Oxford, pp. 187–211.

Madison S (1998) performance, personal narratives, and the politics of possibility. In: S Dailey (ed.) *The future of performance studies: visions and revisions*. National Communication Association, Annandale, pp. 276–286.

Mattingly C (1998) *Healing dramas and clinical plots: the narrative structure of experience*. Cambridge University Press, Cambridge.

Mezirow J (1981) A critical theory of adult learning and education. *Adult Education* 32:3–24.

Mishler EG (1990) Validation in inquiry-guided research: the role of exemplars in narrative studies. *Harvard Educational Review* 60:415–442.

Morgan R (2005) *Realising transformational leadership*. Unpublished dissertation, MSc in Leadership in Healthcare Practice. University of Bedfordshire, Bedfordshire.

Newell M (1992) Anxiety, accuracy, and reflection: the limits of professional development. *Journal of Advanced Nursing* 17:1326–1333.

Okri B (1997) *A way of being free*. Phoenix Books, London.

Parahoo K (1997) *Nursing research: principles, process and issues* (first edition). Palgrave Macmillan, Basingstoke.

Reason P and Rowan J (1981) Issues of validity in new paradigm research. In: P Reason and J Rowan (eds.) *Human inquiry*. John Wiley, Chichester.

Rich A and Parker D (1995) Reflection and critical incident analysis: ethical and moral implications of their use within nursing and midwifery education. *Journal of Advanced Nursing* 22:1050–1057.

Richardson L (2000) Evaluating ethnography. *Qualitative Inquiry* 6:253–255.

Rolfe G (2002) Reflexive research and the therapeutic use of self. In: D Freshwater (ed.) *Therapeutic nursing. Improving patient care through self-awareness and reflection*. Sage, London, Chapter 10.

Sandelowski M (1993) Rigor or rigor mortis: the problem of rigor in qualitative research revisited. *Advances in Nursing Science* 16:10–18.

Schön D (1983) *The reflective practitioner*. Avebury, Aldershot.

Schön D (1987) *Educating the reflective practitioner*. Jossey-Bass, San Francisco.

Simon R and Dippo D (1986) On critical ethnographic work. *Anthropology and Education Quarterly* 17:195–202.

Smith J and Deemer D (2000) The problem of criteria in the age of relativism. In: N Denzin and Y Lincoln (eds.) *Handbook of qualitative research* (second edition). Sage, Thousand Oaks, pp. 877–896.

Spry T (2001) Performance ethnography: an embodied methodological praxis. *Qualitative Inquiry* 7:706–732.

Steele R (1986) Deconstructing histories: toward a systematic criticism of psychological narratives. In: T Sarbin (ed.) *Narrative psychology: the storied nature of human conduct*. Praeger, New York.

Webb C (1993) Feminist research: definitions, methodology, methods and evaluation. *Journal of Advanced Nursing* 18:416–423.

Weinsheimer J (1985) *Gadamer's hermeneutics. A reading of truth and method*. Yale University Press, New Haven.

Weir A (1995) Toward a model of self-identity: Habermas and Kristeva. In: J Meehan (ed.) *Feminists read Habermas: gendering the subject of discourse*. Routledge, London.

Wheatley MJ (1999) *Leadership and the new science*. Brett-Koehler Publishers, San Francisco.

Whitehead J (2000) How do I improve my practice? Creating and legitimating an epistemology of practice. *Reflective Practice* 1:8–13.

Whitman W (1855/2005) *Leaves of grass – introduction by H Bloom*. Penguin, New York.

Wilber K (1998) *The eye of spirit: an integral vision for a world gone slightly mad*. Shambhala, Boston.

Woolf V (1928) *A room of one's own*. Penguin, Hardmondsworth.

Woolgar S (1988) *Science: the very idea*. Tavistock, London.

Chapter 16

An accidental tourist

Lei Foster

I have before me the publicity picture of the movie *The Accidental Tourist*, which stars William Hurt, Kathleen Turner and Geena Davis. The movie is predictably enough based on the book by Anne Tyler; and I have not read the book nor watched the movie. However I am attracted to the idea of 'the accidental tourist' – what makes the idea relevant for me is that the publicity photo, which was ubiquitous at the time of the movie's release in 1988, features a man (Hurt) as the eponymous hero.

For me the notion of the accidental tourist is of someone who unexpectedly finds themselves placed in the position of a tourist. This means either that (i) they have physically found themselves suddenly and unexpectedly in a strange land or (ii) what were familiar surroundings have suddenly and unexpectedly become strange. I have not physically travelled to a strange land (as this land – nursing practice – is the one I have always inhabited); so that the latter definition is most apt. It describes my experience of auto-ethnography, which was most succinctly summed up by Noy (2003) as being a positioning of oneself ('auto') as the subject of a larger social or cultural inquiry ('ethno') through writing ('graphy').

For me this is precisely where narrative comes in. For my study to be 'research' requires me to write about how I have (unexpectedly – 'accidentally') become a 'tourist', and what my experiences are as I wander up and down the once-familiar streets of nursing practice. These things must be written down, for then precious moments of practice and awakening are captured. The process of reflexivity, which according to Freshwater and Rolfe (2001) is a 'turning back on oneself', leads me further and further into layers of narrative (Johns 2009) as I walk up and down, up and down well-trodden paths, retracing my steps, becoming more and more a stranger as each time I ponder the significance of each retracing. These layers of narratives are what I write down each time, on each retraced journey, I keep going back as if I have forgotten something, have this nagging feeling that something's not right, that things simply shouldn't be taken at face value.

I no longer know my own home; nor the city that lunges at me when I open the front door. In order for me to understand what is happening, to try to make sense to me, to try to represent it to the reader, I tell my story, I write my narrative, each time a slightly different tale about the same thing with, surprisingly enough, occasionally different endings too. This is why narrative is so exciting: I never know how the story that I tell is going to end: I never know what insights the story as it unfolds in the telling is going to give me or you, the reader.

You see, for many years in my practice I had a nice comfortable penthouse that over-looked the river. I think it is a situation that anyone desires, not only practitioners. Then one day – through reflection – I wondered, as the popular song declares, 'Is that all there is?', almost as though I was becoming bored with the view.

For our monthly narrative group I had planned to write a narrative as a sort of post-script to a previous narrative experience; but then I thought how there isn't such a thing as a postscript to an experience because you can't ever say 'this experience is now complete, here's what happened afterwards'. Even if you go back and look upon it, it's different because although the experience is in some sense static having happened in the past you have moved on so you don't look back on it the same way. You can't change what happened in the past but you *can* change the way you feel about it, so it is said.

Re-visiting, it is called. As if the experience was not mine to begin with and I am a visitor in returning to it. Or perhaps I look back upon it with a sense of privilege and of honour. This was when my image of the accidental tourist first became real to me, sham-bling about the city streets between tall buildings, battered suitcase in hand, handkerchief on head and dressed in a Hawaiian shirt wet with sweat, wide eyed at the sights that everybody living in the city takes for granted because they live there. The clatter and clang of car horns that accompany my disorderly stroll down the high street in the direc-tion of the town square. This must be my own version of alienation – part fantasy, part dissimulation. The *Financial Times* journalist Rick Owens earned a place in *Private Eye*'s notorious 'Pseud's corner' (*Private Eye* 2007) for declaring his excitement of his alien-ation living in Paris because he was unable to speak French.

That Owens learned the language (and feels he doesn't need to as an Englishman writing for an English publication) is his way of preserving the excitement of alienation, the sense of strangeness (and his own identity as an Englishman, perhaps afraid to immerse himself in the local culture for fear of losing the nationalism whereby he identi-fies himself, and that gives him succour in the strange land in which he finds himself). Paradoxically (or perhaps not) I have always found myself most prolific in writing when I feel alienated, estranged.

I feel alienated and estranged from – but like Owens excited by – having learned the language of nursing practice but having stood back from it and realised that the language I have learned is not in fact appropriate; my excitement comes from realising that the language I have been using for long only signifies – 'names' – other things (language itself is of course symbolic). I have realized that what I 'see' – what has been given to me by clinical governance, by the public health organisation that employs me, the norms and values I acculturate that grant me membership of the community of nursing – are *not* what 'is', are *not* natural. As the *Holy Bible* (Matthew 27:50–51) describes the death of the Christian Messiah as the renting of the veil in two (that is, the destruction – and supersedence – of the mystification of reality made by the ancient Jewish religion); and as Marx's study of commodity fetishism in *Das Capital* revealed to me that instead of seeing a television set, for example, the enlightened subject would 'see' the relations of production that made it – the ethnographer sees 'through' or, better put, 'beyond' appar-ent reality. Cudmore and Sondermeyer (2007) use the analogy of Lewis Carroll's story *Alice Through the Looking Glass* to describe the ethnographic feeling – once Alice enters a very ordinary house she very quickly finds out that appearances were in fact quite deceptive. In reflection we see more than merely that which is reflected back to us, we see beyond (or behind) the two-dimensional image that mimics us. In the analytical process of reflection we wonder, 'What has made up the image projected back at me? What makes up the image of my practice I wish to project?'

I find myself an *accidental* tourist because here I was a citizen of this fair land believing I lived on a plateau, whereas in fact I was an inhabitant of the swampy lowlands (Schön 1983) of practice. I laboured under an everyday *illusion* of practice; and through critical reflection I found myself what Gerrish (1997) describes as a 'marginal native': that is I am 'native' but *not quite*. This is of course one of the great dangers of ethnography, that the researcher 'goes' native (fully becomes a member of the group under study) so that, presumably, remaining on the margins of native-ness guards against this. Lee and Roth (2003) describe this sense as 'legitimate peripheral participation', i.e. that I 'should be there' anyway (and am entitled to be as a registered nurse). What is interesting here is that I already *am* perceived by my colleagues as being 'native' and could return to fully being so if I so wished. Or a 'border ethnographer' – 'the in-between space of clinician/ academic … one who inhabits the slash rather than the territory on either side' (Walker 1997 in Cudmore and Sondermeyer 2007:28).

I like Cudmore and Sondermeyer's (2007:32) comical description of the ethnographic researcher who 'grabs' the data from the field and 'runs' with it back to the safety of their own familiar 'world' … ; This image concurs with my own as the nurse-(auto) ethnographer being a sort of guerrilla who makes regular 'smash 'n' grab' raids into practice and scurries back home to study them. We stand outside a jeweller's shop, back to the window, balaclava muzzling our anxious breath, looking about ourselves urgently to see whether we are observed – then a quick, backward jab of the elbow that smashes the plate glass behind, and amidst the clangour of the emergency alarm, we grab the jewel and run before the raid has been noticed by the patrolling jack-booted troops of clinical governance. However I think this image is disingenuous since even the ethnographer's own 'world' (the thief's own home) is no longer familiar: once you have embarked upon the ethnographic journey, even in your own homeland you accidentally become a tourist. I prefer Alsop's (2002) description of the ethnographic researcher being at home and being away (*heim* and *heimat* in her own native German tongue) at the same time. I could say to my colleagues – 'I am one of you but I am not'; what Roberts (2007:20) describes as the 'ethical hangover' of fearing that you betray those you work with by 'researching' them (Cudmore and Sondermeyer 2007). I think that, to the contrary, service users in fact *expect* some sort of distancing by me from a common humanity in my role as a nurse; as was revealed to me when one service user who had requested time with me to talk asked, 'This isn't "therapy", is it?'

Likewise Madison (2004) notes the importance of what he calls the 'positionality' of the researcher; that is where do I position myself – to quote Alsop (2002:para 1), in relation to the 'shifting (of) one's notion of center and periphery and coping with the complexity of multiple centers with multiple peripheries'? (Alsop 2002:para 1).

Some time I will have to admit I had an agenda when I started this, although I don't think I am quite ready to turn embarrassment into honesty quite yet. Originally I had a vague idea of what I wanted to do: reflect on my practice in order to bring the whole bourgeois edifice of public health care down. An ambitious and incredibly naïve project, the sort of narcissism highlighted by Laughlin (1995) to which the ethnographer is vulnerable if unchecked – and, as is so often the case with radicalism, presenting nothing with which to take its place. I wanted to be *noticed,* like one of Crawford *et al.*'s (2008) nurses who hanker for the 'would-be celebrity, recognition, appreciation and the sense that one's efforts will lead to one being discovered (that) are crucial to the enacted professional identity'.

But if I am honest about it for a long time I didn't know what I was doing. I can remember the joy I felt at hearing a lecturer during his lecture on qualitative study retort,

'If you don't know what you're doing, that's okay – you're not supposed to!' I remember him now leaning forward, his bearded face puce with intent, his hands spread flat on the yellow Formica-topped table as he roared. I can remember how uncomfortable the room was, small and stuffy, crammed with students of many nationalities. I knew I would never see most of those people ever again, there from that cramped room set in a converted red brick basilica at the back of town.

I don't know when I decided to abandon my penthouse …

… but suddenly here I am. Having discovered a path after chopping maniacally at undergrowth for the past 15 months.

Postscript

It looked easy: I would write reflectively about my transformation from everyday nursing practice to ideal practice. And my writing about that, and my reflections, and how my reflections improved my practice still further (i.e. reflexively) comprised a sort of research on myself, of why I think the way I do, and why I do what I do. And with a flourish I will end my thesis with a clarion of glory because I will have achieved ideal practice. At the end of my struggle I would be a hero. I would be what Crawford *et al.* (2008) sardonically refer to as 'a celebrity practitioner'.

My journey to ideal practice was going to be like that of Hegel's journey of Spirit in his philosophical tome named *The Phenomenology*, which achieves the Absolute (Salih 2002). It is not for nothing that this is known as idealism: I alone would carry the authentic Spirit of mental health Recovery to its realisation as ideal practice. However, and this is the paradox, during my reflective study I often felt that my practice as a mental health practitioner was more often that of Hegel's Unhappy Hero.

> The Spirit (or 'Geist') progresses by negating everything that falls its way without ever being certain that a happy ending ultimately awaits it, and it is only once it has passed through the successive stages that Hegel describes – sense-certainty, perception, force and understanding, self-certainty, stoicism, scepticism, unhappy consciousness, reason, logic, psychology, reason, and so on – that it finally reaches its destination of absolute knowledge. (Salih 2002:24)

In other words, I *am* the 'hero' of my story – of this transformation towards ideal practice – but not a happy, celebrated one. For it has not been a straightforward journey, causing me to feel unhappy. In reality my journey has turned from idealism when I started out to cynicism and despondency by the time I have reached the stage at which I write now. I recognise in myself Fleming and Spicer's (2002, 2003) suggestion of the cynic as a sort of self-styled hero, one who believes that they have retained their virtue despite the colonisation of the System in which they find themselves. Pointedly the same authors make the case that in fact cynicism doesn't change anything, and that organisations should be encouraged to tolerate cynicism as it distracts workers from effective agitation (Fleming and Spicer 2002, 2003). The contemporary philosopher Slavoj Zizek remarks that in fact cynicism disguises depression and despondency and feelings of helplessness in the individual (Zizek 2008).

During the course of my study, my work became increasingly shot through with cynicism, disguised as satire, in my creation of defamiliarised (Shlovsky 1965) short plays that described aspects of my practice. To 'defamiliarise' something means to think of it in terms of images (Shlovsky 1965). In the small supervision group in which they were read by group members taking different parts, my satires achieved local notoriety and laughter. One supervisor, Amanda, observed that they were reminiscent of tired acts in creaky old music halls just as that era was coming to an end. (Interestingly just at the inception of the National Health Service (NHS), in which I work.)

It was an accidental metaphor – if there can be such a thing, for it will necessarily have arisen from deep within my own subconscious. Something, somewhere, some time ago, took root in my soul. As a child I watched televised music hall acts hosted by the late Roy Hudd, and so perhaps something stuck from then. I also like the various visual adaptations of *Alice in Wonderland*, which informed my characterisation of the team manager as like the capricious and contradictory Queen of Hearts, and Douglas Adams' creation of Slartibartfast in *The Hitch Hikers' Guide to the Galaxy* (Adams 1979) and of Reg in *Dirk Gently's Holistic Agency* (Adams 1988), both of whom informed my character of the chief executive, and of Abbot and Costello, whom I thought of when I depicted the two estates workers Bob and Dave.

I now realise two things. First, that my idea of the ethnographer being compared to an *accidental* tourist is disingenuous. Autoethnography is itself an intensely conscious act, a decision, riddled with the guilt and concerns summarised above by Cudmore and Sondermeyer (2007). I didn't expect myself to be drawn to the idea of autoethnography as a sort of tourism, by which the familiar becomes unfamiliar. It is a part of a conscious (and reflexive) process; but the image of the tourist fits. It is only accidental in the sense that the metaphor is unexpected and suits so well; and that I did not predict the effect that assuming the role of pseudo-autoethnographer would have upon me.

Second, I now realise that I was unhappy working in an in-patient unit for the four years that was the length of my study. Just as the MPhil part of my study was drawing to a close, the residential unit in which I worked was closed down by the organisation, ostensibly for refurbishment, and I resisted redeployment to the local acute mental health unit instead obtaining a secondment in the community. Since this move, I have realised that my inpatient work was clouding my perspective, much like a battery hen knows only its cage and in frustration pecks itself. I wonder whether there is perhaps a significant difference for those who work in the community or in-patient care. A friend who is a community mental health practitioner described herself as feeling she is 'self-employed'.

So then everything is accidental but not so. It is still, however, curious to me that the unit closed down *at the same time as I ended the MPhil part of my study and came to write my thesis up*. Needless to say I had nothing to do with the closure. However, as Brown and Majomi (2006) remark, the tradition of lament in the NHS assumes the gravity of bardism, and the bard is one who puts this misery into narrative and into song. One aspect of the bard is that they are considered to have mystical power – to be a 'weaver of magic and spells' and to have a particularly gifted and perspicacious knowledge of the oppressor. So I was a bard (although as Amanda pointed out, a self-styled one because it was without the assent of my peers) who weaved their magic and spells and got the unit that led to such universal (and farcical) misery and suffering being closed (which is extremely unlikely). In fact the unit closing was probably good for all of the team, and even the service users, some of whom had been there for two or three years.

It was accidental. The dictionary definition of an accident is of an unexpected event. Several unexpected events and feelings and thoughts took place in the four years of my research study. I have heard it said that there are some people who will always end up landing on their feet should disaster (or at the very least precipitated change) befall them. Well, perhaps I am one of those and, like them, I have miraculously 'come up smelling of roses'. Perhaps also this is the next stage of my research study: time to haul up my rucksack and travel again. ...

References

Adams D (1979) *The hitchhiker's guide to the galaxy.* Pan Macmillan, London.

Adams D (1988) *Dirk Gently's holistic detective agency.* Pan Macmillan, London.

Alsop CK (2002) Home and away: self-reflexive auto-/ethnography. *Forum: Qualitative Social Research* 3:3. Available at: www.qualitative-research.net/fqs-texte/3-02/3-02alsop-e.htm (accessed 19 November 2007).

Brown B and Majomi P (2006) *The archaeology of the tongue: bardic lament in the UK's 'New NHS'.* Unpublished paper. Available at: www.academicarmageddon.co.uk/prog/ bardiclament2006.htm (accessed 30 May 2009).

Crawford P, Brown B and Majomi P (2008) Professional identity in community mental health nursing: a thematic analysis. *International Journal of Nursing Studies* 45(7):1055–1063.

Cudmore H and Sondermeyer J (2007) Through the looking glass: being a critical ethnographic researcher in a familiar nursing context. *Nurse Researcher* 14:25–35.

Fleming P and Spicer A (2002) Workers' playtime? Unravelling the paradox of covert resistance in organizations. In: SR Clegg (ed.) *Management and organization paradoxes.* Advances in Organization Studies, Volume 9. John Benjamins, Amsterdam, pp. 65–86.

Fleming P and Spicer A (2003) Working at a cynical distance: implications for power, subjectivity and resistance. *Organization* 10:157–179.

Freshwater D and Rolfe G (2001) Critical reflexivity: a politically and ethically engaged research method for nursing. *Nursing Times Research* 6(1):526–537.

Gerrish K (1997) Being a 'marginal native': dilemmas of the participant observer. *Nurse Researcher* 5:25–34.

Johns C (2009) *Becoming a reflective practitioner* (third edition). Wiley-Blackwell, Oxford.

Laughlin MJ (1995) The narcissistic researcher: a personal view. *The Qualitative Report* 2:2. Available at: www.nova.edu/ssss/QR/QR2-2/laughlin.html (accessed 20 November 2007).

Lee S and Roth WM (2003) Becoming and belonging: learning qualitative research through legitimate peripheral participation. *Forum: Qualitative Social Research* 4:2. Available at: www. qualitative-research.net/fqs-texte/2-03/2-03leeroth-e.htm (accessed 29 August 2007).

Madison DS (2004) *Critical ethnography: method, ethics, and performance.* University of North Carolina, Chapel Hill, North Carolina.

Noy C (2003) The write of passage: reflections on writing a dissertation in narrative methodology. *Forum: Qualitative Social Research* 4(2) Available at: www.qualitative-research.net/index.php/ fqs/article/view/712/1542 (accessed 3 March 2010).

Private Eye (2007) 1195:27.

Roberts L (2007) Ethnography and staying in your own nest. *Nurse Researcher* 14:15–24.

Salih S (2002) *Judith Butler: essential guides for literary studies.* Routledge Critical Thinkers series. London: Routledge.

Schön D (1983) *The reflective practitioner. How professionals think in action.* Temple Smith, London.

Shlovsky C (1965) Art as technique. In: LT Lemon and MJ Reis (eds.) *Russian formalist criticism: four essays.* University of Nebraska Press, Lincoln, pp. 3–24.

Zizek S (2008) Tolerance as an ideological category. *Critical Inquiry* 34:660–682.

Chapter 17

Reflections

Christopher Johns

> Our lives have become narrow enough. Our dreams strain to widen them, to bring to our waking consciousness the awareness of greater discoveries that lie just beyond the limits of our sights. We must not force our poets to limit the world any further. (Okri 1997:4–5)

'All the world's a stage …' – famous lines often quoted and yet ring a truth. Practitioners no matter what disciplinary persuasion perform narrative day to day. Life is the ultimate teacher and its lessons learned through experience (Remen 1996) if we are mindful enough to pay attention. So much of we is wrapped up in the past or projected into a future. Very few of us are here present *now*. Very few of us pay attention to the mundane fabric of our lives simply because it is taken for granted. It is normal and outside the scope of our gaze. Reflection then enables us to pay attention, to become mindful, to take nothing for granted.

In constructing narratives we become the poets of our own lives. We stir ourselves from our complacency to open the shutters of our lives to reveal the full landscape of our practice. This is the beauty and great gift of a carefully constructed narrative, to reveal the world, not as something to view but to experience. If you choose to research self through narrative as self-inquiry and transformation, you become a poet and contribute to a new way of researching and writing grounded in the passion, beauty and terror of everyday practice, no matter the colour and ilk of your practice.

Texts that are prescriptive of how we should think, feel and act are no longer tenable, for health care practice is a creative act interpreted within the unfolding moment. We need inspirational texts written by poets to challenge us, to take us on journeys where the mundane becomes profound, simply because our practice makes a difference to peoples' lives. We need such texts like we need breath.

This second edition of this book is a further personal landmark, a re-gathering of fragments of ideas that influence my approach to constructing narratives of self-inquiry and transformation towards self-realisation. The shift of emphasis from realising a vision as a lived reality to self-realisation is as significant as it is subtle. Subtle because it says the same thing differently and yet significant because it does, a least in my mind, strengthen the ontological focus. Realising a vision is looking out from self whereas self-realisation is looking more in at self, and no matter what we seek to realise, it is who I am that is most vital.

Through the narratives, I have endeavoured to open a space of clearing, to show practitioners the possibilities of narratives of self-inquiry to explore themselves.

I wonder what I would have done differently if I had had this book to guide me when I first tentatively stepped out to construct my first narratives. I think that part of me would have held it tight for security while another part would have pushed it aside as stifling my own imagination and creativity. So, as with all theory, treat the book with respect because it is deeply written, yet view it with curiosity. Now – how does this book inform my practice? Where do these ideas come from? I trust you to respond wisely.

What is the value of the narrative and performance?

- Narrative enable the development of the practitioner's personal knowing, a knowing that is subjective and contextual within the particular situation, and evolving in new patterns in response to new situations within the reflexive spiral of being and becoming.
- Narrative inform other practitioners who may experience similar scenarios as those set out within the narratives. The reader can more easily relate to this knowing because such knowing is contextual rather than abstract. Each narrative is a snapshot of practice that reveals its subtlety and complexity that can never be adequately dealt with in more conventional abstract theoretical texts.
- Narrative illuminates the context or the background of the practitioner's experience highlighting the ever-shifting relationship between foreground and background and the way practice is patterned as a complex and chaotic whole.
- In their revelation of everyday contradictions, narratives critically expose and understand those conditions that constrain self-realisation as a focus for change – conditions grounded in tradition, force and embodiment. As the narratives portray, such conditions are not so easily shifted despite rhetoric of patient-centred care. Such contradiction lies thick on the surface.
- The narratives integrate extant theory within personal knowing in ways that illuminate the relevance of theory to inform practice and in ways that test the value of theory to inform practice. In doing so extant theory is transcended.
- The narratives illuminate the development of insights and ideas as a product of co-creating meaning, the effort to make sense of unfolding situations. Such ideas and insights become available to readers to utilise in their own particular circumstances.
- Narratives are experiential of the journey of self-inquiry and transformation towards self-realisation. Each one tests, expands and deepens the ground, offering new insights into narrative journey around such issues as co-creating meaning, dwelling with the text, the depth of the cues of the Model for Structured Reflection, coherence, reflexivity, narrative form, constraining forces, ethics – how these factors synchronise and pattern within the hermeneutic spiral towards self-realisation. Such understanding is vital in order to be mindful of *narrative discipline*. Wilber (2000) emphasises that in such a relative world cutting free from some anchoring point is inevitably a descent into nihilism and narcissism where anything goes, where discipline breaks down. Self-inquiry might be open to a criticism of narcissism by researchers or readers locked into modernity, because it does focus on self – 'What makes you so special?'. The world is viewed as relational and dynamic, unfolding in non-linear patterns. It is not static or predicable, but does have patterns of universal truths within it. As Wilber sees it – a world of 'universal deep features and local surface features' (2000:288). The narratives weave the patterns of the universal and local within the uniqueness of the unfolding situation.
- Collectively narratives offer multiple voices on discrete phenomena such as leadership. John-Marc's narrative is one of 40 similar narratives that focus on realising

transformational leadership in a transactional world – enabling a tentative theory to be constructed around this idea. The nature of the struggle to realise transformational within the contextual transactional organisational world can be analysed. The nature of leadership is also revealed, giving meaning to the ideals espoused within the theories.

- Performance and narrative enable the author to show, not tell, opening the audience to an embodied learning experience that moves people to realise their own insights, and in doing so, trajecting them into social action.

References

Okri B (1997) *A way of being free*. Phoenix House, London. Text extracts used with permission of The Marshall Agency.
Remen R (1996) *Kitchen table wisdom: stories that heal*. Riverhead Books, New York.
Wilber K (2000) *Sex, ecology, spirituality: the spirit of evolution*. Shambhala, Boston.

Appendices

Appendix 1

The question – How might the narrative be reflexively 'marked' or plotted?
Four key frameworks used in the narratives are:

- The Being available template (Johns 2009)
- Capacities for transformational leadership (Schuster 1994)
- Development of participatory competence (Kieffer 1984)
- Construction of voice (Belenky *et al*. 1986)

Being available template

The being available template was constructed inductively by analysing patterns within practitioners' reflections shared in guided reflection sessions. This analysis involved 500 shared experiences over a four-year period (Johns 1998). All the shared experiences in some way reflected the practitioners' striving to realise holistic practice. As such, I sought to construct an adequate framework so the nature of holistic practice might be patterned as a guide and marker of realisation. The nature of holism is essentially the idea of wholeness, that the whole is greater then the sum of its parts. So whilst I could draw out lists of attributes or parts, I needed to capture the irreducible essence of holism.

At its core is the irreducible quality of being available template is *the practitioner being available to work with the (whole) person requiring help in order to help them find meaning in their health event experience, to help them make best decisions about their life, and to assist them as necessary to meet their health needs*. Of course, such description of holistic practice is open to conjecture.

I then explicated from shared experiences six fundamental and inter-related qualities that seem to determine the extent the practitioner can be available (Box A.1). These cannot be viewed in isolation from each other in that they form a pattern of being. Since 1994, this framework has been continuously tested and refined, leading to an ever-deepening appreciation of what it means to be and know oneself as a holistic practitioner. Editions of my book *Becoming a reflective practitioner* (Johns 2009) have been extensively organised around the template. For example, it can be argued that the goal of any holistic practitioner is to ease suffering. If so, what might be the proper focus of the plot – easing suffering or becoming a holistic practitioner?

Box A.1   The six fundamental qualities

The extent the practitioner can be available to the person is determined by the extent:

- She holds the intent to realise her vision of practice – given that we are more likely to realise those things we mindful intend;
- She is concerned for and compassionate – given we pay attention to things and people because they matter to us;
- She appreciates the person's life pattern – given that we can only nurse what the person reveals to us;
- She can effectively grasp situations, make effective clinical judgement, respond with appropriate and skilful action to meet the diversity of the person's (whole) health needs – the nature of aesthetic knowing;
- She is poised – given that unless the practitioner is mindful of her own limitations and can manage her own concerns she will not be available to the other;
- She can create and sustain an environment where being available is possible – given that the practitioner is socialised into organisations where her ability to be available is always compromised by issues such as resources, tradition, force and her own embodiment of ways of being that are not conducive to holistic practice.

Perhaps the being available template should reflect easing suffering in its core therapeutic? As such, it could read:

> The core therapeutic of holistic practice is the practitioner being available to the person to help appreciate and ease that person's suffering.

This rendition gives a stronger focus to clinical outcome – easing suffering, whereas the former format emphasised the process *of working with the person to meet their health goals*. The focus on meeting their health goals is paramount and would inevitably reduce their suffering. Hence meeting their health needs is a more encompassing plot than easing suffering. Either way, the six inter-related factors that determine the extent the practitioner can be available would not change.

Frameworks, such as the being available template, must be sensitive enough to portray the nuances, subtleties, complexities and contradictions of everyday practice, yet robust to reflect the practitioner's journey of realisation in ways the reader can follow the trail and be convinced of its authenticity.

A risk with any theoretical framework, is to fit understanding within the framework rather than use the framework creatively to inform understanding. To offset this risk requires a sceptical attitude to challenge the adequacy of the framework to inform and frame development. Developmental frameworks can only be guides to frame development, not a rigid structure to force-fit experience.

Schuster's capacities of transformational leadership (1994)

The students on the MSc in Leadership in Healthcare Practice, University of Bedfordshire, often choose to use Schuster's 13 capacities of transformational leadership framework (Box A.2) to frame and mark the emergence of their leadership. Other approaches can be constructed from diverse leadership theories.

Box A.2 The 13 capacities

- The practitioner holds a vision for the organisation that is intellectually rich, stimulating and rings true;
- She is honest and empathetic. People feel emotionally safe and trust that she has their interests at heart;
- Her character is well developed, without the prominent dark side of ego power – her behaviour aligns with her words;
- She sets aside her own interests in looking good and getting strokes, instead making others look good and giving others power and credit;
- She evinces a concern for the whole (not just her organisation) reflected in her passionate and ethical voice being heard when necessary;
- Her natural tendency is to develop others to become engaged, deepen perspectives and be effective;
- She can share power with others – she believes sharing power is the best way to tap talent, engage others, and to get work done in optimal fashion;
- She takes risks, experiments and learns. Information is never complete;
- She has a true passion for work and the vision. That's evident in commitment of time, attention to detail, and ability to renew her energy;
- She effectively communicates, both listening and speaking;
- She understands and appreciates management and administration. They appreciate that – she moves towards shared success without sacrifice;
- She celebrates the now. At meetings or wherever, she sincerely acknowledges accomplishment, staying in the moment before moving on;
- She persists in hard times. That means she has the courage to move ahead when she is tired, conflicted and getting mixed signals.

Each capacity is underpinned by deep thinking (head), empathy (heart) and congruent action (hand). Schuster cautions against viewing these attributes as a simple list, realising the risk of imposing an authoritative prescription of transformational leadership. Schuster acknowledges that leadership is much greater than the sum of these parts (the reductionist threat).

Development of participatory competence (Kieffer 1984)

Whether the practitioner's journey of self-inquiry and transformation is concerned with leadership, holistic practice or education, a core attribute is becoming empowered to take action to resolve contradiction so as to be more able to shift the conditions of self and practice to realise one's vision as a lived reality. Empowerment is also at the very core of reflective practice – first understanding, second empowerment, third transformation.

Kieffer plotted the development or empowerment of community leaders through four eras of involvement: era of entry, era of advancement, era of incorporation and era of commitment.

The era of entry is characterised by a sense of one's integrity being violated and that it cannot be tolerated. In terms of narrative, it sets the plot – a journey to overthrow the forces that violate until self emerges triumphant in realising desirable practice.

Era of entry	It is only when a practitioner's sense of integrity is violated (to the extent of overcoming one's own subjection) can people respond (the provocation of empowerment). Moving through this initial phase demands especially that each practitioner alters her sense of relation to long-established symbols and systems of authority
Era of advancement	This era has three major aspects: (a) Centrality of a mentoring relationship; (b) The enabling impact of supportive peer relationships within a collective organisational structure; (c) Cultivation of a more critical understanding of social and political relations (the more they understand the more motivated they are to continue). Over time, through ongoing effort, people construct more viable strategies for political action, more effective mechanisms for collective expression and support, and more sophisticated capacity for social analysis and resource development
Era of incorporation	In this era, self-concept, strategic ability, and critical comprehension substantially mature. Through continuing struggle, practitioners confront and learn to contend with the (seeming) permanence and painfulness of barriers to self-determination – a growing sense of being-in-the-world.
Era of commitment	Those practitioners who develop a fully realised participatory competence are those who succeed in reconstructing their sense of personal mastery and awareness of self in relation to the political world. Practitioners commit themselves to adapting their empowerment to continuing proactive community mobilisation and leadership.

The narratives of Jane Groom (Chapter 12) and Yvonne Latchford (Chapter 7) used Kieffer's framework as a marker of self-development.

Voice as metaphor

Another approach to marking empowerment is the work of Belenky *et al.* (1986) using *voice* as a metaphor for empowerment. The majority of practitioners I have worked with in guided reflection are women, and as such, it is crucial to pay attention to the struggle women have within patriarchal-dominated organisations such as the health care service (Watson 1990) to have their voice heard and valued. This is, of course, resonates with the theme of a critical social science; the struggle to throw off the forces of oppression that deny 'voice' and realisation of self's best interests.

Belenky *et al.* (1986) identified five stages of developing voice from listening to the experiences of groups of women; silence, received voice, subjective voice, procedural voice (connected and separate), and constructed voice. The level of *silence* represents women who have no voice, dominated by the authoritative voices of others. Reflection gives the person a *potential* voice to write her journal or share her story, to ask self 'who am I?'. Potential, because the forces that keep women/practitioners silent may shut off even this possibility. I have often asked people to write a brief description of a recent experience and it is beyond them to do this. I have noted two reasons why practitioners struggle with this activity. The first is a technical reason – they do not know how to reflect, reflecting the way they can only speak with the voices of others to the extent they deny their own intuitive sense. The second is more profound – they do not know who they are and have no way of expressing self. Of course this raises all sorts of dilemmas in using reflection as a developmental process in that the very tool of empowerment may serve to disempower (Johns 1999). Aileen's story (Chapter 6) is included in the book as an exemplar of her struggle to find a voice to reflect. It is an important story because she is a mature and intelligent woman, yet found herself feeling increasingly helpless and powerless to change her predicament and also unable to express this predicament in any coherent way. She had descended into self-alienation whereby she felt she was clinging on to remnants of her real self. She felt she was going to fragment. Her brief narrative plots her journey to recover herself.

The level of *received voice* is listening and speaking with the voice of others. Women conceive themselves as capable of receiving, even reproducing knowledge from all knowing external authorities but not capable of creating knowledge of their own, reflected in the way the practitioner speaks as if filled with the words of others yet without any critical understanding. It is profoundly difficult to reflect on this level because the person cannot respond to the reflective cues beyond simple description. They lack the resources to be critical of self. Reflection is experienced as confrontational and threatening. At this level practitioners want a didactic style off guidance that fits with the experience of being filled up. Yet they also resist being emptied because the words of others have become embodied. On this level reflection proceeds with a gentle inquiring light to plant the seeds of doubt. The typical response of the received knower is 'don't know'. 'Why do you feel that way?' – 'I don't know.' 'Could you respond in different ways?' – 'I don't know', etc.

At the level of *subjective* voice reflection is perceived as permission to have and voice opinions and feelings, to express outrage, to shed tears, to rant against injustice, and most importantly to connect with others and form a caring community where people, perhaps for the first time, can express themselves with a sense of freedom. On this level, feminist strategies such as the PEACE and Power feminist process (Wheeler and Chinn 1991) offer practitioners a mirror to see themselves within this process. The group process is explicitly about valuing self and taking power yet in peaceful ways. However, at the subjective level, the practitioner's voice is unsubstantiated.

At the level of *procedural* voice the practitioner is able to realise self within the simultaneous and complementary processes of separate and connected knowing. Separate knowing is the ability to critically apply theory to practice in meaningful ways. Connected knowing is the ability to know and connect self with the experiences of others. In other words, in order to know the other, one has to know self so connection can be made in terms of the meanings the other gives to a situation rather. People who experience self as predominantly separate tend to espouse a morality based on impersonal procedures for establishing justice whilst people who experience the self as predominantly connected tend to espouse a morality based on care.

The level of *constructed* voice is the weaving of the subjective and procedural voices into a coherent whole whereby the practitioner can speak with an informed, passionate and assertive voice. From this perspective women view all knowledge as contextual, experience themselves as creators of knowledge and value both subjective and objective strategies for knowing. Developing the practitioner's *constructed voice* is always the intent of guided reflection expressed in narrative form.

References

Belenky M, Clinchy B, Goldberger N and Tarule J (1986) *Women's ways of knowing: the development of self, voice and mind.* Basic Books, New York.

Johns C (1998) *Becoming an effective practitioner through guided reflection.* PhD thesis. Open University.

Johns C (1999) Unravelling the dilemmas within everyday nursing practice. *Nursing Ethics* 6:287–298.

Johns C (2009) *Becoming a reflective practitioner* (third edition). Wiley-Blackwell, Oxford.

Kieffer CH (1984) Citizen empowerment: a developmental perspective. *Prevention in Human Services* 84:9–36.

Schuster JP (1994) Transforming your leadership style. *Association Management* 46:39–42.

Watson J (1990) Moral failure of the patriarchy. *Nursing Outlook* 38:62–66.

Wheeler CE and Chinn PL (1991) *Peace and power: handbook of feminist process*. National League of Nursing, New York.

Appendix 2

Narrative structure

Chapter 1 – Beginnings or background	In this chapter the practitioner/researcher positions self in context of their narrative to enable the reader to see where the practitioner is coming from, is at now, and where she is heading. Utilising Heidegger's (1964) concept of fore-structure gives this chapter structure: • Forehaving – something we have in advance from our past that has shaped 'who we are'– our family upbringing, our professional association, key experiences, life events; • Fore-sight – something we have now as we begin the journey which influences us now – issues of role, context, values; • Forconception – something we see in advance that gives direction to the narrative- ideas of what self-realisation might mean, vision, agendas; Heidegger M (1964) *Being and time* (transl. Macquarrie J and Robinson E). Harper and Row, New York.
Chapter 2 – Narrative construction	In this chapter, the practitioner tells the story of how they constructed the narrative (chapters 3/4). It combines what traditionally is divided into methodology (the philosophical approach to the research) and method (how the research was conducted and analysed). The most favoured approach is to structure this chapter through the six dialogical movements (see Fig. 2.1) woven with the practical application of philosophical ideas.
Chapter 3 – The narrative	In this chapter, the practitioner presents her reflexive narrative structured through a series of (reflected-on) experiences that were insightful towards self-realisation. Issues such as what self-realisation means and changes, and barriers that constrain will be woven through the narrative. This chapter might be split into several chapters that mark eras of the research (for example year 1, 2, 3 etc)
Chapter 4 – Significance	In this chapter, the practitioner draws out her key insights in moving towards self-realisation and highlights their significance in terms of what has been learnt/new knowledge gained. For doctoral work, this is most vital. The practitioner also draws conclusions for the wider significance of her self-inquiry, moving into the sixth dialogical movement where the narrative is viewed as an opening a dialogical space in terms of clinical practice, education, research and society.
Chapter 5 – Reflection	On another level of reflection, the guide and practitioner consider the congruence of the research, notably dilemmas and contradictions they faced within the process.

Index

Page numbers in *italics* represent figures or boxes, those in **bold** represent tables.